Professional Nursing
Concepts and Challenges

Professional Nursing

Concepts and Challenges

Kay Kittrell Chitty, Ed.D., R.N.

Associate Professor, School of Nursing
University of Tennessee at Chattanooga
Chattanooga, Tennessee

W.B. Saunders Company
Harcourt Brace Jovanovich, Inc.
Philadelphia   London   Toronto
Montreal   Sydney   Tokyo

W.B. SAUNDERS COMPANY

Harcourt Brace Jovanovich Inc.

The Curtis Center
Independence Square West
Philadelphia, PA 19106

Library of Congress Cataloging-in-Publication Data

Professional nursing: concepts and challenges / [edited by] Kay
  Kittrell Chitty.
      p.   cm.
    1. Nursing—Vocational guidance.   2. Nursing—Social aspects.
  I. Chitty, Kay Kittrell.
    [DNLM: 1. Nursing.   WY 16 P9644]
  RT82.P755   1993
  610.73'06'9—dc20
  DNLM/DLC   92–49443

ISBN   0–7216–4061–3

PROFESSIONAL NURSING: Concepts and Challenges

Printed in United States of America

Last digit is the print number: 9   8   7   6   5   4   3   2   1

To my family—Charlie, Katherine, and Chuck—who have lovingly supported me in all my professional endeavors, including the preparation of this book. Thank you for saving me from total obsession with "The Book"; for never asking, "Why?"; and for accepting my need to always have a major project under way.

Reviewers

**Connie S. Austin, M.A.Ed.,
M.S.N., R.N.**
Azusa Pacific University
  Azusa, California

Penny S. Brooke, M.S., R.N., J.D.
University of Utah
Salt Lake City, Utah

Mary de Meneses, Ed.D., R.N.
Southern Illinois University at
  Edwardsville
Edwardsville, Illinois

Sue E. Elster, Ph.D., R.N.
University of Illinois
Chicago, Illinois

Filomena C. Flores, Ph.D., R.N.
California State University, Fresno
Fresno, California

Jane H. Freeman, Ed.D., R.N.
Jacksonville State University
Jacksonville, Alabama

**Isabelita Z. Guiao, Ph.D., R.N.,
C.S.**
The University of Texas Health
  Science Center at San Antonio
San Antonio, Texas

Dolores Hilden, Ph.D., R.N.
Teikyo Marycrest University
Davenport, Iowa

**Judith Ann Kilpatrick, M.S.N.,
R.N.C.**
Widener University
Chester, Pennsylvania

Eloise R. Lee, Ed.D., R.N.C.
Cedar Crest College
Allentown, Pennsylvania

Mary E. O'Donnell, M.A., R.N.
College of Staten Island
Staten Island, New York

Gloria R. Perry, Ph.D., R.N.
Southern Illinois University at
  Edwardsville
Edwardsville, Illinois

**Karen A. Piotrowski, M.S.N.,
R.N.C.**
D'Youville College
Buffalo, New York

**Bonna Stover Powell, M.A.,
R.N.C., P.N.P.**
Teikyo Marycrest University
Davenport, Iowa

Mary E. Sampel, M.S.N., R.N.
Saint Louis University
Saint Louis, Missouri

**Sheri H. Smith, M.S.N., R.N.,
C.E.T.N.**
Jacksonville State University
Jacksonville, Alabama

Joyce K. Soehnlen, M.S.N., R.N.
Walsh College
North Canton, Ohio

**Maureen L. Thompson, Ph.D.,
R.N.**
Syracuse University
Syracuse, New York

**Laura Daly Williams, M.N., R.N.,
C.R.R.N., C.S.**
University of Southwestern Louisiana
Lafayette, Louisiana

Doris I. Young, Ed.D., R.N.
Widener University
Chester, Pennsylvania

Contributors

Virginia Trotter Betts, M.S.N., J.D., R.N.
Research Associate Professor and Senior Research Associate
Vanderbilt University
Nashville, Tennessee
and
President, American Nurses Association

Marilynn K. Bodie, Ph.D., R.N.
Assistant Professor for the Practice of Nursing
School of Nursing
Vanderbilt University
Nashville, Tennessee

Carol T. Bush, Ph.D., R.N.
Professor
Nell Hodgson Woodruff School of Nursing
Emory University
Atlanta, Georgia
Acting Chief
Human Resources Planning & Development Branch
Division of State & Community Systems Development
Center for Mental Health Services
Substance Abuse and Mental Health Services Administration
Bethesda, Maryland

Pamela S. Chally, Ph.D., R.N.
Academic Dean, West Suburban College of Nursing
Oak Park, Illinois

Kay K. Chitty, Ed.D., R.N.
Associate Professor, School of Nursing
University of Tennessee at Chattanooga
Chattanooga, Tennessee

Nancy L. Davis, M.S., C.R.R.N.
Director, Nursing Services
Siskin Hospital for Physical Rehabilitation
Chattanooga, Tennessee

Catherine J. Futch, M.N., R.N., C.N.A.A.
Associate Professor
Nell Hodgson Woodruff School of Nursing
Emory University
Deputy Director of Nursing
Grady Memorial Hospital
Atlanta, Georgia

Leslie B. Himot, M.S., R.N.
Associate Professor
Department of Nursing
Kennesaw State College
Marietta, Georgia

Pamela J. Holder, D.S.N., R.N., O.C.N.
Acting Director
School of Nursing
The University of Tennessee at
  Chattanooga
Chattanooga, Tennessee

Jennifer E. Jenkins, M.B.A., R.N., C.N.A.A.
Adjunct Faculty
Vanderbilt School of Nursing
Nashville, Tennessee
Consultant
Jenkins and Associates
Memphis, Tennessee

Judith K. Leavitt, M.Ed., R.N., F.A.A.N.
Political and Educational Consultant
Upstate Coordinator
Geraldine Ferraro for U.S. Senate,
  1992
Ithaca, NY

Carolyn Maynard, Ph.D., R.N.
Assistant Professor of Nursing
University of North Carolina at
  Charlotte
Charlotte, North Carolina

Elaine F. Nichols, Ed.D., R.N.
Associate Dean, Undergraduate
  Program
Associate Professor of Nursing
The University of Akron
Akron, Ohio

Barbara R. Norwood, M.S.N., R.N.
Assistant Professor
School of Nursing
The University of Tennessee at
  Chattanooga
Chattanooga, Tennessee

Barbara K. Redman, Ph.D., R.N., F.A.A.N.
Executive Director
American Nurses Association
Washington, D.C.

Frances I. Waddle, M.S.N., R.N.
Health Facilities Consultant
Oklahoma State Department of
  Health
Executive Director
Oklahoma Nurses Association
Oklahoma City, Oklahoma

Acknowledgments

No project such as the preparation of a textbook is completed without the assistance of many people. First, I would like to express my thanks to all the students who encouraged me to share my ideas about becoming a professional nurse, and to my colleagues who supported me during the many months of writing and editing. Particular thanks are due to Grayson Walker, who encouraged me to balance the day-to-day pressures of administration with my academic interests and provided me with the freedom to do so.

Gratitude is due to my nurse colleagues across the country who contributed chapters, to the reviewers whose constructive and insightful suggestions guided both the content and organization of this book, and to the many nurses who shared their own experiences, thus enriching its content.

The assistance of my incomparable secretary Mary Lee Hudson, research assistants Judith Gift and Eleanor Sudderth, and reference librarian Ray Hall were all invaluable. Special thanks to Beth Craig, Sue Goodwin, Nora Burke, and Michael Quinn for their assistance in preparing the manuscript.

Finally, my warmest appreciation goes to Thomas Eoyang, Editor-in-Chief, Nursing Books, W.B. Saunders Company, for sharing my vision for this book and giving me the chance to turn vision into reality.

Preface

Professional Nursing: Concepts and Challenges is a student-centered book that addresses the nonclinical aspects of nursing and introduces the concepts underlying professionalism. Professional nursing is far more than "doing"; it is a process of "becoming." Therefore, this book focuses both on content about nursing as a profession and on self-development. To that end, self-development activities and personal inventories are integrated throughout the book to assist learners in self-awareness, which provides the basis for professional nursing practice.

This book unabashedly promotes nursing's professional values. Students of nursing need to understand and appreciate what the profession stands for and what nurses collectively believe in and prize about our profession. Readers are encouraged to take an active role in shaping their own educational experiences rather than being passive recipients of knowledge.

This is a "user-friendly" book. We hope that it engages the reader, presents information in an understandable and interesting manner, and is visually appealing. Although this is a contributed book, the chapters are organized consistently. The chapter format includes objectives; vocabulary words; text supplemented by boxes, tables, and figures highlighting important points; review/discussion questions; references; and, for most chapters, suggested readings. The review questions often suggest topics appropriate for classroom discussion, in-class activities, or out-of-class assignment. Key terms appear in boldface at the point of introduction in the text. The Glossary defines these terms.

Several chapters contain research notes designed to demonstrate the relevance of research to nursing. Numerous chapters are highlighted by interviews with nurses who share their activities, insights, and excitement to bring various concepts to life. Patient vignettes and case studies also contribute to the realism and animation of the text.

The term **patient** is used throughout the text in preference to the popular "client" terminology. This choice was an editorial decision designed to promote consistency and is intended to make no statement about the autonomy of the patient/client or the nature of the nurse–patient/client relationship. A serious attempt has been made to avoid gender-specific pronouns. When pronouns could not be avoided, the potential for sex-role stereotyping was carefully scrutinized. The cultural diversity of both nurses and patients has been explored, and the challenge to nurses of knowing, respecting, and incorporating patients' cultural beliefs in their care is emphasized.

Professional Nursing: Concepts and Challenges was written to serve as a flexible resource for two audiences: students new to nursing and registered nurses (R.N.s) pursuing bachelor of science in nursing (B.S.N.) degrees. Program diversity makes a review of previous nursing concepts desirable, and the format of this book encourages that process. While the book presupposes no prior knowledge of health care and nursing, it contains sufficiently challenging content in the areas of nursing philosophies, theory, research, ethics, legal, and political aspects to stimulate discussion at many levels. The reading level is manageable for most of today's college students.

Since it is intended as a resource for survey courses, the book introduces a wide array of topics. The impact of historical events on modern nursing practice is reviewed, various definitions of nursing are explored, and philosophies of nursing are examined. Students are encouraged and assisted to begin developing their own philosophies of nursing. The integration of nursing research, theory, and practice is emphasized, and an array of practice options and roles is examined. The nursing process is explored as a means of critically analyzing patients' needs. Legal and ethical aspects of nursing practice are reviewed, and perspectives on the future of nursing are projected. Readers are encouraged to become politically active.

The book is designed to encourage students from diverse backgrounds to view nursing as a profession, to develop a common language, to understand what is meant by "professional," and to develop a conceptual framework upon which to build a professional curriculum. Its 23 chapters may be used independently and in any order, depending on course objectives and the level of the learners.

Chapters 1 through 5 describe the evolution of nursing from ancient times to the present, including educational patterns and the social forces shaping nursing and nursing's professional associations. Chapters 6 through 8 focus on defining professional nursing and professional socialization of nurses. Chapters 9 and 10 describe beliefs about nursing and explain the foundational concepts of person, environment, and health. Chapters 11 and 12 review the interaction between theory and research and describe the research process. Chapters 13 through 15 describe how health care is delivered and financed and review traditional and innovative methods of nursing care delivery. Chapters 16 and 17 explain the scientific method and the nursing process, whereas Chapters 18 and 19 explore the impact of illness on patients and families and how nurses use themselves as therapeutic agents. And Chapters 20 through 23 focus on the ethical, legal, and political challenges professional nursing faces and predict challenges that nurses of the future will encounter.

Preparing this textbook has reminded me of what a proud tradition we have in nursing and what wonderful opportunities yet await our attention. Never before in history has the nursing profession been in such a powerful position to affect the health care of the nation. The goal of this book is to combine professional knowledge and self-knowledge and thus to equip learners with an unbeatable combination of abilities that will assist them in taking the nursing profession to its next higher level of development.

Kay K. Chitty

Contents

Chapter

History of Nursing

Catherine J. Futch

CHAPTER OBJECTIVES

What students should be able to do after studying this chapter:

1. Describe the ancient origins of nursing.

2. Discuss the influence of religious orders on the development of nursing.

3. Describe Florence Nightingale's influence on nursing practice and nursing education.

4. Describe the early nursing schools in the United States.

5. Identify key nursing leaders who shaped the profession in this country and tell their accomplishments.

6. Trace the history of black nurses and black schools of nursing in the United States.

7. Explain the relationship between wars and the development of nursing in the United States.

VOCABULARY BUILDING

People and terms to know:

Clara Barton	Mary Breckinridge	Dorothea L. Dix
Mary Ann Ball/"Mother Bickerdyke"	Namahyoke Curtis	Lavinia Dock
	Deaconess Institute at Kaiserswerth	Francis Reed Elliott
		"famous trio"

1

Martha Franklin
Frontier Nursing
  Service
Goldmark Report
Annie Goodrich
Henry Street
  Settlement
holism
Hippocrates

Mary Eliza Mahoney
Florence Nightingale
Mary Adelaide
  Nutting
Lucille Petry
Linda Richards
Isabel Hampton Robb
Margaret Sanger
Jessie Sleet Scales

Spellman Seminary
Susie Taylor
Sojourner Truth
Harriet Tubman
Lillian Wald
Yale School of
  Nursing

*N*ursing has a fascinating history that parallels the history of humankind. For as long as there has been life, so has there been the need to seek care and comfort from illness and injury. "From the dawn of civilization, evidence prevails to support the premise that nurturing has been essential to the preservation of life. Survival of the human race, therefore, is inextricably intertwined with the development of nursing" (Donahue 1985, p. 2).

The Journey

In looking at the historical development of nursing as a profession, we see that cultural and societal changes have shaped the profession of nursing as we know it today. This chapter will trace the development of nursing from ancient times to the present.

Nursing from Ancient Times to the Nineteenth Century

"Nursing has been called the oldest of the arts and the youngest of the professions" (Donahue 1985, p. 2). The word *nurse* evolved from the Latin word *nutricius,* which means "nourishing" (Kalisch and Kalisch 1986, p. 1). The roots of medicine and nursing are intertwined and found in mythology, ancient cultures, religion, and reasoned thinking.

ANCIENT CIVILIZATIONS

The ancient Egyptians created a very advanced civilization. Their medical practices were equally impressive. The Egyptian Imhotep is known as the first physician. He is believed to have lived around 2700 B.C. and was later worshiped as the god of healing.

Egyptian physicians are believed to have specialized in certain diseases (such as internal diseases, fractured bones, and wounds), and they wrote textbooks of

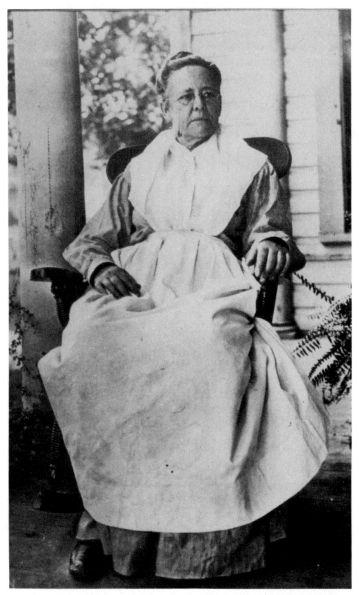

Annie Davis Baker, first head nurse, Scott and White Hospital, Temple, Texas.
(Courtesy of Sarah Parisi M.S.N., R.N., subject's great, great grandaughter.)

medicine as it was practiced at that time. They also hired women, later known as midwives, to assist with childbirth. These women were the first recorded nurses.

The ancient Hebrews practiced preventive medicine as long ago as 1200 to 600 B.C. The Hebrews isolated people with contagious diseases and actively quarantined contaminated wells. Their religious laws forbidding the eating of pork supported the avoidance of food-borne diseases such as trichinosis, which was transmitted by consuming infected pork.

Eastern cultures also influenced the practice of early medicine. As early as 800 B.C., Indian physicians performed amputations and sophisticated procedures such as plastic surgery. Traditional Chinese medicine taught that disease results from an imbalance of the two life forces, yin and yang. To control the flow of these forces and thus cure disease, Chinese physicians inserted very fine needles into specific body parts. This practice, acupuncture, is still in use today.

GREECE AND THE ROMAN EMPIRE

Belief in Apollo, the Greek god of healing, and Asclepius, the Greek god of medicine, predominated in the Greek civilization, which reached its peak around 400 B.C. The Greeks prayed to Apollo and Asclepius for magical cures for their illnesses.

Belief in gods and magical cures gave way to understanding through the work of early scientists such as the Greek physician **Hippocrates** (400 B.C.). Hippocrates believed that disease had natural, not magical, causes. His work marked the separation of medicine from religion for the first time in history.

After 300 B.C. the Roman Empire dominated the ancient world, conquering Egypt and Greece. Roman noblewomen, including the wives of emperors, cared for the sick. Early Roman physicians built on the groundwork of their Egyptian and Greek predecessors.

The Romans are best known for advances in the health of the public. They constructed an impressive network of aquaducts and sewers that provided Rome with both a continuous supply of fresh water and a waste disposal system, making a high level of sanitation possible.

Galen, a Greek physician living in Rome about 100 B.C., performed numerous experiments on animals to learn about anatomy and disease. Although Galen's influence lasted hundreds of years, many of his animal experiments led to erroneous conclusions when applied to human beings.

Although some of their information was later proved inaccurate, these early scientists began erasing the mystique surrounding the human body's processes and replacing it with knowledge.

THE MIDDLE AGES

Progress in Western civilization's quest for knowledge about disease and the human body slowed during the early part of the Middle Ages, known as the Dark Ages, which lasted from A.D. 400 to 900. In the Muslim empire of southwest and central Asia, however, advances continued.

Avicenna, an Arab physician, wrote a volume called the *Canon of Medicine* that outlined all the diseases and treatments known at that time. This book was used by physicians for hundreds of years. In western Europe, deep in the antiin-

tellectualism that characterized the Dark Ages, "scientific medicine survived . . .
chiefly through the efforts of Jewish physicians who translated Greek and Arabic
medical treatises into Latin and who circulated Greco-Arabic medical knowledge throughout Christendom" (Kalisch and Kalisch 1986, p. 7).

Following the Dark Ages, interest in care of the sick was sparked by the
effects of poverty, disease, the ravages of war, and a renewed quest for knowledge. There were massive epidemics of diseases such as leprosy and bubonic
plague. From 500 to 1400, 25 percent of the population of Europe died in
epidemics. Widespread disease stimulated the building of hospitals. The oldest
known hospital was the Hôtel-Dieu (House of God), built in Lyons, France, in
542. Medical schools multiplied rapidly, and books were written describing
smallpox, measles, and other infectious diseases.

Around 1060, Constantinus Africanus established a university at Salerno,
Italy. This university was a dominant western European force in medical education until well into the twelfth century. It was particularly important to nursing
because it provided women with the opportunity to study nursing and midwifery. A midwife named Trotula wrote a famous twelfth-century obstetrical
treatise entitled *Trotulae curandanum aegritudinum muliebrum* [Trotula on the
cure of diseases of women].

RELIGION'S INFLUENCE

In 1099 the first separate military-nursing order was formed. Known as the
Knights Hospitalers of St. John of Jerusalem, they "soon became famous and
highly esteemed, providing thousands of pilgrims and crusaders in the Holy City
with hospitality and care" (Kalisch and Kalisch 1986, p. 9). This group is the first
identifiable organization of nurses. Eventually, in addition to their commitment
to the care of travelers, those who were ill, and those who were impoverished,
they also became known as a powerful military order.

> During the later Middle Ages, lasting from 900 to 1500, religious orders contin-
> ued their interest in nursing. St. Benedict's Rule decreed that every monastery
> have a hospital, and although care for the ailing was at first directed mainly to-
> ward members of the order, workers on church-owned estates were eventually
> included. The masses, however, still had to depend on their womenfolk for treat-
> ment and care during illness. (Kalisch and Kalisch 1986, p. 11)

Much nursing care during this period was provided by monks and nuns who
were members of Catholic nursing orders. The care was segregated by sex, with
women caring for women and men caring for men.

Many monasteries were closed due to the rise of Protestantism during the
Protestant Reformation of the fifteenth century. Only the hospitals were left as
places to care for the poor sick. The wealthy never used hospitals, preferring to
be cared for at home. It is little wonder, since sanitation in hospitals was unknown, and conditions were often desperate.

> In a typical hospital of the 1400s, the daily work of the nurses began at 5:00 A.M.,
> when, after rising and washing, they went downstairs to church service. Then the
> sister nurses went about their work in areas such as the laundry, the wards, and

the hall for admittance. When the patients were awake, each nurse would make the rounds with a basin in one hand and a towel in the other. Later, while beds were being made, the healthier patients were allowed to get up while the more seriously ill were moved to vacant beds. Each bed, a straw-filled mattress suspended on cords stretched from four corner posts, held at least two and in many cases three patients. . . . Sister nurses were forbidden to witness childbirths, to help with gynecologic examinations, or even to diaper boy babies. Close contact with male patients, such as administering enemas, was also prohibited, as was the care of patients suffering from venereal diseases. Servants were employed to carry out these tasks. (Kalisch and Kalisch 1986, p. 17)

THE DARK PERIOD

In the sixteenth and seventeenth centuries, plague and pestilence again wrought havoc throughout the civilized world. The few medicines in existence were herbs or concoctions consisting of "urine, animal excreta, powdered earthworms, and the like" (Kalisch and Kalisch 1986, p. 17). Such factors as an incomplete understanding of how the human body functioned, lack of basic hygiene, and no understanding of the role of yet-to-be-discovered microorganisms in illness resulted in millions of additional deaths from measles, leprosy, typhus, bubonic plague, and other infectious diseases.

The years from 1600 to 1850 have been described as the darkest period of nursing history. Hospitals were charitable institutions staffed by untrained women of the lower classes, many of ill repute. Nurses and physicians themselves often contracted and died of the same diseases they were treating in others.

By the middle of the eighteenth century, life expectancy was still short, infant mortality was still high, and crowded conditions in city slums continued to breed disease. Most nursing care was provided in the home, and those who were exposed to hospital care were often at great risk. Max Nordau wrote of a late-eighteenth-century European hospital:

In one bed of moderate width lay 4, 5, or 6 sick persons beside each other, the feet of one to the head of another. . . . In the same bed lay individuals infected with infectious diseases beside others only slightly unwell; on the same couch, body against body, a woman groaned in the pains of labor, a nursing infant writhed in convulsions, a typhus patient burned in the delirium of fever, a consumptive coughed his hollow cough, and a victim of some diseases of the skin tore with furious nails. (Kalisch and Kalisch 1986, p. 24)

Medical education in the eighteenth century was better than it had been and more plentiful, but not enough was known to make a difference. Although scientists had suspected that "seeds" created disease, it was not until the late 1800s that Louis Pasteur and Robert Koch demonstrated that microorganisms caused disease. This was a turning point for health care worldwide.

Nursing in America from Colonization to Independence

As America was colonized, the same health care problems were encountered here that occurred throughout Europe. The first hospital built in the colonies was located in what later became known as New York. Its doors opened in 1658 (Selavan 1984). Most patients suffering from contagious diseases, however, were placed in what were called "pest houses" such as those in Boston, New York, Philadelphia, and Charleston. By 1776, Virginia had two private hospitals as well as a hospital for the insane. Philadelphia had Pennsylvania Hospital, owing, in part, to the influence of Benjamin Franklin.

Early American physicians were prepared through courses of study in Europe and a variety of apprenticeships. Untrained and uneducated nurses provided "care" to those unfortunate enough to be hospitalized. Physicians were not required to have a license to practice medicine. There were

> . . . no medical libraries, medical journals or medical societies. Most doctors prepared their own medicine from herbs which they often grew themselves. Of the 3,500 practitioners in America at the beginning of the Revolution, only 400 held M.D. degrees. . . . Anyone could practice medicine and almost everyone did. (Selavan 1984, p. 19)

Female members of each household continued to be the primary providers of nursing care.

THE AMERICAN REVOLUTION'S INFLUENCE

Soldiers who fought in the new nation's American Revolution (1775–1783) were more apt to die from disease or the effects of their care than they were from the wounds of battle. "Purging, blistering, and bleeding" were the treatments of choice, and when wounds became infected, amputation was the only option. They also had to contend with pneumonia, dysentery, lack of adequate food, impure water, and unclean camps and hospitals (Selavan 1984, p. 19).

Two major health care victories emerged from the American Revolution. The first was the routine innoculation of troops against smallpox, which greatly decreased the spread of smallpox in the nation. The second was the recognition that the United States Army needed clean hospitals and nurses to participate in supervising the care provided in them.

In spite of the absence of army hospitals, the names of paid nurses did appear on military payrolls and pension lists, and "women who acted as nurses were entitled to the same rations as soldiers" (Selavan 1984, p. 21). Gen. George Washington was reportedly tempted to replace male wartime attendants with female nurses and even suggested that "women be enlisted for the same money paid to soldiers" (Selavan 1984, p. 21). The general's army was strong on paper, but the number of healthy men able to fight at any given time was much lower, owing to poor nutrition and lack of medical care.

Toward the end of the war, leaders recognized that military veterans, often grievously wounded, needed special facilities to care for them. These peacetime military hospitals were never realized, but the seeds were planted—physicians and generals had recognized the value of proper nursing care for soldiers in combat.

The Dawn of Modern Nursing: Florence Nightingale

From the late 1700s through 1853, the manner in which the sick were cared for in America remained essentially unchanged. In Europe, however, the dawn of nursing was under way. "The **Deaconess Institute at Kaiserswerth**, Germany, was established in 1836 by Pastor Theodor Fliedner" (Donahue 1985, p. 234). By 1842 the work of Pastor Fliedner and his followers resulted in a large hospital and planned training program for the deaconesses who believed that their duty lay in the care of the sick and the provision of social services (Donahue 1985, p. 234).

> The program in nursing included a rotation in hospital clinical services (experience on wards for men, women, and children as well as those for communicable disease, convalescents, and sick deaconesses), instruction in visiting nursing, theoretical and bedside instruction in the care of the sick, instruction in religious doctrine and ethics, and enough pharmacy to pass the State examination for pharmacists. Their program of study took three years. An interesting principle was enforced in that the nurses were required to follow the physician's orders exactly, and the physician alone was responsible for the outcome. (Donahue 1985, p. 235)

Graduates of the Kaiserswerth program spread their influence throughout the world. By 1849, four of the deaconesses were in Pittsburgh, Pennsylvania, where they assumed responsibility for the Pittsburgh Infirmary, later known as Passavant Hospital.

THE YOUNG FLORENCE

Meanwhile, in England, **Florence Nightingale** was coming of age (Fig. 1–1) Miss Nightingale, born to an upper-class English family, was shaped by three major influences in her life. First, she was dissatisfied with what she viewed as the dull, routine life-style of the upper-class women of her day. She had an active mind and an interest in her surroundings beyond household and social events.

Second, she had received "a classical education equal to that of most men of her day" (Smith 1984, p. 9). This education provided her with an understanding of the circumstances of the world in which she lived. This fueled her desire to secure the necessary financial and political influence to make a difference—to create lasting changes in the provision of health care.

Third, she became aware of the inadequate care being provided in hospitals as she accompanied her mother on visits to the ill. What she saw in those hospitals intrigued her and made her want to become more involved.

NIGHTINGALE AT KAISERSWERTH

In spite of the concerns of parents and friends, she began to visit and care for the sick both in her own family and in her community. Out of her experiences came the recognition that nurses required knowledge, training, and discipline if they

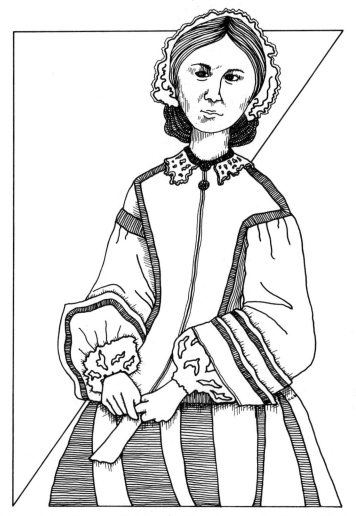

Figure 1–1   Florence Nightingale. (Drawing by Cathy Campbell Beahm.)

were to be effective. She discussed her beliefs with her friend Elizabeth Fry, herself an advocate for more humane treatment in prisons. Through her, Nightingale learned about and sought admission to the school at Kaiserswerth.

The three months of training she received were not only rigorous; in addition, they helped her clarify what was lacking in the current training of English nurses. Upon her return to England, to the great consternation of her family and friends, she embarked on a career that would have lasting impact on nursing in England, in the United States, and throughout the world.

IN THE CRIMEA

Miss Nightingale's work began in earnest during the Crimean War (1854–1856). She and a small band of untrained nurses went to the British hospital at Scutari in Turkey, where she wanted to make a difference in the care of British soldiers. What she found was a hospital "so crowded that patients lay on the floor, still in bloody uniforms. Bath equipment, sheets, cutlery, and laundry facilities were either non-existent or nearly so" (Smith 1984, p. 10). With great compassion and in spite of the unwelcoming attitude of the military officers with whom she worked, she set about the task of organizing and cleaning the hospital and providing care to the wounded soldiers.

Through her efforts and the help of others she enlisted to assist with her causes, Florence Nightingale introduced numerous improvements in the military hospital care of this period. Her efforts were largely responsible for dramatic reductions in the wartime death rate of British soldiers from 42 percent to 2 percent.

AFTER THE WAR

Following Scutari, Florence Nightingale almost single-handedly tried to change health care in her native England. She

> protested against the corridor system of hospitals and fought for pavilions (1850); printed her extensive octavo on the health of the Army (1858); issued the anonymous blue book on military sanitation in which she demonstrated the frightful but preventable mortality of the recent Crimean War (1859); showed the relationship of sanitary science to medical institutions (*Notes on Hospitals*, 1859); established the Army Medical School at Fort Pitt, Chatham, and chose its faculty (1860); and founded the first training school for nurses (St. Thomas's Hospital, London, 1860). Florence Nightingale epitomized her life work when she wrote in a private note: "I stand at the alter of the murdered men, and, while I live, I fight their causes." (Robinson 1946, p. 129)

In addition to being a great war nurse, Nightingale also was the founder of modern nursing education. Through the publication of countless articles and papers, she shared her ideas about nursing and nursing education. Her most famous written document, *Notes on Nursing*, was published in 1863. Miss Nightingale was the first to mention "**holism**" (treating the whole patient) in nursing and the first to clearly state that a unique body of knowledge was required of those wishing to practice professional nursing. Although she never set foot on American soil, her work served as a catalyst for the development of the foundations of American nursing.

Nursing in America: The Civil War, 1861–1865

While Florence Nightingale was involved with the founding of her training school for nurses at St. Thomas's Hospital, the United States was moving toward a civil war that would divide the nation and result in huge casualties and loss of life for both sides.

Neither North nor South was prepared to care for large numbers of sick and injured soldiers, but as war became imminent, women once again mobilized an effort to care for those they loved. Black and white, rich and poor, married and single women cared for sick and wounded soldiers in hospitals, provided clothing and food for soldiers, developed aid societies, and secretly sheltered fugitive black slaves. The care provided by women during America's Civil War was profoundly influenced by what they had learned of the work of Florence Nightingale in the Crimea.

As a result of an 1861 meeting between Dr. Elizabeth Blackwell of New York, President Abraham Lincoln, and the acting surgeon general of the United States, Lincoln created the United States Sanitary Commission. This commission was given responsibility for planning the care of the war's wounded.

THE INFLUENCE OF DOROTHEA DIX

Dorothea L. Dix, a Boston schoolteacher who had devoted herself to the care of the mentally ill, volunteered her services to the newly formed United States Sanitary Commission. She was immediately appointed superintendent of Women Nurses of the Army (Austin 1984, p. 22).

Miss Dix listed the following criteria for the selection of army nurses: "age, at least 30 and not over 50; good health and endurance; matronly demeanor, with experience and good character; plainly dressed, with no ornaments, and no hoops" (Austin 1984, p. 22). Miss Dix's selection process was directed toward excluding those women she judged too pretty, too popular, or too fun loving to serve as effective nurses. Many women who did not meet her stringent criteria, however, provided active and valuable service during the war. Soon 100 young women who met the Dix qualifications went to Bellevue and New York Hospital for a month's training by hospital staff physicians to prepare them to supervise care of the wounded.

In the South, volunteers provided care in hospitals or in their own homes. With the establishment of a medical department under Confederate Surgeon General Samuel Preston Moore, "Richmond, Virginia, became a vast hospital center for the South. . . . Some hospitals like the Chimborazo Hospital in Richmond were large, having several divisions with 'lady' nurses in charge" (Austin 1984, p. 24).

CONTRIBUTIONS OF BLACK NURSES

Many black women, both free and slave, made contributions during the Civil War. Most famous are **Sojourner Truth**, **Harriet Tubman**, and **Susie Taylor.**

Born a slave in New York State and freed by the New York State Emancipation Act of 1827, Sojourner Truth (1797–1881) was not only a famous abolitionist and underground railroad agent, itinerant preacher and lecturer, women's rights

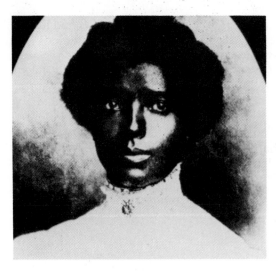

Figure 1–2 Sojourner Truth: a nurse in the Civil War. (Courtesy of Joyce A. Elmore.)

worker, and humanitarian, but also a nurse during the Civil War and immediately thereafter. (Carnegie 1986, p. 6)

Having changed her name from "Isabella" to "Sojourner" after her emancipation in 1827, she spent her life as her name implied, traveling and telling about slavery wherever she went (Fig. 1–2). After the war, she continued her work in the Washington, D.C. area as a nurse/counselor for the Freedmen's Relief Association. She helped find homes and jobs for freed men and worked in Freedmen's Village, caring for the ill in the hospital. She gathered together a group of women to clean the Freedmen's Hospital because of her concern about the unhygienic conditions there.

Harriet Ross Tubman (1820–1913) was an abolitionist who was sometimes called "Conductor of the Underground Railroad." Tubman "made 19 secret trips below the Mason and Dixon line, leading more than 300 slaves to freedom. She served as a nurse in the Sea Islands off the coast of South Carolina, caring for the sick and wounded without regard to color" (Carnegie 1986, p. 9). Miss Tubman was later commended by Acting U.S. Assistant Surgeon General Henry K. Durrant for her "kindness and attention to the sick and suffering" (Carnegie 1986, p. 9).

Susie King Taylor (1848–1912) was a young black girl who learned to read and write in secret. When Fort Pulaski, South Carolina, fell to Union troops, a Union officer assigned the 14-year-old Susie to teach black refugee children to read and write. Following her marriage, she was employed by Company E of the First South Carolina Volunteers as a laundress but continued her work as a teacher and nurse in her free time.

At Beaufort, South Carolina, during the summer of 1863, Susie King Taylor met Clara Barton, later to be the great "moving spirit" in the founding of the American Red Cross. She frequently accompanied Miss Barton, who treated her very cordially, on rounds in the hospitals at the front. (Carnegie 1986, p. 11)

Working as a volunteer nurse, she served the Union for more than four years.

"THE LITTLE LADY IN BLACK SILK" AND "MOTHER BICKERDYKE"

Clara Barton (1821–1912), perhaps the most well-known Civil War nurse, was called the "little lone lady in black silk" (Donahue 1985, p. 294). She was, however, a little lady of iron will. Preferring to act on her own and free from the direction of others, Miss Barton

> . . . independently operated a large scale war relief operation in which she arranged for huge quantities of supplies to be furnished to the Army and the hospitals. . . . She nursed in Federal hospitals and with the armies on the battlefield and cared for the wounded of the Confederate Armies. Her impartiality was expressed in the nursing care she extended to both whites and blacks, Northerners and Southerners. . . . On more than one occasion, bullets made holes in her dresses and she became one of the most prominent figures among the lay nurses of the Civil War. Her work embodied the ideals now characteristic of the Red Cross and became the foundation of her later success in the development of the American Red Cross in 1881. (Donahue 1985, p. 294)

A final Civil War woman known for her nursing skill was **Mary Ann Ball** (1817–1901). She answered the call for women to help in caring for the wounded and dying. A widow with two small sons, she was affectionately called **"Mother Bickerdyke."** She

> . . . served under fire in nineteen battles from Fort Donelson in Tennessee to Savannah, Georgia. She organized diet kitchens, laundries, and an ambulance service. She supervised the nursing staff and distributed supplies. At night she often walked through the abandoned battlefields, afraid that someone who was still alive would be left uncared for. She became known as one of the greatest nurse heroines of the Civil War." (Donahue 1985, p. 302)

Throughout the Civil War, laywomen (i.e., women who were not nurses) in both the Union and the Confederacy were empowered by their patriotism, caring, and Nightingale's Crimean example to do more than they dreamed they could do.

The Birth of a Profession: 1870–1900

With the final shots of the Civil War still ringing, the stage was set for the birth of organized nursing in America. Florence Nightingale had broken the ground, and many who knew of her work recognized the wisdom of her efforts. Those who had served in the war and recognized the need for trained nurses were poised to lead the way.

The years following the Civil War saw a number of events merge to support the founding of training schools for nurses. In 1869 Dr. Samuel Gross recommended to the American Medical Association that large hospitals should begin the process of developing training schools for nurses. He proposed that the students in these schools would be taught by medical staff and resident physicians. Simultaneously, members of the United States Sanitary Commission who served during the war began to lobby for the creation of nursing schools. Support for their efforts gained momentum as supporters of social reform reported the results of their visits to existing hospitals.

While intended to be helpful in the overall goal of establishing training schools for nurses, the recommendations of Dr. Gross and his colleagues were often in direct opposition to the teachings and recommendations of Miss Nightingale, who believed nurses should be trained and supervised by other nurses. These conflicting viewpoints heralded the beginning of a long and heated conflict between medicine and nursing regarding the proper education and supervision of nurses.

During this postwar time, society was also changing. Immigration, industrialization, and urbanization were altering the face of America. More and more people were in need of care that could no longer be provided by family members because many families were separated by immigration and migration from farms to cities.

Women, out of both economic necessity and the wish to leave the confines of home, were entering the workplace. They sought jobs in factories and workshops and as teachers, clerks, seamstresses, and untrained nurses in hospitals and homes. Societal changes and the movement to provide formal training for nurses dovetailed at this point in history.

The movement to formalize nurses' training found an advocate in Sarah J. Hale, editor of *Godey's Lady's Book and Magazine* for more than 30 years. She published an editorial entitled "Lady Nurses" in the February 1871 issue:

> Much has been lately said of the benefits that would follow if the calling of the sick nurse were elevated to a profession which an educated lady might adopt without a sense of degradation, either of her own part or in the estimation of others. . . . There can be no doubt that the duties of sick nurse, to be properly performed, require an education and training little, if at all, inferior to those possessed by members of the medical profession. To leave these duties to untaught and ill-trained persons is as great a mistake as it was to allow the office of surgeon to be held by one whose proper calling was that of a mechanic of the humblest class. The manner in which a reform may be effected is easily pointed out. Every medical college should have a course of study and training especially adapted for ladies who desire to qualify themselves for the profession of nurse; and those who had gone through the course, and passed the requisite examination, should receive a degree and a diploma, which would at once establish their position in society. The "graduate nurse" would in general estimation be as much above the ordinary nurse of the present day as the professional surgeon of our times is above the barber-surgeon of the last century. (Donahue 1985, p. 310)

THE FORMATION OF TRAINING SCHOOLS FOR NURSES

Training schools for nurses did evolve but not exactly in the manner Mrs. Hale had envisioned. In 1872 the New England Hospital for Women and Children established a training school for nurses. The hospital's newly formed training school was opened with a class of five students. The course of training lasted one year, and on October 1, 1873, Melinda Ann **(Linda) Richards** (1841–1930) completed the program of study and received a certificate of graduation. She is known as the first "trained nurse" in the United States.

In that same year, 1873, three more schools opened; the Bellevue Training School (May), the Connecticut Training School (October), and the Boston Training School (November) were all established. Known as the "**famous trio**," these schools were to have been patterned after the Nightingale Plan. There were few actual similarities. Dolan (1984), who studied the early programs, reported a number of obvious differences between these three schools and the Nightingale Plan. She found that the major similarity "was that nurses were in charge of the programs, the teaching (at least the bedside part of it), and the students." The separation of nursing education from the control of the medical profession had begun. A detailed discussion of the basic principles of Nightingale schools is found in Chapter 2.

The nurse training schools of the 1870s brought about slow but gradual change in the practice of nursing. The impact of these early training schools was seen in the gradual creation of order and cleanliness out of the confusion and filth that had existed:

> By 1879 there were eleven training schools in the United States. By the turn of the century there were no less than 432 schools, and most of these had expanded their programs to two or three years. The standards, however, varied greatly among the schools. . . . The function of the hospitals slowly changed from refuges of the destitute to institutions for the care of the sick and injured. The value of trained nurses had finally been proven, and this resulted in a growing demand for trained nurses. (Donahue 1985, p. 324)

BLACK NURSES' TRAINING

On August 1, 1879, **Mary Eliza Mahoney** (1845–1926) completed the 16-month course of training at the New England Hospital for Women and Children and became America's first black "trained nurse." At the time, only a few token admissions to training schools for nurses were granted to black or Jewish applicants. With segregation by law in the South and by choice in the North, it followed that black schools of nursing would have to be opened if black women were to enter the profession in large numbers.

In 1886, **Spellman Seminary** in Atlanta, Georgia, started the first nursing program for blacks. It was followed in 1891 by Dixie Hospital Training School in Hampton, Virginia, and in 1892 by Tuskegee Institute in Alabama. (The Tuskegee program became the first baccalaureate program in a traditionally black institution in 1948 [Carnegie 1986].) These programs were responsible for the nursing education of generations of black nurses.

THE DEVELOPMENT OF NURSING ORGANIZATIONS

In 1893, **Isabel Hampton (Robb)** presented a paper at the International Congress of Charities, Correction, and Philanthropy at the Chicago World's Fair

Box 1–1   Lillian Wald's Awakening

From the schoolroom where I had been giving a lesson in bed-making, a little girl led me one drizzling March morning. She had told me of her sick mother, and gathering from her incoherent account that a child had been born, I caught up the paraphernalia of the bed-making lesson and carried it with me.

The child led me over broken roadways . . . between tall, reeking houses . . . past odorous fish stands for the streets were a market-place, unregulated, unsupervised, unclean, past evil-smelling, uncovered garbage cans, and perhaps worst of all, where so many little children played. . . .

The child led me on through a tenement hallway, across a court where open and unscreened closets were promiscuously used by men and women, up into a rear tenement, by slimy steps whose accumulated dirt was augmented that day by the mud of the streets, and finally into the sickroom.

All the maladjustments of our social and economic relations seemed epitomized in this brief journey and what was found at the end of it. The family to which the child led me was neither criminal nor vicious . . . and although the sick woman lay on a wretched, unclean bed, soiled with a hemorrhage two days old, they were not degraded human beings. . . . It would have been some solace if by any conviction of the moral unworthiness of the family, I could have defended myself as part of a society which permitted such conditions to exist. . . . miserable as their state was, they were not without ideals for the family life, and for society, of which they were so unloved and unlovely a part.

That morning's experience was a baptism of fire. Deserted were the laboratory and the academic work of the college. I never returned to them. . . . To my inexperience it seemed certain that conditions such as these were allowed because people did not *know*, and for me there was the challenge to know and tell. When early morning found me still awake, my naive conviction remained that, if people knew things,— and "things" meant everything implied in the condition of this family,—such horrors would cease to exist, and I rejoiced that I had training in the care of the sick that in itself would give me an organic relationship to the neighborhood in which this awakening had come.

"protesting the lack of uniformity of instruction in training schools and the completely inadequate education being provided" (Christy 1984, p. 38). Her presentation resulted in the formation of the American Society of Superintendents of Training Schools for Nurses. This society changed its name in 1912 to the National League of Nursing Education (NLNE); in 1952 it was again reorganized and given its current name, the National League for Nursing (NLN) (Christy 1984).

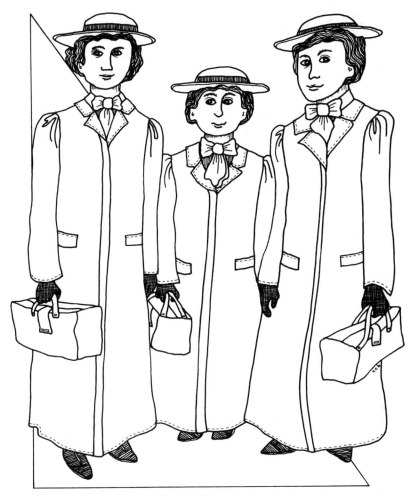

Figure 1–3   Henry Street Settlement Nurses. (Drawing by Cathy Campbell Beahm.)

In that same year, 1893, another nursing influential, **Lillian Wald**, underwent a transformational experience that changed the direction of nursing profoundly. Her graphic description of this event in her life is reprinted in Box 1–1.

As a result of this experience, Lillian Wald and her colleague, Mary Brewster, moved into a tenement on New York's Lower East Side. With the help of private philanthropists, they provided care to their neighbors and established the **Henry Street Settlement** and public health nursing in the United States (Christy 1984, p. 38) (Fig. 1–3). Wald later formed the National Organization of Public Health Nurses (1912), marking the beginning of specialization in nursing.

Isabel Hampton Robb recognized the need "to unite practitioners of nursing." She had already been instrumental in the formation of the National League for Nursing Education. In 1896 she was again successful in her efforts, founding the Associated Alumnus of the United States and Canada, which in 1911 became officially known as the American Nurses Association (ANA) (Christy 1984, p. 38). Nurses were getting organized for the work ahead.

EDUCATIONAL REFORM

October 1899 marked the culmination of some four years of work by the American Society of Superintendents of Training Schools for Nurses. Isabel Robb had chaired a committee to "investigate a means to better prepare nurses for leadership in schools of nursing. Teachers College, which had opened in New York ten years earlier for the training of teachers, seemed the logical choice. The program was originally designed to prepare administrators of nursing service and nursing education. It was established as an eight-month course in hospital economics" (Donahue 1985, p. 335).

Mary Adelaide Nutting came to Teachers College in 1907 to be "the first nursing professor in the world. . . . Under her direction, the department progressed and became a pioneer in education for nurses. The school became known as the 'Mother-House' of collegiate education because it fostered the initial movements toward undergraduate and graduate degrees for nurses" (Donahue 1985, p. 335).

In October 1900, following the dedicated work of Robb, Nutting, Dock, and others, the first issue of the *American Journal of Nursing* was published (Christy 1984, p. 39). Nursing now had an organized means of communication among the members of the profession.

MILITARY NURSING ESTABLISHED

The Spanish-American War (1898) provided the first opportunity for trained nurses to be accepted in military hospitals. It also marked the first time a trained black nurse, **Namahyoke Curtis**, was employed as a contract nurse by the War Department. Her efforts and the efforts of all graduate nurses involved in this war emphasized the importance and need for military nurses. This realization led to the formation of the Army Nurse Corps (1901) and the Navy Nurse Corps (1908).

Organized nursing in America had moved out of its infancy. By 1900 there were some 1200 trained nurses in addition to 109,000 untrained nurses practicing in homes, public health settings, hospitals, and the military (National League for Nursing 1990). While much was left to be accomplished, the trained nurse was destined to make a difference.

Nursing in the Twentieth Century—In Step with a Changing Society

From its humble beginnings, nursing during the twentieth century grew into a respected profession, the development of which continued to parallel that of the country.

1900–1920: SOCIAL AWAKENING, WORLD WAR I

The period from 1900 to 1920 was both a period of social awakening and a period of continued social injustices. The invention of the telephone, the airplane, and the automobile created more and faster avenues for communication and travel. Yet women still could not vote, and minorities were left to pave their own way in this changing society.

In 1900 **Jessie Sleet (Scales)** became the first black public health nurse. In 1908 the National Association of Colored Graduate Nurses (NACGN) was founded by **Martha Franklin**, but in 1916, some state nurses' associations barred black nurses from membership. This barrier also prevented them from being eligible for membership in the ANA. Undaunted by this barrier, **Francis Reed Elliott** became the first black nurse accepted by the American Red Cross Nursing Service in 1918.

Though minority groups in nursing were struggling, the profession as a whole continued to expand and establish new standards for the fledgling profession. In 1903 the first four state nursing licensure laws were passed in North Carolina, New Jersey, New York, and Virginia. These laws marked nursing's first successful efforts to become self-regulating and paved the way for licensing examinations nationwide. Progress in this era also included the 1912 establishment of the Town and Country Nursing Service by the American Red Cross and the opening of the first birth control clinic in America by **Margaret Sanger** in 1916. Sanger's clinic was the forerunner of Planned Parenthood.

In April 1917, the United States entered World War I. Destined to become the bloodiest war of all time because of new weapons and military technology, the nation once again mobilized its resources. Young men were drafted into the armed services in large numbers; the Army Nurse Corps and Navy Nurse Corps made concentrated efforts to expand their forces. With too few nurses available to meet both civilian and military needs, controversy raged about how best to meet the critical nursing shortage. In spite of almost insurmountable pressure from all sides to create a quick solution, calmer heads prevailed, and the Army School of Nursing was formed in 1918. Designed to quickly but competently meet the military's increased need for nurses, the school was headed by **Annie Goodrich**, then president of the ANA and an assistant professor of nursing at Teachers College.

The war effort was severely hampered by the great influenza epidemic of 1918–1919. Physicians and nurses as well as troops and civilians were struck with influenza. "The death toll in the United States alone for the last four months of 1918 and the first six months of 1919 was 548,452–five times greater than the total World War I American military deaths" (Kalisch and Kalisch 1986, p. 361). Health care resources were decimated by the epidemic. Because of the severity of the situation, 18 black nurses were ultimately accepted by the military, representing a breakthrough for this minority group. They were never actually able to participate in the war effort, however, because the war ended soon after their appointment.

The year 1919 marked the passage of the Nineteenth Amendment to the U.S. Constitution. That amendment extended voting privileges to women.

Women's suffrage had been under active consideration for 40 years before it was approved, and nursing organizations had formally voted to support the amendment on a number of occasions before it was actually passed. **Lavinia Dock** was a well-known early twentieth-century nurse who was actively involved in women's rights issues and the suffragette movement (Fig. 1–4). Dock, affectionately called "Little Dockie," was a small, red-haired woman whose appearance belied her leadership abilities. In 1925, looking back at the evolution of nursing and its involvement with societal issues, Lavinia Dock and Isabel Stewart wrote:

> When we consider the whole movement of social progress, the breaking down of the spirit of hatred and prejudice, the promotion of kindlier and more humane relations between human beings, the organization of practical and effective measures for reducing human suffering and distress, it would be hard to find any group of workers who have contributed more to the sum total of social effort than have nurses. (Donahue 1985, pp. 13–14)

Trained nurses *had* been involved, even to the point of marching in public parades to support the causes they believed in, such as women's suffrage.

1920–1929: THE ROARING TWENTIES

The decade of the 1920s saw the beginning of unheard of freedom for women. Shortened hairstyles, rising hemlines, and the use of cosmetics were all part of the "flapper" era of the 1920s. Hospitals continued to expand, as did schools of nursing, yet they often did not employ their own graduates, preferring to staff the hospital with student nurses because student help was less expensive.

In 1923 the findings of a nursing report entitled *Nursing and Nursing Education in the United States* were published. Called the **Goldmark Report**, "this document emphasized the desirability of establishing university schools of nursing to train nurse leaders. It pointed out the fundamental faults in hospital training schools, and identified the primary obstacle to higher standards as the lack of funds set apart specifically for nursing education" (Kalisch and Kalisch 1986, p. 374). There were at this time some 25 colleges and universities offering a bachelor's degree in nursing. Even so, the combined enrollment in all of these schools totaled only 368 (Kalisch and Kalisch 1986).

> The year 1924 marked another first in nursing education when the **Yale School of Nursing** was opened as the first in the world to be established as a separate university department with an independent budget and its own dean, Annie W. Goodrich . . . . It demonstrated its effectiveness so markedly that in 1929, the Rockefeller Foundation assured the permanency of the school by awarding it an endowment of one million dollars" (Kalisch and Kalisch 1986, p. 379).

Despite opposition by physicians, hospital-based training schools, and veteran nurses, collegiate nursing programs were under way.

During the 1920s, nursing was also progressing on another front—rural midwifery. Responding to the lack of maternity care for rural women, **Mary Breckinridge** founded the **Frontier Nursing Service** in 1925. Although untrained women had served as midwives for centuries, the Frontier Nursing Ser-

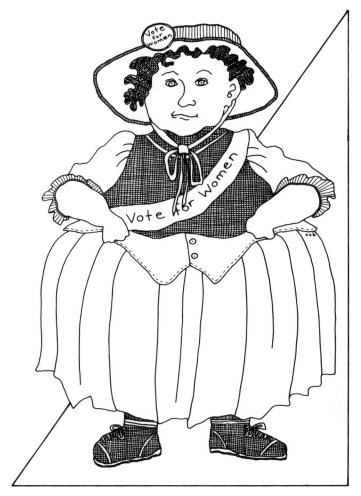

Figure 1–4 Lavinia Dock. (Drawing by Cathy Campbell Beahm.)

vice provided "the first organized midwifery service in this country" (Donahue 1985, p. 350).

1929–1937: THE DEPRESSION

By 1927 there were some 2286 schools of nursing in the United States, most of which were hospital based (Kalisch and Kalisch 1986, p. 369). The prosperity of the nation was waning in these early days leading up to the Great Depression. The use of private-duty nurses declined as family resources diminished. There was insufficient funding for visiting nurse services. Soon there were too many trained nurses, and unemployment nationwide was on the rise. The stock market crash of 1929 marked the beginning of a long period of economic decline and further unemployment in the United States.

During the 1930s the country struggled to emerge from the economic depression that caused devastating hardships. Nursing unemployment hit an all-time high. Yet even in this time of economic depression, medicine made a number of advancements. As medical technology advanced and nurses demonstrated that they were well trained in the care of the sick, hospitals rapidly became the primary setting for health care. Health insurance plans evolved, Social Security was passed in 1935, and labor movements brought renewed attention to working conditions and child labor.

The labor movement forced hospitals and training schools to look more closely at the way in which they utilized student nurses. Training schools reduced the long duty schedules of student nurses, and hospitals actively recruited graduate nurses, which served to reduce nursing unemployment. The shift in employment of graduate nurses from homes to hospitals coincided with increasing hospital admissions and a decline in home-based care that was to last until the 1980s.

1937–1945: THE WAR YEARS

The decade of the 1940s found the country emerging from a major economic depression, preparing for war, fighting the war, and recovering from it. It was also a time of prosperity and progress for nursing.

The 1941 Lanham Act supported the need for additional trained nurses by allocating funds for additions to dormitories, libraries, classrooms, and other physical facilities (Donahue 1985, p. 413). Through the efforts of Frances Payne Bolton, federally funded support for nursing education came with the passage of the Appropriations Act for 1942 (Donahue 1985, p. 412). It was followed by the Nurse Training Act of 1943, which was also sponsored by Mrs. Bolton. Later this act became known as the Bolton Act and resulted in the creation of the United States Cadet Nurse Corps. It was administered by the U.S. Public Health Service, Division of Nurse Education, led by **Lucille Petry**. (In 1949, Miss Petry became the first woman appointed to the position of assistant surgeon general of the United Public Health Service. At that time, this was the highest post ever held by a nurse.) By the war's end, some 65,000 nurses had enlisted and graduated from the Cadet Nurse Corps (National League for Nursing 1990), and nearly 69,000 nurses were serving in the Army and Navy Nurse Corps (Donahue 1985, p. 415).

World War II served as a catalyst for significant advances in medical science and in care given by nurses and physicians. Such advances as blood transfusions, early antibiotics, improved treatment for malaria, trauma care, rehabilitation, and other techniques were discovered out of the need to treat those ravaged by war. Science, medicine, and nursing were changing, expanding, and becoming more proficient. Nurses, along with their physician colleagues and military corpsmen, were present on every battlefront—on the land, at sea, and in the air. Some were wounded, some died, and some were captured and placed in prisoner-of-war camps. Once again, nurses played an instrumental role during wartime.

The first Nurse Draft Bill was introduced late in the war, but the war's end made the bill unnecessary. Nurses who served in the war were officers and, when discharged following the war, had access to further education through the GI Bill of Rights. They entered undergraduate and graduate programs to earn advanced degrees in nursing. Many, however, chose to return to more traditional, nonworking female roles following the war.

The postwar economic boom and the "baby boom" both served to stimulate the construction of hospitals. The nursing shortage once again became painfully acute in hospitals, and two new categories of workers emerged in response to the shortage. They were the nursing assistant (NA) and the licensed practical nurse (L.P.N.). One-year practical nursing programs, begun during the war as an expedient way to supplement the numbers of registered nurses, became institutionalized with licensure of L.P.N.s.

As with any labor shortage, working conditions in hospitals became increasingly difficult, with long hours, low pay, large work loads, and insufficient help. Many nurses were unhappy with both their working conditions and the quality of nursing care they were able to provide in these adverse conditions. In 1946 the ANA authorized its state units to form collective-bargaining units, and another conflict arose—to strike or not to strike. Heated debates throughout the country defined the ethical dilemma of nursing professionals: the duty to care for patients and the personal duty to care for oneself.

Discrimination against black nurses continued throughout the years surrounding the war. In 1940 in Mississippi, for example, there were 3 black public health nurses and 1 million black people. This disproportion was typical of the barriers blacks faced in entering all professional fields.

1945–1965: THE POSTWAR ERA AND TECHNOLOGICAL EXPLOSION

In the 20 years following World War II, the United States experienced an explosion of technology that profoundly affected health care. A vast store of medical knowledge and technical advances resulted from World War II, and within two decades, the nation was engaged in two more wars—Korea and Vietnam (Fig. 1–5). With each war, medical advances were made. As science and technology moved to the forefront of health care, the size, number, and distribution of hospitals rapidly expanded. Changes took place within nursing as well.

During the 1950s, a shorter educational route to becoming a nurse, the associate degree program, was added to the degree and diploma programs already in existence. The *Journal of Nursing Research* was founded in 1952 as the pace and quality of nursing research rapidly expanded. Military corpsmen entered nursing programs, and the number of male nurses increased. More nurses sought advanced degrees. State units of the ANA accepted black nurses for membership, as did the ANA itself. The NACGN was dissolved in 1951 but was followed in 1972 by the formation of the National Black Nurses Association.

Health insurance plans expanded, creating a great demand for more health services. The Civil Rights Movement, which began in the early part of the 1960s,

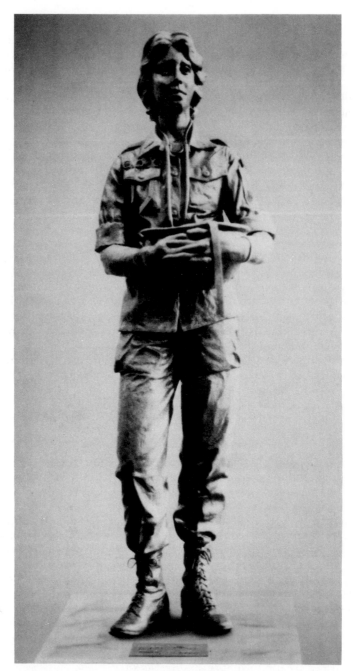

Figure 1–5 Vietnam nurse. (© 1984 Rodger M. Brodin Studios, Inc. All rights reserved. Used by permission.)

moved the country into an era of social justice that broke down some barriers of inequality of the races and the sexes. Technological advances resulting from space exploration impacted medical science and nursing practice even further. Undreamed of life-saving drugs and life-prolonging technologies were developed. Trauma care and care of premature babies saved thousands of lives that formerly would have been lost. To keep up with the new technologies, critical care nursing evolved as a specialty area of practice.

1965–1990: HEALTH CARE BOOM AND ESCALATING COSTS

The next 25 years saw unparalleled growth of hospitals and other health care agencies. Medical technology reached previously unheard of heights with astounding new medical, surgical, and diagnostic techniques. Not unexpectedly, the costs of health care also rose steadily. Nursing's political agendas during this time centered around parity with medicine and autonomy in practice (National League for Nursing 1990).

Civil rights and the women's movement continued to be major social issues. The assassinations of John F. Kennedy, Martin Luther King, and Robert F. Kennedy shocked and saddened the nation but heightened the need for continued social reform.

Nursing specialization continued and with it developed specialty-focused professional organizations. The nurse practitioners' role evolved to meet changing health care needs and eventually paved the way for increasingly collaborative relationships between nursing and medicine. However, it also created conflict in some areas of the country as physicians and nurses battled over the right to practice.

Lyndon B. Johnson's "Great Society" reforms reflected the prevailing social climate and demand for improved living conditions and access to health care. In 1965, Medicare and Medicaid were made law. Access to health care for the nation's elderly, poor, and disabled seemed assured. Shortly thereafter, however, health care costs began to rise dramatically. In response, major legislative acts were passed to curtail these costs. Chapter 14 will discuss this legislation in some detail.

Large numbers of nurses were employed outside hospitals: in business, industry, law, government, education, the military, and the community. Entrepreneurship prevailed as nurse-owned and -operated businesses emerged. These new opportunities contributed to continued periodic nursing shortages, however.

By 1990 the face of both nursing and health care had changed. Hospitals cared predominantly for the acutely ill, as patients moved away from the hospital and back into community-care settings and the home. Major health care issues centered around the uninsured, the elderly, the homeless, the disadvantaged, and the AIDS (acquired immunodeficiency syndrome) epidemic. As they had done throughout their history, nurses continued to reach out and provide care to the needy wherever they happened to be. Minority nurses continued to seek recognition for their accomplishments, and the nursing profession continued to grow and adapt to the rapidly changing health care needs of society.

1990s: THE ERA OF COST CONTAINMENT—NURSING LEADS THE WAY

The decade of the 1990s will be characterized by efforts toward cost containment and heightened efficiency in health care. By 1992, the need for major health care reform was recognized by many Americans. Organized nursing had assumed a major leadership role in the reform effort by submitting its *Agenda for Health Care Reform.* The plan for reform, discussed more fully in Chapter 4, was comprehensive and focused on restructuring the nation's health care system, reducing costs, and improving accessibility to all who are in need of care. A number of the challenges faced by the nursing profession in the decade of the 1990s are covered in Chapter 23.

CHAPTER SUMMARY

The history of nursing is rich, filled with struggle, neglect, missed opportunities, vision, courage, and victory. Margretta Styles, a contemporary nursing leader, wrote "A Biblical Fable on Our Origins," from which the following is excerpted:

> In the beginning, God created nursing. He (or she) said, "I will take a solid, simple significant system of education and an adequate, applicable base of clinical research, and on these rocks will I build My greatest gift to mankind—nursing practice." On the seventh day He threw up his hands. And has left it up to us. (Donahue 1985, p. 434)

And we have not done too badly! After years of apprenticeship learning and exploitation of students in the workplace, we now have a significant system of nursing education. After using research findings from other disciplines, we now have our own rapidly growing base of clinical research and a pool of nurses educated to pursue nursing research. After decades of basing our professional actions on theories from psychology, sociology, education, and medicine, we now are developing nursing theories on which to base our practices. And we have strong, caring, committed practitioners, educators, and leaders who give nursing life, shape, and vitality. The words of Florence Nightingale are as appropriate today as when she wrote them:

> Nursing is an art; and if it is to be made an art, it requires as exclusive a devotion, as hard a preparation, as any painter's or sculptor's work; for what is the having to do with dead canvas or cold marble, compared with having to do with the living body—the temple of God's spirit? It is one of the Fine Arts; I had almost said, the finest of the Fine Arts. (Donahue 1985, p. 469)

Nurses have significant impact on the practice and profession of nursing. They can be the driving force in shaping health care in the twenty-first century and improving the quality of life for all humankind.

REVIEW/DISCUSSION QUESTIONS

1. What influence did the involvement of early religious groups in caring for the sick have on modern nursing?

2. How did Florence Nightingale's Crimean experience affect American nursing?

3. Cite the forces leading to the establishment of training schools for nurses in America.

4. How was the development of nursing in the United States influenced by the medical profession?

5. What were the contributions of early black nurses?

6. Wars have often been the driving force in creating social change. How did wars influence the profession of nursing?

REFERENCES

Austin, A. L. (1984). Nurses in American history: Wartime volunteers—1861–1865. In *Pages from nursing history: A collection of original articles from the pages of Nursing Outlook, the American Journal of Nursing and Nursing Research.* New York: American Journal of Nursing.

Carnegie, M. E. (1986). *The path we tread: Blacks in nursing, 1854–1984.* Philadelphia: J.B. Lippincott.

Christy, T. E. (1984). Nurses in American history: The fateful decade, 1890–1900. In *Pages from nursing history: A collection of original articles from the pages of Nursing Outlook, the American Journal of Nursing, and Nursing Research.* New York: American Journal of Nursing.

Dolan, J. (1984). Nurses in American history: Three schools—1873. In *Pages from nursing history: A collection of original articles from the pages of Nursing Outlook, the American Journal of Nursing, and Nursing Research.* New York: American Journal of Nursing.

Donahue, M. P. (1985). *Nursing: The finest art, An illustrated history.* St. Louis: C.V. Mosby.

Kalisch, P. A., and Kalisch, B. J. (1986). *The advance of American nursing* (2nd ed.). Boston: Little, Brown.

National League for Nursing. (1990). *Nursing in America: A history of social reform* (videotape). New York: Author.

Robinson, V. (1946). *White caps: The story of nursing.* Philadelphia: J.B. Lippincott.

Selavan, I. C. (1984). Nurses in American history: The revolution. In *Pages from nursing history: A collection of original articles from the pages of Nursing Outlook, the American Journal of Nursing, and Nursing Research.* New York: American Journal of Nursing.

Smith, F. T. (1984). Florence Nightingale: Early feminist. In *Pages from nursing history: A collection of original articles from the pages of Nursing Outlook, the American Journal of Nursing, and Nursing Research.* New York: American Journal of Nursing.

Wald, L. D. (1915). *The house on Henry Street.* New York: Henry Holt.

SUGGESTED READINGS

Baer, E. D. (1990). Editor's notes for *Nursing in America: A history of social reform* (videotape). New York: National League for Nursing.

Benson, E. R. (1990). An early 20th century view of nursing. *Nursing Outlook,* 38(6), 275-277.

Kampen, N. B. (1988). Before Florence Nightingale: A prehistory of nursing in painting and sculpture. In A. H. Jones (Ed.), *Images of nurses: Perspectives from history, art, and literature.* Philadelphia: University of Pennsylvania Press.

Maggs, C. (Ed.). (1987). *Nursing history: The state of the art.* U.K.: Croom Helm.

Palmer, I. S. (1984). Nightingale revisited. In *Pages from nursing history: A collection of original articles from the pages of Nursing Outlook, the American Journal of Nursing, and Nursing Research.* New York: American Journal of Nursing.

Parsons, M. E. (1984). Mothers and matrons. In *Pages from nursing history: A collection of original articles from the pages of Nursing Outlook, the American Journal of Nursing, and Nursing Research.* New York: American Journal of Nursing.

Rosenberg, C. E. (1987). *The care of strangers: The rise of America's hospital system.* New York: Basic Books.

Chapter

Educational Patterns in Nursing

Elaine F. Nichols

CHAPTER OBJECTIVES

What students should be able to do after studying this chapter:

1. Trace the development of basic and graduate education in nursing.
2. Discuss the significance of three national nursing studies.
3. Explain the difference between licensure, certification, and accreditation.
4. Discuss the traditional and alternative ways of becoming a registered nurse.
5. Differentiate between licensed practical nurses and registered nurses.
6. Differentiate between academic credit and continuing education credit.
7. Discuss the significance of the ANA position paper.
8. Discuss program options for registered nurses and students with baccalaureate degrees in nonnursing fields.

VOCABULARY BUILDING

Terms to know:

accreditation	ANA position paper	Brown Report
advanced degrees	articulation	certification
alternative	associate degree	CEU
educational	baccalaureate degree	continuing education
programs	basic programs	(CE)

diploma program	licensure	NCLEX-PN
external degree	Lysaught Report	NCLEX-RN
generic master's degree	mandatory continuing education	practical nurse R.N.-to-B.S.N. education
Goldmark Report	Mildred Montag	

*D*iversity is the major characteristic of nursing education today (Fig. 2–1). Influenced by a variety of factors—societal changes, efforts to achieve full professional status, women's issues, historical factors, public expectations, expectations of nurses themselves, legislation, national studies, and constant changes in the health care system—many differing types of nursing education programs exist.

In 1991, there were 1607 **basic programs** preparing beginning registered nurses (R.N.s) in the United States. Of these, 51 percent were associate degree programs, 40 percent were baccalaureate programs, and 10 percent were diploma programs (Division of Research 1990). In addition to the basic registered nurse programs, there were also 182 accredited master's programs, 54 doctoral programs, and 1048 practical nursing programs. Also included in the educational system of nursing are a large number of continuing education programs and advanced-practice certification programs.

This chapter provides an orientation to the multiple educational patterns in existence in nursing today. It covers the history behind these educational programs, descriptions of the various programs, and trends and future issues.

The Development of Nursing Education in the United States

As seen in Chapter 1, Florence Nightingale is credited with founding modern nursing and creating the first educational system for nurses. After hospitals came into existence in western Europe and prior to the influence of Florence Nightingale, hospital care was given by women such as prisoners and prostitutes, who

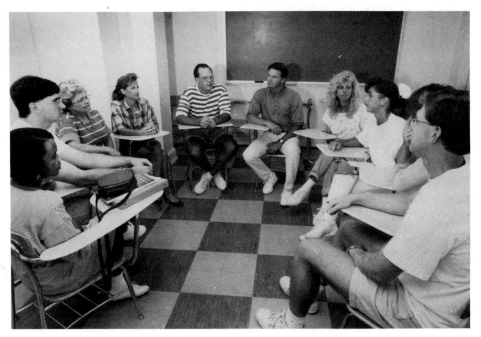

Figure 2–1 There were 1607 programs preparing beginning registered nurses in 1991. Students entering nursing today are a widely diverse group.

were held in very low regard by society. These women learned to give care by doing it. There was no organized program to educate nurses.

Nightingale stressed that nursing was not a domestic, charitable service but a respected occupation requiring advanced education. She opened a school of nursing at St. Thomas Hospital, London, in 1860 and established the following basic principles for the school:

1. The nurse should be trained in an educational institution supported by public funds and associated with a medical school.
2. The nursing school should be affiliated with a teaching hospital but independent of it.
3. The curriculum should include both theory and practical experience.
4. Professional nurses should be in charge of administration and instruction and should be paid for their instruction.
5. Students should be carefully selected and should reside in nurses' houses that form discipline and character.
6. Students should be required to attend lectures, take quizzes, write papers, and keep diaries. Student records should be maintained (Notter and Spalding 1976).

Miss Nightingale also believed that the nursing schools should be separate financially and administratively from hospitals where the students trained. This was not the case, however, when nursing schools were first established in the United States.

Following the 1873 establishment of the "famous trio" of nursing schools at Bellevue in New York, in Connecticut, and in Boston, other schools rapidly developed. By 1900, there were 432 hospital-owned and -operated **diploma programs** in the United States (Fondiller 1986). These early training programs differed in length from six months to two years, and each school set its own standards and requirements. The primary reason for the schools' existence was to staff the hospitals. The education of students was not always the primary concern.

Early Studies of Nursing Education

Nursing leaders of the early 1900s were concerned about the poor quality of the nurse training programs. They initiated studies about nursing and nursing education in order to prompt changes. In 1912, Adelaide Nutting conducted an investigation, "The Educational Status of Nursing," that focused on the living conditions of students, the material being taught, and the teaching methods being used (Christy 1969).

As mentioned in Chapter 1, a major study was published in 1923. Titled "The Study of Nursing and Nursing Education in the United States" and referred to as the **Goldmark Report**, it focused on the clinical learning experiences of students, hospital control of the schools, and the lack of prepared teachers (Kalisch and Kalisch 1986).

In 1934, another study entitled "Nursing Schools Today and Tomorrow" reported the number of schools in existence, gave detailed descriptions of the schools, described their curricula, and made recommendations for professional collegiate education (Committee on the Grading of Nursing Schools 1934).

In 1937, *A Curriculum Guide for Schools of Nursing* was published outlining a three-year curriculum. This document influenced the structure of diploma schools for many years after its publication (National League of Nursing Education 1937).

Although spread over a number of years and undertaken by different groups, these studies consistently made five recommendations:

1. That nursing education programs be established within the system of higher education.
2. That nurses be highly educated.
3. That students not be used to staff hospitals.
4. That standards exist for nursing practice.
5. That all nurses meet certain minimum qualifications upon graduation.

These early studies set the stage for the development of the educational programs that exist today.

Educational Pathways to Becoming a Registered Nurse

Today, preparation for a career as a registered nurse can begin in one of three ways: in an associate degree program, in a baccalaureate degree program, or in a hospital-based diploma program. Following the completion of a basic program for registered nurses, graduates are eligible to take the National Council Licensing Examination for Registered Nurses (NCLEX-RN). Upon successful completion of the licensing examination, graduates may legally practice as registered nurses and use the initials "R.N." after their names.

Having three different educational routes to licensure for registered nurses is confusing to the public and to nurses themselves. Each type of program will therefore be described with its history, unique characteristics, and special issues. The basic programs will be discussed in the order in which they appeared in nursing education history.

The Diploma Program

The hospital-based **diploma program** was the first type of nursing education begun in the United States. At the peak of diploma education in the 1920s and 1930s, approximately 2000 programs existed, with numerous programs in almost every state. Diploma programs produced many outstanding nurses, but since the peak in the first third of the century, their numbers have decreased steadily (Conley 1973).

In the last 30 years there has been a dramatic decline in diploma programs as nursing education moved into collegiate settings where other professionals are educated. In 1960, there were approximately 800 diploma programs in the United States. By 1980 that number had decreased to approximately 300. And by 1990 there were only 152 diploma programs located in 26 states. Half the states had no diploma programs.

In 1990 the largest number of diploma schools (34) remained in Pennsylvania, with two other states, New Jersey and Ohio, having 17 and 15, respectively (Council of Diploma Programs 1990). Although the number of diploma programs has significantly decreased, the majority of nurses practicing today received their basic nursing educations in diploma programs.

In the late 1800s and early 1900s, diploma programs provided one of the few avenues for women to obtain formal education and jobs. Most of the early programs followed a modified apprenticeship model. Lectures were given by physicians, and clinical training was supervised by head nurses and nursing directors. Nursing courses paralleled medical areas and included surgery, obstetrics, pediatrics, and operating room experience. Students were sometimes sent to affiliated institutions where they could obtain experiences that were not available at the home hospital.

The schedule was very demanding, with classes being held after patient care assignments were completed. Critics charged that students were used as inexpensive labor to staff the hospitals and that education was a lower priority. The truth of those charges varied from hospital to hospital, but there is no question that early nursing students literally ran the hospitals.

Programs lasted three years, and at graduation, students were awarded diplomas in nursing. Today, most diploma programs are about 24 months in length.

A problem that many diploma graduates have faced is that hospitals are not recognized as part of the higher education system in this country. Most colleges and universities do not recognize the diploma in nursing as an academic credential and have often refused to give college credit for courses taken in diploma programs, regardless of the quality of the courses, students, and faculty. In recent years, diploma schools have established agreements with colleges and universities that enable diploma students to take regular college courses in English, psychology, and the sciences.

The decline in the number of diploma programs is due to several factors: the growth of associate degree and baccalaureate degree programs in nursing; the inability of hospitals to continue to finance nursing education; accreditation standards that have made it difficult for diploma programs to attract qualified faculty; and the increasing complexity of health care, which has required nurses to have greater scientific preparation. Today, diploma programs represent only 10 percent of the total number of basic nursing education programs in the United States.

During the depths of the most recent nursing shortage, which occurred in the middle 1980s, diploma programs experienced increased enrollments. Some hospitals began admitting students to programs that had previously been destined to be phased out. Even though the number of programs overall is generally diminishing, existing programs and practicing diploma graduates are still influential in health care settings and professional organizations.

The Baccalaureate Program

Nursing leaders, armed with early studies of nursing education, wanted nursing education to move into the mainstream of higher education, that is, into colleges and universities where other professionals are educated. Their belief was that nurses needed the **baccalaureate degree** to qualify nursing as a recognized profession and to provide leadership for administration, teaching, and public health nursing.

By the time the first baccalaureate nursing program was established in 1909 at the University of Minnesota, diploma programs were numerous and firmly entrenched as the system for educating nurses. This first baccalaureate program was part of the School of Medicine and followed the three-year diploma program structure. Despite its many limitations, it was the start of the movement to bring nursing education into the recognized system of higher education.

Seven other baccalaureate programs in nursing were established by 1919 (Conley 1973). Most of the early baccalaureate programs were five years in length. This structure provided for three years of nursing education and two years of liberal arts. The growth in the numbers of these programs was slow due both to the reluctance of universities to accept nursing as a theoretical discipline and to the power of the diploma programs. The theoretical, scientific orientation of the baccalaureate program was in contrast to the "hands-on" skill and service orientation that was the hallmark of diploma education and was often questioned.

INFLUENCES ON THE GROWTH OF BACCALAUREATE EDUCATION

National studies of nursing and nursing education stated and restated the need for nursing education and practice to be based on knowledge from the sciences and humanities. Chief among these studies was Esther Lucille Brown's report *Nursing for the Future.* Published in 1948, the **Brown Report**, as it was called, recommended that basic schools of nursing be placed in universities and colleges and that efforts be made to recruit large numbers of men and minorities into nursing education programs. This report, sponsored by the Carnegie Foundation, was widely reviewed, discussed, and debated.

Another major influence on the growth of baccalaureate education occurred in 1965 when the American Nurses Association (**ANA**) published a **position paper** on *Educational Preparation for Nurse Practitioners and Assistants to Nurses.* This paper, which created conflict and division within nursing, represented the most significant influence on the growth of baccalaureate education in nursing. In preparing the position paper, the ANA studied nursing education, nursing practice, and the trends in health care. It concluded that baccalaureate education should become the basic foundation for professional practice.

The position paper made four major recommendations:

1. Education for all those who are licensed to practice nursing should take place in institutions of higher learning.
2. Minimum preparation for beginning professional nursing practice should be baccalaureate education in nursing.
3. Minimum preparation for beginning technical nursing practice should be the associate degree in nursing.
4. Education for assistants in the health service occupations should consist of short, intensive preservice programs in vocational education institutions rather than in on-the-job training programs (American Nurses Association 1965).

In spite of tremendous opposition from proponents of diploma and associate degree education, the ANA, in 1978, further strengthened its resolve by proposing three additional positions:

1. By 1985 the minimum preparation for entry into professional nursing practice should be the baccalaureate in nursing.
2. Two categories of nursing practice should be identified and a mechanism to devise competencies for the two categories established by 1980.
3. There should be increased accessibility to high-quality career mobility programs that use flexible approaches for individuals seeking academic degrees in nursing (American Nurses Association 1979).

The controversy created by the initial ANA position paper and the additional 1978 resolutions continued for many years and is not yet fully resolved. Practicing nurses across the United States, who were mainly diploma program graduates, as well as hospitals that supported diploma programs, vehemently protested the recommendations.

In 1970 the National Commission for the Study of Nursing and Nursing Education published its report entitled *An Abstract for Action*. Also known as the **Lysaught Report**, it made recommendations concerning the supply and demand for nurses, nursing roles and functions, and nursing education. Among the priorities identified by this study were (1) the need for increased research into both the practice and education for nurses and (2) enhanced educational systems and curricula (Lysaught 1970).

In the early 1980s, the National Commission on Nursing published two reports that suggested that the major block to the advancement of nursing was the ongoing conflict within the profession about educational preparation for nurses. These studies recommended establishing a clear system of nursing education including pathways for educational mobility and development of additional graduate education programs.

The latest major national nursing group to support the baccalaureate as the entry credential was the National League for Nursing (NLN). The organization's membership is made up of nurses, faculty members, health care agencies, nursing programs, and nonnursing citizens who are supportive of nursing. After much debate, in 1982 the NLN board of directors approved the *Position Statement on Nursing Roles: Scope and Preparation,* which affirmed the nursing baccalaureate degree as the minimum educational level for professional nursing practice and the associate degree or diploma as the preparation for technical nursing practice (National League for Nursing 1982).

BACCALAUREATE PROGRAMS TODAY

Today baccalaureate programs provide education for both basic students who are preparing for licensure and those registered nurses returning to school to obtain a bachelor of science in nursing (B.S.N.). Baccalaureate programs for registered nurses will be discussed later in the chapter. This discussion will focus on the program characteristics of prelicensure baccalaureate education, sometimes called generic programs.

Basic baccalaureate programs combine nursing courses with general education courses in a four- or five-year curriculum in a senior college or university. Students may be admitted to the nursing program as entering freshmen or after completing certain liberal arts courses. Students meet the same admission requirements to the university as other students and often must meet additional requirements to be admitted to the nursing major.

Courses in the nursing major focus on nursing science, communication, decision making, leadership, and care to persons of all ages in a wide variety of settings. Because this education takes place in senior universities, nursing students interact with the larger student population, which promotes diverse thinking, cultural awareness, and broader socialization.

Faculty qualifications in baccalaureate programs are usually higher than in other basic nursing programs. Often a doctorate in nursing or a related field is required. This requirement ensures that nursing faculty are able to meet the teaching, research, and service requirements of universities (Council of Baccalaureate and Higher Degree Programs 1990a).

Baccalaureate graduates are prepared to take the **NCLEX-RN** and, after **licensure**, assume beginning practice and ultimately leadership positions in any health care setting, including community health. Graduates are also prepared to move immediately into graduate programs in nursing or clinical certification programs. Today, there is great demand for B.S.N.s, and they enjoy the greatest career mobility of all basic program graduates (Fig. 2–2).

An early and continuing criticism of baccalaureate preparation involved the perception that new BSN graduates were less clinically skillful than their diploma-educated counterparts. A number of contemporary B.S.N. programs have responded to this concern by increasing students' time in clinical practice. Preceptorships, in which students are paired with practicing R.N.s and work inten-

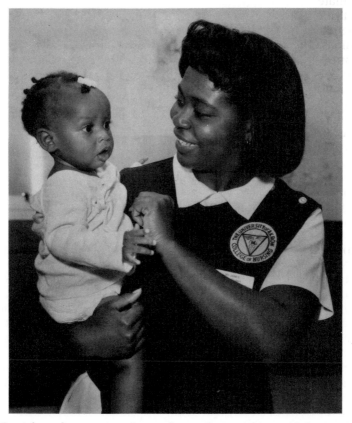

Figure 2–2   A baccalaureate nursing student enjoys working with her patient. (Courtesy of the University of Akron.)

sively in clinical settings, have been a successful method for improving the clinical skills of B.S.N. students.

The Associate Degree Program

Associate degree education in nursing represents the newest form of basic preparation for registered nurse practice. Begun in 1952 as a result of research conducted by **Dr. Mildred Montag**, and fueled by the community college movement of the 1950s, associate degree programs are now the most common type of basic nursing education program in the United States.

In 1991, 812 (51 percent of all basic programs) programs offered the associate degree (Division of Research 1990). The popularity of this program is due to several features: accessibility of community colleges, low tuition costs, shorter length of programs, graduates' eligibility to take the licensure examination for registered nurses, and the availability of jobs. According to Schwirian (1984), students in associate degree programs are more likely to be older, married, and studying part-time than students in other basic nursing programs. In the 1990s, however, these trends are also seen in diploma and baccalaureate students.

Originally, associate degree programs were designed to prepare nurse technicians to function under the supervision of professional nurses. Associate degree nurses were to work at the bedside, performing routine nursing skills for patients in acute and long-term care settings. The original associate degree program, as outlined by Montag (1951), had general education courses in the first year and nursing courses in the second year.

Dr. Montag originally viewed the associate degree as a terminal degree, not a stepping stone to the baccalaureate degree in nursing. Montag's original conceptions of associate degree programs have been modified in actual practice. Associate degree curricula now contain more nursing credits than she suggested. They also include content on leadership and clinical decision making, abilities that Montag did not foresee in technical nurses.

Another departure from Montag's plan is that owing to additions to the curriculum, few students can complete associate degrees in only two years. Most can graduate in three or fewer years, however. In spite of the shortened curriculum, as a group, associate degree graduates tend to perform exceedingly well on licensing examinations.

Associate degree graduates are employed in a wide variety of settings and function autonomously alongside baccalaureate and diploma graduates. In the educational system of nursing today, the associate degree can be a step in the progression to the baccalaureate degree.

Like other nursing programs, associate degree programs are currently undergoing review and revision. In 1990 the NLN Council of Associate Degree Programs prepared a document entitled *Educational Outcomes of Associate Degree Nursing Programs: Roles and Competencies*. This document was in response to a national effort to differentiate the competencies of the associate degree nurse from the competencies of the baccalaureate nurse. The document identified associate degree competencies in three roles: provider of care, manager of care, and member within the discipline of nursing. The further development of these competencies will have a direct effect on associate degree programs in the future.

Alternative Programs

In addition to the three basic programs leading to entry-level nursing practice, several **alternative educational programs** also exist.

BACCALAUREATE PROGRAMS FOR REGISTERED NURSES

After nursing organizations publicly advocated for the baccalaureate degree as the minimum education level for professional practice, the demand for the degree increased. Employers of nurses recognized that broadly educated nurses matched well with the increasing complexities of health care. As a result, they supported the B.S.N. as a requirement for career mobility. Diploma and associate degree graduates returned to school in ever-increasing numbers.

R.N.s with diplomas and associate degrees were not always welcomed into baccalaureate programs. Many were required to take courses that they felt they had already mastered. For a number of years it was difficult for these nurses to complete their B.S.N.s. In the past decade, however, many baccalaureate programs recognized the legitimacy of **R.N.-to-B.S.N. education** and developed alternative tracks to accommodate the unique learning needs of the registered nurse student. **B.R.N.** is also used to refer to R.N.-to-B.S.N. education.

Some B.S.N. programs for registered nurses are offered by universities that also offer a basic baccalaureate program for nonnurses. The R.N. students may be integrated with the basic students, or they may be in a separate or partially separate sequence. Other B.S.N. programs for R.N.s are found in colleges that do not have a basic baccalaureate nursing program.

These programs are increasingly offered owing to the demand for higher education by large numbers of associate degree nurses. In 1980–1981, 8416 R.N. students graduated from baccalaureate programs. There were 292 basic programs that also admitted R.N.s and 95 programs that admitted R.N.s only. By 1990, there were 11,546 R.N. graduates from 488 basic baccalaureate programs and 150 R.N.-only baccalaureate programs (Division of Research 1990).

Most four-year colleges and universities allow the transfer of general education credits from junior and community colleges. Often, some transfer credit is given for nursing courses as well, or there is the option of receiving credit for previous nursing courses through testing.

For diploma graduates, transfer credit is usually given for previous college courses, such as English, if they were included as part of the diploma program and taught by college faculty. Challenge examinations, in which students demonstrate mastery of specific content, may be an option for advanced placement of diploma graduates in B.S.N. courses.

Unresolved issues surrounding B.R.N. programs include the philosophy of some baccalaureate faculty that diploma and associate degree programs should not be stepping stones to baccalaureate degrees and therefore courses taken in those programs should not transfer to baccalaureate credit. There is a continuing concern about maintaining standards and protecting the integrity of the baccalaureate degree while facilitating the progression of R.N. students. There are also problems associated with evaluating previous learning and granting credit for that learning. An additional concern is that educational methods appropriate for basic students may not be useful for the midcareer registered nurse student.

However these issues are ultimately resolved, it is clear that the demand for the B.S.N. by large numbers of associate degree and diploma graduates will continue into the forseeable future.

EXTERNAL DEGREE PROGRAMS

Another alternative program is the **external degree** in nursing. The major difference between the external degree and traditional education is that students awarded an external degree attend no classes and follow no prescribed methods of learning. Learning is independent and is assessed through highly standardized and validated examinations. Students are responsible for arranging their own clinical experiences in accordance with established standards.

The New York Regents External Degree Nursing Program is the most well-recognized external degree model and has both general education and nursing requirements. General education requirements include humanities, social sciences, natural sciences, and mathematics. The nursing categories represent five areas: health, commonalities of nursing care, differences in nursing care, occupational strategy, and performance. The performance examination can be challenged only after successful completion of the other four categories (Wozniak 1973).

The New York Regents External Degree Nursing Program received NLN accreditation in 1981 through the Council of Baccalaureate and Higher Degree Programs. In that same year, the California State University Consortium instituted a statewide external degree baccalaureate program in nursing. In contrast to the prelicensure program in New York, the California program is for registered nurses holding current licenses to practice in the state ("Cal State" 1982).

ARTICULATED PROGRAMS

Another educational pattern created in response to the demand for educational mobility for nurses is a system that provides direct **articulation**, or movement, between programs. The purpose of articulation is to facilitate opportunities for nurses to start and stop at various points and keep moving up the educational ladder. For example, students in an articulated L.P.N./A.D.N./B.S.N. (licensed practical nurse/associate degree in nursing/bachelor of science in nursing) program would spend the first year preparing to be an L.P.N. and the second year completing the associate degree. If desired or necessary, students can "stop out" of the program at the end of the first year, take the licensure examination for practical nursing, and return to the associate degree program at a later time. Or they could continue school after the two initial years to earn a baccalaureate degree (Rapson 1987).

Multiple-entry, multiple-exit programs are difficult to develop. A tremendous amount of joint institutional planning is needed to work out equivalent courses and to keep the programs congruent with each other. A change in one curriculum dictates changes in all the others. Unless mandated by the state, as was done in California, voluntary fully articulated programs are unlikely to become commonplace.

OPTIONS FOR NONNURSING POSTBACCALAUREATE STUDENTS

A recent trend is an increase in the number of students entering nursing programs with baccalaureate degrees in other fields. The educational system in nursing has begun to respond to this group of students by offering options to the traditional basic baccalaureate education. Some baccalaureate programs offer these students an accelerated sequence, which results in a second baccalaureate degree. Many individuals with one degree, however, prefer to pursue a graduate degree.

This desire for graduate degrees led to the development of an accelerated master's degree in nursing for individuals with nonnursing bachelor's degrees. These programs, known as **generic master's degree** programs, usually require about three years to complete. Graduates take the R.N. licensure examination after completing the generic master's program.

Another educational track for students with baccalaureate degrees in other fields is the generic doctorate (N.D.). A program offering the doctorate as the first professional degree was begun at Case Western Reserve University in 1979. This program was based on the philosophy—not shared by all—that professional nursing education should begin at the postbaccalaureate level. Following graduation, N.D. graduates take the registered nurse licensure examination. Graduates are prepared to function as advanced clinical specialists or nurse practitioners and to initiate clinical research utilization studies (*Peterson's Guide* 1992). The generic doctorate is presently offered by three universities: Case Western Reserve in Cleveland, Rush University in Chicago, and the University of Colorado in Boulder.

Practical Nursing Programs

Nursing education includes a large number of programs preparing **practical nurses**. Practical nurses are differentiated from registered nurses by education and licensure and have a limited scope of practice. L.P.N.s, or licensed vocational nurses (L.V.N.s), as they are called in California and Texas, are considered technical workers in nursing.

Practical nursing programs became a significant component of the nursing field during World War II. They were created to satisfy the demand for programs that could produce nurses quickly. The first planned curriculum for practical nursing was developed in 1942. The NLN has an accrediting council for practical nursing programs, but of the 1048 L.P.N. programs in 1991, only 159 had NLN accreditation (Council of Practical Nursing Programs 1990).

Practical nursing education is typically 12 months in length and takes place in a variety of settings: vocational/technical schools, community colleges, and high schools. Many L.P.N. programs now offer credit for prior learning to health care workers such as hospital aides, orderlies, paramedics, emergency medical technicians, and military corps personnel. These individuals often enter nursing through practical nursing programs.

Graduates of practical nurse programs must pass the National Council Licensing Examination for Practical Nursing (**NCLEX-PN**) in order to become licensed. The scope of their practice focuses on basic patient needs in hospitals, long-term care facilities, and homes. They practice under the supervision of a physician or registered nurse.

For many students enrolled in practical nurse programs, the goal is to become a registered nurse. A significant number of newly licensed R.N.s were previously licensed as practical nurses. According to the 1990 new-nurse survey *Licensed to Care*, almost 33 percent of all newly licensed nurses have practiced as L.P.N.s (National League for Nursing 1990a, p. 14).

There is increasing pressure on L.P.N. programs to expand and upgrade. This expansion is usually discussed in terms of phasing out practical nurse programs or converting them to associate degree programs. As long as the demand for nurses is greater than basic registered nurse programs can meet, however, practical nurse programs will flourish.

Accreditation

The concept of **accreditation** of educational programs in nursing is very important. Prospective nursing students should inquire about the accreditation status of any nursing program they are considering. Employers of nurses are usually only interested in hiring nurses who are graduates of accredited programs. And acceptance into graduate programs in nursing is usually dependent on graduation from an accredited baccalaureate program.

Accreditation refers to a voluntary review process of educational programs by a professional organization. The organization, called an *accrediting agency,* is invited to compare the educational quality of the program with established standards and criteria.

The NLN is the official accrediting agency for master's, baccalaureate, associate degree, diploma, and practical nursing programs. The accrediting program is conducted through four NLN councils: the Council of Associate Degree Programs, the Council of Diploma Programs, the Council of Baccalaureate and Higher Degree Programs, and the Council of Practical Nursing Programs. Each council develops its own accreditation program and criteria and revises them periodically (Division of Education and Accreditation 1990).

Accreditation of nursing schools grew out of concern repeatedly expressed by members of the profession about the quality of and standards for nursing education. An accredited program voluntarily adheres to standards that protect the quality of education, public safety, and the profession itself. Accreditation provides both a mechanism and a stimulus for programs to initiate periodic self-examination and self-improvement. It assures students that their educational program is accountable for offering quality education for future practice.

Areas generally scrutinized in accreditation reviews are administration and governance, finances and budget, faculty, students, curriculum, and resources. Criteria, or standards, are established in each area. Programs under review prepare reports, known as self-studies, that show how the school meets each criterion. The self-study is reviewed by a volunteer team composed of nursing educators, and an on-site program review is made by the same team. Following the site visit, the visitors' report and the program's self-study are reviewed by the appropriate NLN council, and a decision is made regarding accreditation.

Once accredited and in good standing, continuing accreditation reviews take place every eight years. Programs that do not meet standards may be placed on warning and given a specific time period to correct deficiencies. Accreditation can be withdrawn if deficiencies are not corrected within the specified time.

Graduate Education in Nursing

A variety of economic, educational, and professional trends are fueling the demand for R.N.s with **advanced degrees**. The rapidly changing health care system requires nurses to possess increasing knowledge, clinical competency, greater independence, and autonomy in clinical judgments. Trends toward community-based nursing centers, private case management, complexity of home care, increasingly sophisticated technologies, and society's orientation to health and self-care are all rapidly raising the educational needs of nurses.

According to projections made by the federal government, 200,000 additional master's and doctorally prepared R.N.s will be needed by the year 2000 (Allen 1990, p. 74). Nurses who have advanced education can become researchers, nurse practitioners, clinical specialists, educators, and administrators. Many open their own clinics where they provide direct care and serve as consultants to businesses and health care agencies. Chapter 5 describes some of the opportunities open to nurses with advanced degrees.

A Data Base for Graduate Education in Nursing (American Association of Colleges of Nursing 1990, p. v) reported that both master's and doctoral students expected to achieve higher status, professional growth/knowledge/skill, autonomy in practice, increased self-esteem, and a sense of personal achievement as a result of their additional education. Certainly having highly educated nurses will further strengthen the profession.

Master's Education

The purpose of master's education is to prepare persons with advanced nursing knowledge and clinical practice skills in a specialized area of practice. Teachers College, Columbia University, is credited with initiating graduate education in nursing. Beginning in 1899, the college offered a postgraduate course in hospital economics, which prepared nurses for positions in teaching and hospital administration. From this limited beginning, there has been consistent growth in the number of master's programs in the United States.

Over the last two decades the growth in numbers of master's programs has been dramatic. In 1970 there were 70 programs; in 1980, 142 programs; and in 1990, 212 programs. Of the 212 master's programs in 1990, 182 were accredited (Council of Baccalaureate and Higher Degree Programs 1990b).

Most individuals in the 1950s and 1960s viewed the master's degree in nursing as a terminal (final) degree. The master's degree was considered the highest degree nurses would ever need. Early master's programs were longer and more demanding than most other master's degrees. Master's programs in the 1950s and 1960s prepared students for careers in nursing administration and nursing education.

With the rapid development of doctoral programs in the 1970s, however, the master's was no longer considered a terminal degree. Programs were shortened to the approximate length of master's study in most other disciplines, and clinical specialization was added as an emphasis. Master's programs in nursing are most often found in senior colleges and universities that have basic baccalaureate programs in nursing. They may also seek voluntary accreditation from the NLN's Council for the Accreditation of Baccalaureate and Higher Degree Programs.

Entrance requirements to master's programs in nursing usually include the following: a baccalaureate degree from an NLN accredited program in nursing, licensure as a registered nurse, completion of the Graduate Record Examination (GRE) or other standard aptitude test, a minimum undergraduate grade point average (GPA) of 3.0, at least one year's recent work experience as a registered nurse in an area related to the desired area of specialization, and specific goals for graduate study.

The average program length is 12 to 18 months of full-time study. The curriculum includes theory, research, clinical applications, and courses in other disciplines related to the student's selected area of specialization and role development. Students are often required to write a comprehensive examination and/ or to complete a thesis (Anastas 1988). The majority of contemporary master's students are preparing for advanced clinical practice. Almost two thirds of recent graduates surveyed had studied for advanced clinical practice, 22 percent for administration/management, and 13 percent for teaching (Division of Research 1990).

Nine broad specialty areas are represented in most nursing master's curricula: adult health, child health, community/public health, gerontology, nurse anesthesia, nursing administration, nurse midwifery, psychiatric/mental health, and nursing education (American Association of Colleges of Nursing 1990). Newer options are being added. Recent additions include nursing information systems, oncology, early intervention, and neonatal nursing (Fig. 2–3).

The master of science (M.S.) and the M.S.N. are the two most common degrees offered (Council of Baccalaureate and Higher Degree Programs 1990b). A new option in master's education is the R.N./M.S.N. track, which allows registered nurses prepared at the associate degree or diploma level to enter a program leading to a master's degree rather than a baccalaureate degree. An-

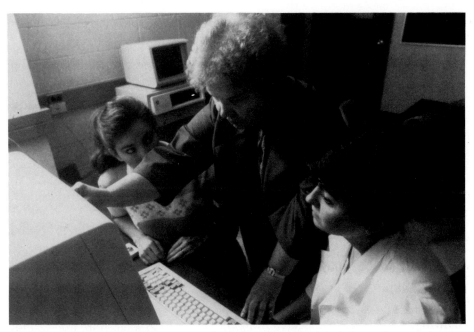

Figure 2–3 Learning to manage multiple sources of patient information requires that today's nurses have well-developed computer skills. (Courtesy of the University of Akron.)

other innovation, the M.S.N./M.B.A. (master of business administration), is also growing. As can be seen, diversity in nursing education extends to the graduate as well as the undergraduate level.

Doctoral Programs

Doctoral programs in nursing prepare nurses to become faculty members in universities, deans of schools of nursing, administrators in large medical centers, and researchers and theorists in nursing. Doctoral programs in nursing offer several degree titles, the most common being the doctor of nursing science (D.N.Sc.) and doctor of philosophy (Ph.D.).

The D.N.Sc., the professional doctorate, is viewed as a practice degree. Conceived as an advanced practice degree with an emphasis on clinical research, the D.N.Sc. is intended to bridge the gap between practice and research (Allen 1990). The Ph.D. is considered the academic degree and prepares scholars for research and the development of theory.

A continuing issue is the relative merit of these two degrees. As currently structured in most universities, the two programs are more similar than different. In the major job market for nurses with doctorates, which is colleges and universities, the Ph.D. is the more prestigious of the two degrees and therefore is favored by many doctorate-seeking nurses. Of 54 programs awarding doctoral degrees in 1991, 77 percent awarded the Ph.D. ("Nursing Doctoral Programs" 1991).

Formal doctoral education began at Columbia University's Teachers College in 1910 with the creation of the Department of Nursing and Health. The first student completed her work for the doctor of education (Ed.D.) with a major in nursing education and was awarded her doctorate in 1932. As of 1991, Teachers College was the only doctoral program in nursing education granting the Ed.D.

In 1934, New York University initiated the first Ph.D. program for nurses. The early programs at Teachers College and New York University provided many of the profession's early leaders who worked over the years for improvement in nursing education (Parietti 1990).

From 1934 to 1954, no new nursing doctoral programs were opened. In 1954 the University of Pittsburgh opened the first Ph.D. program in clinical nursing and clinical research in the country. The American Nurses Association's *Facts About Nursing* (1961) reported that as the 1950s drew to a close, a total of only 36 doctoral degrees had been awarded in nursing (Parietti 1990).

Owing to the limited number of nursing doctoral programs, most nurses earned doctorates in nonnursing fields. Doctoral education for nurses moved into a new phase when the federal government initiated nurse scientist programs in 1962. These programs were created to increase the research skills of nurses and provide faculty for the development of doctoral programs in nursing. The nurse scientist programs were discontinued in 1975 after more universities began offering doctoral programs in nursing.

The 1970s saw a major increase in the number of doctoral programs. Fifteen new doctoral programs were established in that decade alone. Between 1970 and 1980 the number of programs increased to 22. Between 1980 and 1990, the number more than doubled, from 22 to 48 (Parietti 1990). In 1991 the number of doctoral programs stood at 54 ("Nursing Doctoral Programs" 1991). The newest route to a doctorate in nursing is the generic doctorate, discussed earlier in this chapter.

Trends indicate that there is strong support for doctoral education in nursing. Within the last few years the number of requests for admission to these programs has greatly increased. This stems from the requirement of a doctorate for academic advancement and tenure for university nursing faculty. Nurses also desire the doctorate to become competent researchers and to advance the profession as a whole.

It is projected that large numbers of doctorally prepared nurses will be needed in the future as positions requiring the doctorate expand beyond universities. An educational issue now receiving some attention is the differentiation of master's and doctoral education.

Continuing Education

Continuing education, or CE, is a term used to describe informal ways in which nurses maintain clinical expertise during their professional careers. Continuing education for nurses takes place in a variety of settings: colleges, universities, hospitals, community agencies, professional organizations, and professional meetings. Continuing education appears in many forms such as workshops, institutes, conferences, short courses, evening courses, telecourses, and instructional supplements in professional journals.

The ANA Council on Continuing Education was established in 1973. This council is responsible for standards of continuing education, accreditation of programs offering continuing education, transferability of CE credit from state to state, and development of guidelines for recognition systems within states.

In the 1970s the continuing education unit **(CEU)** was created as a method of recognizing participation in nonacademic credit offerings. One CEU was given for every ten hours of participation in an organized, approved, continuing education offering. Today the contact hour has replaced the CEU, and nurses receive one contact hour of credit for each 50 or 60 minutes they spend in a continuing education course.

A major trend currently is **mandatory continuing education**. Any nurse renewing a license in a state having mandatory continuing education has to meet that state's contact hour requirements. This is the government's way of ensuring that nurses are current in their profession before a license is renewed. In 1992, mandatory continuing education as a prerequisite for relicensure was required in 17 states, with 5 more expected to institute requirements in the near future. Table 2–1 lists those states and their current requirements.

Table 2–1   States Requiring Continuing Education for Relicensure

State	Requirement
Alabama	24 hours per two years
Alaska	One of the following: 15 hours of CE, 15 hours of professional activities, or 320 hours of nursing employment per two years
California	30 hours per two years
Colorado	20 hours per two years
Delaware	30 hours per two years
Florida	24 hours per two years
Iowa	45 hours per three years
Kansas	30 hours per two years
Kentucky	30 hours per two years
Massachusetts	15 hours per two years
Minnesota	30 hours per two years
Nebraska	Either 20 hours of CE and 200 hours of nursing employment or 75 hours of CE in two years
Nevada	30 hours per two years
New Hampshire	20 hours per two years
New Mexico	30 hours per two years
Ohio	24 hours per two years (beginning in 1993)
Puerto Rico	36 hours per three years
Texas	20 hours per two years

CE = Continuing education.
(From Mattera, M.D. (Ed.). (1992). *RN presents: Nursing opportunities 1992* (23rd ed.). Montvale, NJ: Medical Economics. Used by permission.)

Certification Programs

Certification is a credential that has professional, but not legal, status. Specialized programs developed to prepare nurses for expanded roles often lead to certification. Some certification programs are part of degree-granting programs such as a master's program, whereas others are considered part of continuing education.

Certification means that a certificate is awarded by a professional group as validation of specific qualifications demonstrated by a registered nurse in a defined area of practice. Certification programs that exist today include nurse practitioner preparation and programs in pediatrics, gerontology, family health, women's health care, nurse midwifery, and nurse anesthesia. These courses provide concentrated study in specific areas and last from several weeks to several months or even years. A comprehensive examination is required to become certified as well as documentation of experience, letters of reference, and other documents.

Certified nurses have greater earning potential, wider employment opportunities, status, and prestige and, in some states, are eligible for insurance reimbursement, just as physicians are. Requirements for admission to certification programs vary, with some requiring only R.N. licensure and others requiring either a baccalaureate or a master's degree.

The American Nurses Credentialing Center (ANCC), a subunit of the ANA, provides a number of certification programs for nurses. Nurses applying for certification through the ANA must demonstrate current practice beyond that required for R.N. licensure. The applicant must take a national examination and submit current evidence of active nursing practice in a specific clinical area. Certificates are awarded for a period of five years, after which the nurse must submit further evidence related to clinical practice and continuing education for renewal of the certificate.

Nurses holding ANA certification at the basic level can be identified by the initials "R.N.,C." (registered nurse, certified) after their names. Those certified as clinical specialists use "R.N., C.S." Box 2-1 lists the areas in which the ANA offers certification.

In addition to the ANA, professional nursing groups offering speciality certification are the Nurses' Association of the American College of Obstetricians and Gynecologists (NAACOG), National Association of Pediatric Nurse Associates Practitioners, American College of Nurse Midwives, and the American Association of Nurse Anesthetists.

Although certification is a desirable concept, there are many problems related to current methods of certification: programs lack uniformity; certificates in different specialties are not equivalent; and not all have similar educational, testing, or practice requirements.

The related questions of how to ensure certification standards and who should be responsible for certification of nurses are major issues in the nursing education system today. The trend is for certification programs to become part of degree-granting nursing programs. If this trend continues, certification will come under accreditation guidelines, which may ensure greater uniformity and equivalency.

Box 2–1   **Areas of Certification Offered by the American Nurses Credentialing Center in 1992**

Clinical Specialist in Community Health Nursing
Community Health Nurse
General Nursing Practice
Adult Nurse Practitioner
Family Nurse Practitioner
School Nurse
School Nurse Practitioner
Gerontological Nurse
Gerontological Nurse Practitioner
Clinical Specialist in Gerontological Nursing
Perinatal Nurse
Pediatric Nurse
Pediatric Nurse Practitioner

Clinical Specialist in Medical-Surgical Nursing
Medical-Surgical Nursing
Clinical Specialist in Adult Psychiatric and Mental Health Nursing
Clinical Specialist in Child and Adolescent Psychiatric and Mental Health Nursing
Nursing Administration
Nursing Administration, Advanced
College Health Nurse
Nursing Continuing Education/Staff Development

(Data from the American Nurses Association.)

The Problem of Reduced Resources in Nursing Education

Hospitals, community colleges, and universities responded to reduced applications to nursing programs during the middle 1980s by downsizing, that is, reducing the number of part-time and nontenured faculty. This resulted in an inability to meet the demand when application numbers rose again in the late 1980s and early 1990s.

Complicating the situation was the poor national economy of the early 1990s, which resulted in lower state budgets and less money for public postsecondary education. Despite enrollment increases for several consecutive years and significant demand for nursing education by qualified students, many could not be accommodated in schools of nursing owing to faculty shortages and other budgetary constraints.

Findings from the National League for Nursing's 1990 biennial census of nurse faculty show that the ten-year trend of decreasing number of full-time faculty continues unabated. In 1990–1991 alone, approximately 2292 prospective qualified baccalaureate degree students were turned away by nursing programs that did not have sufficient resources. "Admission filled" was cited by 70 percent of schools; faculty shortages were listed by more than 56 percent, followed by 54 percent with budgetary constraints, and 36 percent with insufficient clinical space (National League for Nursing 1990b).

Compounding the problem of limited space in the nation's nursing programs is the fact that nursing faculty salaries have not kept pace with those in other settings. It is not uncommon for nursing faculty with advanced degrees and years of experience to see their former students begin their careers at higher salaries than they themselves make. This has created a "brain drain" of nursing faculty leaving education to seek higher-paying positions in hospitals and other settings.

In 1992, an assistant professor of nursing with a master's degree and 14 years' experience in practice and teaching turned down an offer for an additional one-year appointment at a salary of $29,000 for an academic year (9 months) to accept a 12-month position at an area hospital for $45,000. This trend is expected to continue as colleges and universities fail to keep pace with the "market price" of nurses in direct practice today and more and more master's and doctorally prepared nurses reluctantly find it necessary to leave nursing education.

This trend has not gone unnoticed. Enrollment figures in master's programs in nursing show the impact of poor faculty salaries. Of 21 master's students enrolling in 1991 in a new M.S.N. program in a southern state, only 2 registered for role preparation as nurse educators, whereas all the others expressed a preference for nursing administration and clinical specialty preparation.

CHAPTER SUMMARY

The development of nursing education has been influenced by a number of factors leading to a diverse array of program offerings. First provided in hospitals, basic nursing education has evolved into three major types of programs: diploma, baccalaureate, and associate degree, each of which has positive and negative attributes. Alternatives such as the baccalaureate degree programs for R.N.s, external degree programs, and those for postbaccalaureate students further complicate the picture.

Conflict arose when the ANA published a position paper recommending the baccalaureate degree as the minimum preparation for entry-level professional nurses. That issue has not yet been satisfactorily resolved.

Voluntary accreditation by the NLN provides assurance of the quality of nursing education programs. Trends in nursing education include master's and doctoral preparation for nurses and specialty certification.

Lifelong learning through continuing education is considered essential for all professionals. Mandatory continuing education as a prerequisite for relicensure is expected to increase.

In the 1990s, the problem of reduced resources in nursing education is expected to reach crisis proportions. This is a result of underfunding of higher education in general and, in particular, the failure of salaries in schools of nursing to keep pace with those in other settings. Graduate students in nursing are largely uninterested in preparation as nursing educators, and faculties in nursing programs are expected to shrink as a result. This will further compound the shortage of registered nurses in the nation.

REVIEW/DISCUSSION QUESTIONS

1. What factors did you use to determine which type of basic nursing program to enter?
2. How would you advise a high school student interested in nursing to go about selecting a program?
3. What characteristics would be needed for success in an external degree program?
4. Offering complete articulation of all levels of nursing education from practical nursing through doctoral study seems like a logical course of action. Should states mandate articulation? Why or why not?
5. Discuss the merits and drawbacks of mandatory continuing education from the viewpoints of both nurses and consumers of nursing care.
6. What unique contributions to nursing are possible by master's prepared nurses? By doctorally prepared nurses?
7. Explain how the failure of the nation's schools of nursing to remunerate nursing faculty adequately will ultimately result in a critical shortage of nurses.

REFERENCES

Allen, J. (Ed.). (l990). *Consumer's guide to doctoral degree programs in nursing* (Publication No. 15–2293). New York: National League for Nursing.

American Association of Colleges of Nursing. (1990). *A data base for graduate education in nursing: Summary report.* Washington, D.C.: Author.

American Nurses Association. (1961). *Facts about nursing: A statistical summary.* New York: Author.

American Nurses Association. (1965). *Educational preparation for nurse practitioners and assistants to nurses: A position paper* (Publication No. G-83). Kansas City, MO: Author.

American Nurses Association. (1979). *A case for baccalaureate preparation in nursing* (Publication No. NE-6 15M). Kansas City, MO: Author.

Anastas, L. (1988). *Your career in nursing* (Publication No. 14–2216). New York: National League for Nursing.

Brown, E. L. (1948). *Nursing for the future.* New York: Russell Sage Foundation.

"Cal State launches off-campus program for the working R.N." (1982). *American Journal of Nursing, 82,* 893, 904–905.

Christy, T. (1969). Portrait of a leader: M. Adelaide Nutting. *Nursing Outlook, 17,* 20–24.

Committee on the Grading of Nursing Schools. (1934). *Nursing schools today and tomorrow.* New York: National League of Nursing Education.

Conley, V. (1973). *Curriculum and instruction in nursing.* Boston: Little, Brown.

Council of Associate Degree Programs. (1990). *Educational outcomes of associate degree nursing programs: Roles and competencies* (Publication No. 23–2348). New York: National League for Nursing.

Council of Baccalaureate and Higher Degree Programs. (1990). *Graduate education in nursing: Route to opportunities in contemporary nursing 1989–1990* (Publication No. 15–2221). New York: National League for Nursing.

Council of Diploma Programs. (1990). *Education for nursing: The diploma way* (Publication No. 16–1314). New York: National League for Nursing.

Council of Practical Nursing Programs. (1990). *Practical nursing career 1989–1990* (Publication No. 38–1328). New York: National League for Nursing.

Mattera, M. D. (Ed.). (1992). *RN presents: Nursing opportunities 1992* (23rd ed). Montvale, NJ: Medical Economics.

Division of Education and Accreditation. (1990). *Policies and procedures of accreditation for programs in nursing education* (Publication No. 18–1437). New York: National League for Nursing.

Division of Research. (1990). *Nursing data review 1991* (Publication No. 19–2419). New York: National League for Nursing.

Fondiller, S. (1986). Licensure and titling in nursing and society: A historical perspective. In *Looking beyond the entry issue: Implications for education and service* (pp. 3–19) (Publication No. 41-2173). New York: National League for Nursing.

Kalisch, P., and Kalisch, B. (1986). *The advance of American nursing* (2nd ed.). Boston: Little, Brown.

Lysaught, J. (1970). *An abstract for action.* New York: McGraw-Hill.

Montag, M. (1951). *The education of nursing technicians.* New York: Putnam.

National League for Nursing. (1982). *Position statement on nursing roles: Scope and preparation.* New York: Author.

National League for Nursing. (1990a). *Licensed to care: An executive report on the new nurse* (Publication No. 19–2385). New York: Author.

National League for Nursing. (1990b). *Nursing datasource 1990. The registered nurse population: 1988.* Washington, D.C.: Author.

National League of Nursing Education. (1937). *A curriculum guide for schools of nursing.* New York: Author.

Notter, L., and Spalding, E. (1976). *Professional nursing, foundations perspectives and relationships* (9th ed.). Philadelphia: Lippincott.

Nursing doctoral programs in the United States. (1991). *Sigma Theta Tau International Reflections,* 17(2/3), 23–24.

Parietti, E. (1990). The development of doctoral education in nursing: A historical overview. In J. Allen, (Ed.), *Consumer's guide to doctoral degree programs in nursing* (p. 1532) (Publication No. 15–2293). New York: National League for Nursing.

Peterson's guide to graduate programs in business, education, health, and law. (1992). Princeton, NJ: Peterson's Guides.

Rapson, M. (Ed.). (1987). *Collaboration for articulation: RN to BSN* (Publication No. 41–2182). New York: National League for Nursing.

Schwirian, P. (1984). Research in nursing students. In H. H. Werley and J. J. Fitzpatrick (Eds.), *Annual review of nursing research* (vol. 2) (pp. 211–262). New York: Springer.

Wozniak, D. (1973). External degrees in nursing. *American Journal of Nursing*, 73, 1014–1018.

SUGGESTED READINGS

American Association of Colleges of Nursing. (1986). *Essentials of college and university education for professional nursing: Final report.* Washington, D.C.: Author.

Committee for the Study of Credentialing in Nursing. (1979). *Credentialing in nursing: A new approach. American Journal of Nursing*, 79(4), 614–683.

Council of Baccalaureate and Higher Degree Programs. (1990). *Baccalaureate education in nursing: Key to a professional career in nursing* (Publication No. 15-1311). New York: National League for Nursing.

National League for Nursing. (1986). *Interpretive statement on NLN position in support of two levels of nursing practice.* New York: Author.

Chapter

The Social Context for Nursing

Leslie B. Himot

CHAPTER OBJECTIVES

What students should be able to do after studying this chapter:

1. Describe how individuals are socialized.
2. Identify own patterns of socialization and their effect on personal development.
3. Analyze the traditional roles of women and how these have affected the development of the nursing profession.
4. Discuss social trends affecting the development of nursing as a profession.
5. Explain the impact of the media on the image of nursing.
6. Evaluate the continuing development of technology and the implications for nursing.
7. Describe the history and causes of nursing shortages in the United States.

VOCABULARY BUILDING

Terms to know:

androgyny	role	socialization
consumerism	role models	stereotypes
demographics		

*E*very profession is profoundly affected by the society it serves, and nursing is no exception. The social context has shaped nurses attitudes, nursing practice, and the attitudes of the public toward nursing over the years.

Nurses need to understand how nursing is related to society as a whole. What impact does society have on the practice of nursing? Does the fact that nursing is a female-dominated profession have a bearing on the way the profession has developed? How do **demographics** (population trends) affect nursing? How does the public view nurses? Should this image be changed? What causes periodic nursing shortages? This chapter provides an overview of some of the social issues that affect nurses and the development of nursing as a profession.

Social Issues Influencing Nursing

The modern profession of nursing enjoys the talents of both men and women, but it has traditionally been dominated by women. Women continue to make up the vast majority of registered nurses, with males composing only 3.3 percent of all nurses in 1988 (McKibben 1990).

Since women generally share certain societal influences during their development, it is important to look at the development of nursing as a female-dominated profession. Specifically, the process of socialization of women bears exploration.

Traditional Socialization of Women

Socialization is the process whereby values and expectations are transmitted from generation to generation. In Western society, women have generally been socialized to avoid risk taking, to avoid conflict, and to acquiesce to authority. Traditionally, feminine attributes include an orientation toward security, peacekeeping, and submission (Muff 1988).

Women have also been socialized to be self-sacrificing to parents, husbands, and children. When women subordinate their own needs for the sake of others, they can avoid dealing with unpleasantness and conflict. They also avoid the appearance of aggressiveness, for which assertive behavior has often been mistaken in the past (Muff 1988).

To understand more about how the traditional socialization of women operates, let us look at role theory. A **role** is a goal-directed pattern of behavior learned within the cultural setting. People carry out their assigned roles because both society and the individuals themselves expect this behavior.

From very early times, women have been assigned the role of care giver. Chapter 1 reviewed how members of religious orders, deaconesses, noblewomen, and other women were assigned this role over the centuries. In the early nineteenth century, women of the lower classes served as "nurses" in homes and hospitals. After Florence Nightingale influenced nursing, the image became more credible because nurses had training, values, and more hygienic practices. Still, in terms of prestige and power, modern nursing's roots were planted in a labor pool of women with little influence.

Since the attribute of caring was assumed to be women's duty, nursing was a role assigned to women by society. Friedman (1990, p. 2851) found it unsurprising that "what had once been socially expected of women became bound up with what they started to do for a living."

In the early days of modern nursing, then, the roles assigned to women were healer, care taker, and nurturer, none of which was assigned high value by the larger society. The first formal schools of nursing in this country, such as Bellevue Hospital and the Boston Training School, were developed to attract "respectable women" into nursing, which could have added to nursing's value. But by replacing untrained hospital "nurses" with students who worked in the hospital in return for room, board, and training, one powerless labor pool was simply exchanged for another.

Roles are learned, usually from others carrying out the role, who are called "**role models.**" Consider some of the nursing role models in twentieth-century fiction that today's middle-aged women read as girls. Cherry Ames was the heroine of a series of books produced by Grosset & Dunlap, Inc. in the 1940s. These books imparted a strong message of glamour, excitement, and romance that does not exist in real nursing. They also portrayed nurses as rather simple and subservient to male doctors, in whom they were usually romantically interested. Cherry Ames books, widely available and very popular during the postwar years and into the 1950s, were written for, and read almost exclusively by, young adolescent girls.

Sue Barton was another fictional role model of the Cherry Ames era. This sentence from a Sue Barton book entitled *Sue Barton, Student Nurse* demonstrates the role relationships of nurses and doctors during these years: "A nurse must always rise to her feet when addressed by a doctor" (Boylston 1945, p. 23). This practice of standing up or giving up one's seat at the nurses' desk to physicians has gradually diminished over the years but is not entirely extinct.

Although examination of the Cherry Ames and Sue Barton books does not constitute sociological research, it does shed light on the prevailing social attitudes about nursing in the era in which they were written. They clearly demonstrate that women were assigned certain roles by the larger society, which included the care-giver role, and were expected to be self-sacrificing in their duty to others and subservient to doctors.

In a classic piece of nursing literature, "Toward Androgyny," Patricia Geary Dean (1978) argued that social influences on women have resulted in the victimization of nurses. But she also reminded nurses that victimization requires both a victim and an oppressor and exhorted nurses to thwart their oppressors by becoming more assertive. She identified several areas where assertion would be particularly helpful: in establishing practice standards, in resolving the dilemma of multiple educational levels in nursing, in increasing nursing's responsibility for patient care, in improving nursing's image, and in supporting other nurses. Dean argued that pursuing these activities assertively will help nurses develop both feminine and masculine characteristics, which is called **androg-**

Box 3–1   Assertiveness Self-Assessment

In order to be an effective nurse, you must be assertive enough to represent your patients and yourself. Test your Assertiveness Quotient by completing the following questionnaire. Give each question a 1, 2, or 3 based on how comfortable you feel about each item:

1—I feel very uncomfortable
2—I feel moderately comfortable
3—I feel very comfortable

A Q TEST

Assertive Behavior

_____ Speaking up and asking questions at a meeting

_____ Commenting about being interrupted by someone the moment he or she interrupts you

_____ Stating your views to an authority figure (e.g., minister, boss, teacher, father)

_____ Attempting to offer solutions and elaborating on them when others are present

Your Body

_____ Entering and exiting a room where superiors are gathered

_____ Speaking in front of a group

_____ Maintaining eye contact, keeping your head upright, and leaning forward when in a personal conversation

Your Mind

_____ Going out with a group of friends when you are the only one without a "date"

_____ Being especially competent, using your authority and/or power without labeling yourself as "bitchy," impolite, bossy, aggressive, castrating, or parental

_____ Requesting expected service when you haven't received it (e.g., in a restaurant or a store)

Apology

_____ Being expected to apologize for something and not apologizing since you feel you are right

_____ Requesting the return of borrowed items without being apologetic

Compliments, Criticism, and Rejection

_____ Receiving a compliment by saying something assertive to acknowledge that you agree with the person complimenting you

_____ Accepting a rejection

_____ Not getting the approval of the most significant person in your life

_____ Discussing another person's criticism of you openly with that person

_____ Telling someone that she or he is doing something that is bothering you

Saying No

_____ Saying "No"—refusing to do a favor when you really don't feel like it

Box content:

Turning down a request for a meeting or date _____

Manipulation and Countermanipulation

Telling a person when you think she or he is manipulating you _____

Commenting assertively to someone who has made a patronizing remark to you _____

Talking about your feelings of competition with another person with whom you feel competitive _____

Anger/Humor

Expressing anger directly and honestly when you feel angry _____

Arguing with another person _____

_____ Telling a joke

_____ Listening to a friend tell a story about something embarrassing, but funny, that you have done

_____ Responding with humor to someone's put-down of you

If you have mostly 3's and a few 2's, you are assertive enough to advocate for your patients and yourself. If you have a few 1's, write each one down and seek out three occasions to try more assertive behaviors in these situations. If you have five or more 1's, you need an assertiveness course and/or some real work on your part.

(From *The Assertive Woman: A New Look* © 1987 by Stanlee Phelps and Nancy Austin. Reproduced for W. B. Saunders Company by permission of Impact Publishers, Inc., P.O. Box 1094, San Luis Obispo, CA 93406. Further reproduction prohibited.)

yny. By becoming androgynous, asserted Dean, nurses should be able to exceed the limitations of both traditionally female and traditionally male roles. You may want to evaluate your own level of assertiveness by using the "Assertiveness Self-Assessment" in Box 3–1.

Problems Faced by Men in Nursing

Women are not alone in being assigned certain roles by society. Men in nursing frequently encounter prejudice for being members of a "women's" profession. Since their numbers are small, consisting of only 3.3 percent of all nurses practicing in 1988, most members of the general public have not had contact with male nurses. When they do, they often think the male nurses are medical students or medical residents.

The numbers of men in nursing are expected to increase as work conditions and salaries improve. Male nursing students often face discrimination from practicing nurses, physicians, and the public. It is all too common for male students to find themselves unwelcome in prenatal clinics, delivery rooms, and other settings in which male physicians have free access.

One male obstetrician in a midsized southeastern community refused to allow a male nursing student in the delivery suite, explaining, "My patients are

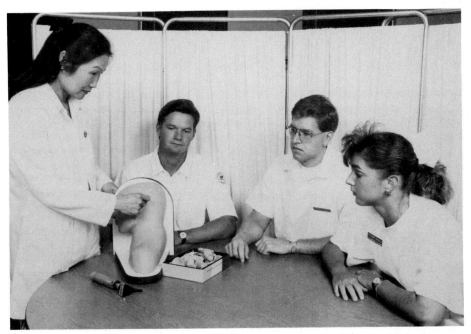

Men are entering nursing in record numbers thereby increasing diversity within the profession.

uncomfortable with a man in the room." The irony of one male health professional restricting the access of another male health professional student based on the student's gender did not escape the notice of the student. Unfortunately, the nurse in charge of the unit chose not to advocate for the student, and the student's clinical instructor was unsuccessful in doing so. He had to transfer to a different clinical group in another hospital to complete his clinical objectives. This type of incident is, unfortunately, not uncommon.

In a book entitled *Women's Issues in Nursing: Socialization, Sexism, and Stereotyping* (Muff 1988), several male nurses related their experiences. One nurse described how many of his middle-aged female patients were "bashful" when being attended by a male, whereas younger women did not seem to mind having a male nurse. He attributed this difference in younger women's attitudes to changes in societal **stereotypes** about male- and female-appropriate employment.

Another obstacle men face is the question of whether they are able to be nurturing enough to be nurses. A male nurse in Muff's book volunteered his belief that men can be "caring and sensitive" enough toward people's needs to fulfill the nursing role (p. 273). He anticipated the question and answered it even before it was asked because it is a question often raised about the appropriateness of nursing as a male occupation.

Another nurse reported how he had to deal with the question of his masculinity from time to time. When he first entered nursing school, people asked, "What kind of man would willingly choose to be a nurse? Don't you really want to be a doctor?" He related that there was often a question about his sexual orientation underlying these comments. He continued, "I dealt with these issues then and continue to do so" (p. 276). As pioneers in a traditionally female profession, questions about men in nursing will continue until the proportion of male nurses increases, their visibility increases, and the public becomes comfortable with their abilities.

The Consumer Movement

Since the late 1960s, the American public's level of satisfaction with goods and services has come under scrutiny. Consumer activist Ralph Nader burst into the public consciousness in 1966 with the publication of his book *Unsafe at Any Speed*, which was an exposé of the safety hazards in General Motors' Chevrolet Corvair (Stewart 1989). The book became a national best-seller, Nader became world famous, and the consumer revolution in this country was under way.

In the late 1960s and early 1970s, "Nader's Raiders," a group of idealistic young people, turned out report after report. These reports exposed large corporations for their inadequate adherence to safety regulations and governmental agencies for failing to enforce the regulations already on the books. Governmental watchdog agencies, such as the Occupational Safety and Health Administration (OSHA), the Environmental Protection Agency (EPA), and the Consumer Product Safety Commission, were all established following the public outcry prompted by reports written by the crusading Nader and his Raiders (Stewart 1989).

Eventually, health care services themselves came under scrutiny. The American public, fueled by the principles of consumerism, criticized the dehumanization of health care. This led to the development in 1972 of the American Hospital Association's (AHA) document "A Patient's Bill of Rights," which guaranteed certain rights and privileges to every hospitalized patient. "A Patient's Bill of Rights" is reprinted in Box 3–2.

Many people believe the AHA document was the first formal declaration of its kind. A little known fact is that in 1959, 14 years before the AHA action, the National League for Nursing (NLN) generated a statement about patients' rights. Until the AHA's "A Patient's Bill of Rights" was published, however, the prevailing attitude in health care was that providers knew best and good patients simply followed directions without asking questions.

The rise of **consumerism** in health care led to the involvement of consumers in pressing Congress for legislation protecting the public from inadequate care, experimental drugs, poor nutrition, and many other health-related issues. More recently, consumer groups have demanded controls on spiraling health care costs and gained participation on boards of health planning agencies, accrediting bodies, and professional licensing boards. Most state boards of nursing have at least one consumer member.

Box 3–2   "A Patient's Bill of Rights"

The American Hospital Association presents a Patient's Bill of Rights with the expectation that observance of these rights will contribute to more effective patient care and greater satisfaction for the patient, his physician, and the hospital organization. Further, the Association presents these rights in the expectation that they will be supported by the hospital on behalf of its patients, as an integral part of the healing process. It is recognized that a personal relationship between the physician and the patient is essential for the provision of proper medical care. The traditional physician-patient relationship takes on a new dimension when care is rendered within an organizational structure. Legal precedent has established that the institution itself also has a responsibility to the patient. It is in recognition of these factors that these rights are affirmed.

1. The patient has the right to considerate and respectful care.
2. The patient has the right to obtain from his physician complete current information concerning his diagnosis, treatment, and prognosis in terms the patient can be reasonably expected to understand. When it is not medically advisable to give such information to the patient, the information should be made available to an appropriate person in his behalf. He has the right to know, by name, the physician responsible for coordinating his care.
3. The patient has the right to receive from his physician information necessary to give informed consent prior to the start of any procedure and/or treatment. Except in emergencies, such information for in-formed consent should include but not necessarily be limited to the specific procedure and/or treatment, the medically significant risks involved, and the probable duration of incapacitation. Where medically significant alternatives for care or treatment exist, or when the patient requests information concerning medical alternatives, the patient has the right to such information. The patient also has the right to know the name of the person responsible for the procedures and/or treatment.

4. The patient has the right to refuse treatment to the extent permitted by law and to be informed of the medical consequences of his action.
5. The patient has the right to every consideration of his privacy concerning his own medical care program. Care discussion, consultation, examination, and treatment are confidential and should be conducted discreetly. Those not directly involved in his care must have the permission of the patient to be present.
6. The patient has the right to expect that all communications and records pertaining to his care should be treated as confidential.
7. The patient has the right to expect that within its capacity a hospital must make reasonable response to the request of a patient for services. The hospital must provide evaluation, service, and/or referral as indicated by the urgency of the case. When medically permissible, a patient may be transferred to another facility only after he has received

complete information and explanation concerning the needs for and alternatives to such a transfer. The institution to which the patient is to be transferred must first have accepted the patient for transfer.

8. The patient has the right to obtain information as to any relationship of his hospital to other health care and educational institutions insofar as his care is concerned. The patient has the right to obtain information as to the existence of any professional relationships among individuals, by name, who are treating him.

9. The patient has the right to be advised if the hospital proposes to engage in or perform human experimentation affecting his care or treatment. The patient has the right to refuse to participate in such research projects.

10. The patient has the right to expect reasonable continuity of care. He has the right to know in advance what appointment times and physicians are available and where. The patient has the right to expect that the hospital will provide a mechanism whereby he is in-

formed by his physician or a delegate of the physician of the patient's continuing health care requirements following discharge.

11. The patient has the right to examine and receive an explanation of his bill regardless of source of payment.

12. The patient has the right to know the hospital rules and regulations that apply to his conduct as a patient.

No catalog of rights can guarantee for the patient the kind of treatment he has a right to expect. A hospital has many functions to perform, including the prevention and treatment of disease, the education of both health professionals and patients, and the conduct of clinical research. All these activities must be conducted with an overriding concern for the patient, and, above all, the recognition of his dignity as a human being. Success in achieving this recognition assures success in the defense of the rights of the patient.

Reprinted with permission of the American Hospital Association, copyright 1972.

Nursing as a profession and nurses as individuals have long been advocates for their patients. The impact of the health care consumer movement has been to promote increased accountability on the part of all health professions, including nursing.

Influence of the Women's Movement

The women's movement, which began in the 1960s, has had a profound effect on society and has both hurt and helped the nursing profession. As women of the 1960s and 1970s sought career opportunities beyond the traditional female ones of teaching and nursing, bright and able women who formerly would have become nurses pursued careers in accounting, architecture, engineering, computer science, and a variety of other fields. This meant that nursing faced more competition for students than it once did.

While this hurt nursing temporarily, the pendulum has now begun to swing back as women realize how natural and good a "fit" nursing is for them. In the 1990s, when women can freely choose any professional field of study, many are again choosing nursing. Deans and directors of the nation's schools of nursing report that applications from women attorneys, computer programmers, accountants, and other "new" fields are soaring. It seems that nursing's appeal is still strong for people who want to make a real difference in the lives of others.

The women's movement helped nursing by bringing economic issues such as low salaries and poor working conditions into the open. The movement provoked a conscious awareness that equality and autonomy for women were inherent rights, not privileges.

Nursing also benefited from the women's movement in more subtle ways. As nursing students were increasingly educated in colleges and universities, they were exposed to campus activism, protest, and organizations that were trying to effect change in the status of women. Learning informal lessons about power and how to effect change has had a positive effect on modern students, who later can use the lessons learned to improve the status of nursing.

In spite of these positive effects, the nursing profession has been slow to internalize the feminist message of self-determination and commitment. Historically, many nurses have looked on nursing as a useful way to occupy themselves until marriage. To others, nursing was a "job" used to supplement the major breadwinner's income or pay for a family vacation, new car, or camp for the kids. Sometimes nurses worked only to tide the family over through temporarily rough economic waters, returning to home and family when the family's financial situation improved. This "stepping in" and "stopping out" of the profession has meant that these nurses' energies and loyalties were split. The result is that nursing has not prospered as it might have if all its members were in for the long haul.

It is unfortunate that many of the nearly 2 million who are registered nurses have not fully accepted the necessity for long-term professional commitment, which not only enhances personal growth but also strengthens the profession from within. With the firm commitment of its members to lifelong full participation, nursing can grow to its maximum potential, expand opportunities for its members, and ultimately contribute to the advancement of women and society at large.

The Graying of America

In 1981 there were approximately 25 million people 64 years of age or older in the United States. They represented 11 percent of the total population. Demographic projections estimate that the proportion of elderly will grow rapidly in the next two decades. The fastest-growing segment of society is those over 85, and by the year 2000 there are expected to be 108,000 Americans 100 years of age or older (Dentzer 1989).

People over 65 have fewer years of schooling and are more likely to be poor, widowed, female, living alone, and suffering from chronic disease than are younger people. Between 1965 and 1983, hospital use by people over 65 grew by more than 50 percent. This is in contrast to a 10 percent increase in hospitalizations for the total population during the same period (Dentzer 1989).

Eighty percent of older Americans have one or more chronic health conditions resulting in limitations in activities of daily living for half of those affected. Another 18 percent are more severely limited, and 5 percent are confined to their homes. In 1988 6.9 million Americans required long term care. As a consequence, the elderly use a disproportionately higher share of health services than other age-groups. They accounted for 29 percent of health care expenditures in 1987. The leading causes of death among the elderly are heart disease, cancer, stroke, arteriosclerosis, diabetes, lung disease, and cirrhosis of the liver.

The oldest "baby boomers," those Americans born between 1946 and 1964, are already in their early to midforties and are entering the "heart attack years" (Dentzer 1989). As these postwar babies age, their large numbers are expected to create additional strain on the health care system.

This "graying of America" has a special impact on the health care system and the nursing profession that will stretch our already-stressed capacity to provide adequate medical and nursing care.

The Impact of Technological Advances on Nursing

Since the first effective antibiotics were discovered in the late 1940s, many infectious diseases that accounted for the deaths of hundreds of millions of

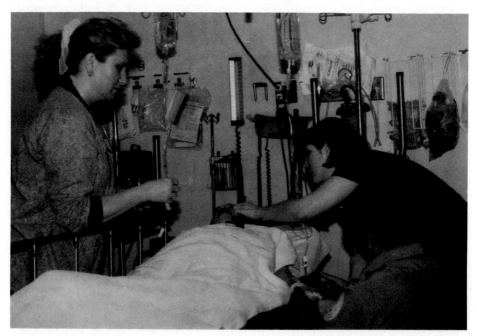

Nurses balance "high-tech" and "high-touch" nursing. (Courtesy of Memorial Hospital, Chattanooga, TN.)

people in preantibiotic days have been controlled. Vaccines to prevent smallpox, typhoid fever, polio, and other killers are available worldwide. As a result, modern medicine has conquered most acute infectious diseases, and life expectancy has increased dramatically as a result.

Today, chronic diseases such as diabetes, cardiovascular disease, cancer, acquired immunodeficiency syndrome (AIDS), kidney disease, and lung diseases represent the most serious health threats. Unhealthy life-style choices such as poor nutrition, smoking, lack of exercise, and alcohol abuse have all been indicated in these disorders, as yet no single clear-cut genetic or environmental factor has been isolated.

In spite of the absence of clearly identified causes or cures for some diseases, many treatments have been developed that enable scores of people, who in previous generations would have died, to live long lives. Such technological breakthroughs as coronary bypass surgery, kidney dialysis, lasers, immune system–boosting drugs, computers, microsurgery, electronic fetal monitoring, and noninvasive diagnostic techniques such as computerized axial tomography (CAT) and magnetic resonance imaging (MRI) are as commonplace today as tonsillectomies once were.

What is the impact of technological advances on nursing and patient care? One of the most widely debated issues is "high-tech" versus "high-touch" nursing. Technological advances now allow nurses to monitor their patients' conditions on computer screens at the nurses' station. Without even entering the patient's room, nurses can gather large amounts of information and make nursing decisions based on that information. Sometimes nurses seem to pay more attention to machines than to patients. Nurses must actively guard against ignoring patients' needs for human interaction as a result of technological advances.

Communication and record keeping in nursing are changing rapidly owing to the use of computers. Whereas nurses used to write out laboratory, supply, and pharmacy slips, send them to the appropriate department, and wait for the service or supplies to be delivered, they can now order supplies electronically. Some hospitals have computers at every patient's bedside, many of which are voice activated. Nurses merely have to talk to the computer, and their assessments and nurses notes are automatically recorded. This frees nurses to spend more time on direct patient care.

Technological progress can have both positive and negative consequences. In Chapter 20, some of the dilemmas created by artificial life support through technology will be explored.

Multiculturalism in Nursing

Despite the fact that the proportion of minorities in the overall population figures is rising, nursing has remained a predominantly white profession. The percentage of nonwhite nurses increased only 0.5 percent between 1980 and 1988, from 8.5 percent to 9 percent. Although patients in the health care system, particularly in large urban areas, are from diverse cultural and ethnic backgrounds, the nurses who care for them are not. The nursing profession must address this discrepancy by actively recruiting more minority students. This is a

"Computer Usage in the Hospital Setting"

"I admit it—I was computerphobic. I received my B.S.N. in 1970 before the information systems invasion. I felt like the commercial on TV that says a cursor is someone who uses bad language, not some pointer on a computer. Now *my unit* is a pilot for the bedside computer system, which offers capabilities for charting vital signs, nursing interventions, and modifications right on a computer at the patient's bedside. I'm teaching others as staff from all over the hospital rotate through this unit. Nurses in the 1990s will benefit from the advanced technology as increased automation assumes a wider role in clinical areas. New graduates take to the computer rather easily, as many have had some exposure to computers in their nursing curricula."

—R.N., JFK Medical Center, New Jersey

long-term solution, however. In the short term, nonminority nurses must be sensitive to the multicultural nature of the patient population and take their special needs into consideration when planning nursing care (Glynn and Bishop 1986). The importance of culturally sensitive nursing care is discussed in Chapter 18.

Nursing's Image Today: Powerless or Powerful?

What the public thinks about nursing influences prospective nurses. Prior to entering school, many nursing students have had no firsthand knowledge of the profession other than what they have seen, read, and heard. They get their ideas largely through the media. The media image of nursing, whether accurate or not, attracts some people to the profession and repels others.

Beatrice and Phillip Kalisch (1982) conducted several studies on the image of nursing during the late 1970s and early 1980s. They looked at the image of nursing as depicted on television and in magazines, movies, and newspapers. They concluded that over a 15-year period the public image of nurses failed to reflect changing conditions within the profession. The Kalisches concluded that the media images of nursing perpetuated a negative image of nurses.

A theme in most of the hospital-oriented television series examined in the study was male-physician dominance. Nurses were seen mostly as part of the hospital "background scenery." The long-running soap opera *General Hospital* continues to portray inaccurate and degrading scenes involving nurses. For example, the gossipy character "Amy Vining, R.N." embodies many negative characteristics that damage nursing's image.

A group of nurses fed up with the negative media images of their profession formed an organization called Nurses of America. They publish the newsletter *Media Watch*, which monitors television's portrayals of nurses. With help from newsletter readers, who fill out media surveillance forms, Nurses of America

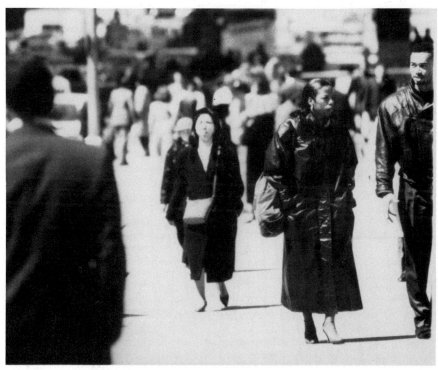

The multicultural nature of American society must be considered in providing nursing care. (Courtesy of *Tennessee Nurse*. Photo by Thomas Sconyers.)

keeps track of how nursing is viewed on television screens across the nation. The surveillance forms ask them to evaluate any type of nursing broadcast, from an appearance by a nurse on a talk show or news broadcast to a fictional nurse character on network programs.

It was the unified power of nurses that launched a successful campaign to eliminate the television program *The Nightingales*. This late 1980s program outraged nurses by its depiction of nursing students as sex objects in demeaning situations. Pressure by nurses on the producers of this series led to the cancellation of the short-lived program.

Another 1980s television series, *China Beach*, depicted nurses as intelligent, autonomous health professionals. This series, which received critical acclaim, was an award-winning drama about nurses in Vietnam. The program was widely praised by nursing groups, and its star became a media spokesperson and advocate for nursing. Unfortunately, the series was canceled, and a letter-writing campaign by Nurses of America calling for the renewal of the series was unsuccessful.

Critics might argue that nurses have more important things to do than worry about how nursing is portrayed in the media. Many nurses disagree, believing

Research Note

For about 20 years there has been a trend in nursing away from wearing the traditional white uniform and cap. It was thought that children and psychiatric patients in particular were more comfortable with nurses dressed in street clothes or colored uniforms. A question that remained unanswered was, "Does the type of uniform a nurse wears affect patients' image of that nurse?"

Sandra Mangum (1991) and her fellow researchers surveyed patients, nurses, and administrators in a regional medical center about the professional image portrayed by different uniform styles. Volunteers consisting of 100 patients, 30 nurses, and 15 administrators from medical-surgical areas and administrative offices were used. They were both male and female and ranged in age from 18 to 70 years.

The subjects were shown pictures of the same nurse in a variety of uniforms and asked to rate her on traits such as confident, competent, attentive, efficient, approachable, caring, professional, reliable, cooperative, and empathic. Results showed that patients' perceptions were significantly different from those of the nurses. Patients rated the nurse in a white dress uniform and

cap significantly higher than did the nurses. Rated second was the nurse in a white pants uniform and cap. The nurse pictured in a colored designer scrub suit was rated low by patients but significantly higher by nurses.

There was general agreement among the three groups regarding the nurse they would like to have care for them. The nurse in the pants uniform with stethoscope was preferred by all three groups. There was also general agreement on which nurses the respondents would least like to have care for them. The nurse in white pants with a colored top, the nurse in colored scrubs, and the nurse in the lab coat over street clothes were least preferred.

The researchers concluded that nurses should consider image and professional presentation as a factor they can utilize to enhance public perceptions about nursing. They suggested that it would "behoove nurses to listen to the patient's opinion and perception of professional image since the nurse is judged primarily by what is worn . . . at the bedside" (p. 130).

(From Mangum, S., et al. 1991). Perceptions of nurses' uniforms. *Image: Journal of Nursing Scholarship*, 23(2), 127–130. Used by permission.)

that when nursing's image is consistently misrepresented to the extent that it negatively affects the way the public thinks about nurses, it is time to take action.

In the official publication of the National Student Nurses Association, *Imprint*, Barbara Smith (1986) suggested that nursing students have an exciting opportunity to improve nursing's image. Smith suggested that nurses take ownership of the image problem and invest themselves in actions designed to improve nursing's image. She specifically recommended developing public speaking skills; dressing professionally; and modeling healthy behaviors such as weight control, regular exercise, and not smoking (Figs. 3–1 and 3–2). Smith

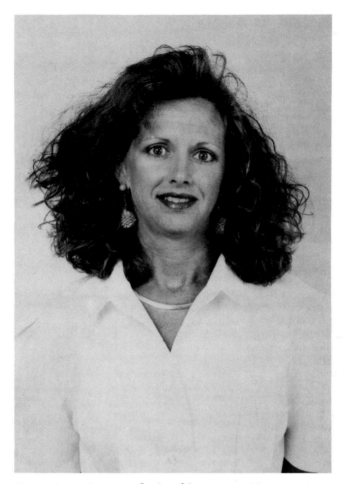

Figure 3–1   An unprofessional image. (Used by permission.)

believes that "nurses who nurture themselves nourish a professional image as they radiate good health and have something to give others" (p. 30).

Although nursing practice has changed a great deal in the past two decades, the public is largely unaware of these changes and the range of services nurses can provide. There are encouraging signs, however, that the American public has gotten the message and that the image of nursing is improving.

The clearest indication of this change in public perceptions came from a 1990 survey commissioned by the NLN and conducted by Peter D. Hart of Research Associates, Incorporated (Hart 1990). According to the study, *A Nationwide Survey of Attitudes Toward Health Care and Nurses,* most Americans view nurses positively. Despite serious concerns about skyrocketing costs and unequal access to health care, 77 percent of the respondents viewed nursing as a con-

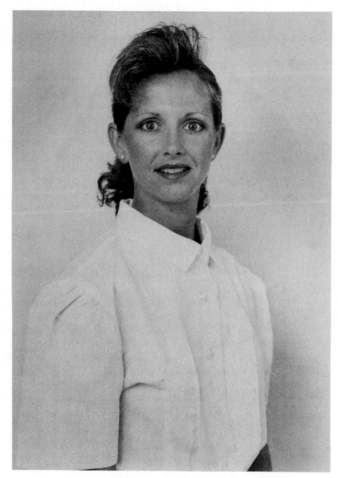

Figure 3-2   A professional image.

structive force in the health care system. Four of five adults (80 percent) characterized their contacts with nurses as either "favorable" or "very favorable." A conclusion drawn by the researchers was that "nurses are far and away the health care provider the public most respects and supports. . . . Nurses are perceived much more positively than the other health care . . . groups tested in the survey" (p. 10).

This type of data can most certainly be used to the advantage of the profession. This favorable image can serve as a catalyst to educate the public regarding expanded nursing roles and the quality of care rendered by nurses. It will serve well in the recruitment of qualified students to the profession.

News Note: **"Big Gain in Nursing Students Lifts Hopes Amid a Shortage"**

Nursing school enrollment rose sharply this year, according to a new study, raising hopes that the four-year-old nursing shortage may be easing.

Preliminary results from the study, by the National League for Nursing, found that about 230,000 students were enrolled in registered nurse programs this fall, a 14 percent increase over last year's enrollment of 201,458. The highest enrollment in the past 20 years was 250,000 students in 1983.

While the current shortage still has many hospitals scrambling to find enough qualified nurses, experts in the field say they expect it to ease gradually over the next few years.

"I think the nursing shortage is beginning to subside, not just because of rising enrollments, but because of increased sensitivity to the idea that nurses are a scarce resource, and should not be used to fill in for orderlies, bookkeepers and dietitians," said Peri Rosenfeld, of the National League for Nursing, a nonprofit research and advocacy group based in New York. "Hospitals are rethinking what nurses should do, and freeing them from other tasks to do real nursing."

She and others said the revamping of nursing jobs, plus rising salaries and an improving image of the nursing profession, had combined to make nursing a more attractive career. . . .

. . . said Judith Huntington, director of governmental affairs at the American Nurses Association in Washington, "It's excellent that enrollment is rising. But with an aging society, the demand for nurses is going to continue to grow, well beyond the year 2000." The Bureau of Labor Statistics has estimated that the health care industry would create 350,000 new jobs for registered nurses by the year 2000.

. . . "I've wanted to be a nurse ever since I was eight," said Kami Zartman, 21, who will graduate from Ohio State University's nursing school in June. "It's a really hard, professionally fulfilling job, and I think we are going to have to do better at getting that image across. . . . "

—Tamer Lewin

Nursing Shortages: Myth or Reality?

There is nothing new about nursing shortages. The first documented reference concerning shortages was in 1915, when nursing leaders expressed concern about the nature of the work in nursing and the effect on the number of people entering the field (Murphy, Belinger, and Johnson 1988). Since World War II, hospitals have been plagued with periodic shortages of nursing ("Breaking the Shortage Cycle" 1987). Each time the shortage of registered nurses became acute, the solution was seen as twofold: increase the supply of nurses and create a new worker to supplement the number of nurses.

Practical nursing programs, which produce graduates in only one year, were created to meet the nation's civilian and military needs during the war years. The nursing shortage of the 1950s stimulated shortened registered nursing programs: Two-year associate degree programs were the result. In the 1960s, shortages led to the creation of the unit-manager role whose job was to take over certain tasks to relieve nurses, who could then concentrate on providing patient care. The 1970s witnessed the emergence of new workers such as emergency medical technicians (EMTs), physician's assistants (PAs), respiratory therapists, and others who took on various aspects of patient care.

As you will learn in Chapter 4, the shortage of the late 1980s witnessed a proposal by the American Medical Association to create yet another "nurse extender" called the "registered care technician." Tired of seeing "solutions" to the nursing shortage that failed to address the real issues of low salaries and poor working conditions, nurses responded quickly and negatively, and that idea has now been dropped.

The nursing shortage of the 1990s is different from previous ones. It is believed that increased demand for nurses is the major cause for the persistence of the current nursing shortage. The American Nurses Association's publication *The Nursing Shortage and the 1990s: Realities and Remedies* (McKibben 1990) cites as evidence the fact that the supply of nurses grew steadily in the 1980s, and more nurses than ever before (16 million in 1988) are employed in nursing. Over the last three decades, schools of nursing have doubled the output of nurses. From 1977 to 1987, for example, the number of employed nurses grew by 49 percent, whereas the growth in the general population was less than 10 percent ("Breaking the Shortage Cycle" 1987).

The demand for nurses to provide care in a variety of settings reflects both the aging of Americans, with the resulting increase in chronic and severe health conditions, and the greater use of nursing-intensive technologies. Longer average life spans and the aging of the baby boomers, the oldest of whom are now middle-aged, herald a continuing demand for general health services and specific needs for nurses far into the future.

Some people believe that shortages are created by nurses leaving hospital work for nonhospital nursing positions. The fact is, hospitals employ about the same proportion of the total pool of registered nurses, two thirds, as they did decades ago, but the ratio of nurses to patients is higher.

It may be surprising to learn that there are more nurses per hospitalized patient than ever before. Over a 14-year period in the late 1970s and 1980s, there was an increase from about 50 nurses per 100 patients to over 90 nurses per 100 ("Breaking the Shortage Cycle" 1987). This is due to two factors. First, more treatment is provided to hospitalized patients because the patients have illnesses and needs that demand greater attention. Lesser needs and treatments are usually fulfilled with outpatient services. Also, to control costs, patients are discharged to home care as soon as possible. There are no longer many hospitalized patients who are recuperating in the hospital and therefore largely able to care for themselves. Second, technological advances such as open heart surgery, organ transplants, and the like, have made special care units, staffed with specialized nurses, necessary. In these units, owing to patient acuity (degree of illness), one nurse cares for only one or two patients.

A factor contributing to the current nursing shortage is that beginning in about 1983 and continuing until about 1987 there was a significant drop in the number of students entering schools of nursing. This coincided with a population dip in the overall number of people of college age, the lowest since World War II. Figure 3–3 shows fluctuations in the college-age population since 1970.

Even the most prestigious schools had to step up recruitment and develop innovative programs to attract a wider range of applicants. These strategies included recruiting more minority students, practical nurses, people with degrees in other fields, and others already in health fields such as EMTs and paramedics.

During the years of low enrollments, a number of schools were closed. Hospitals that had found operating diploma programs quite costly took the opportunity presented by low enrollments to phase out their nursing schools. To be sure, nursing education *is* expensive. Clinical supervision of nursing students by faculty requires a low instructor-student ratio, usually about 1 : 8. Clinical instruction is time-consuming as well, so nursing education is very faculty intensive and therefore costly.

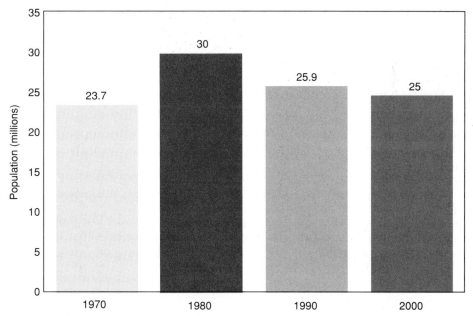

Figure 3–3 College-age (18- to 24-year-old) population. (From U.S. Department of Commerce, Bureau of the Census (1989). *Statistical Abstract of the United States.* Washington, D.C.)

During the downswing in enrollments during the 1980s, some universities closed their nursing programs, citing the expense of nursing education. Others eliminated nontenured and part-time faculty positions. Classes were smaller; there were fewer graduates; and by 1986, a new shortage was described as a national problem ("RN Shortage Suddenly Surfaces" 1986).

A downswing in the national economy in the early 1990s resulted in an increase in applications to schools of nursing nationwide. Whereas just a few years earlier there were vacancies in most schools, by 1992 many programs were turning qualified applicants away because of full classes and inadequate numbers of faculty to provide clinical instruction. And limitations on state funding for higher education made it impossible for colleges and universities to respond quickly to the increased demand.

Unless there is continued high interest by prospective students and a dramatic change in funding to schools of nursing, it is projected that by the year 2000 there will be a shortage of 600,000 baccalaureate- and graduate degree–prepared nurses (McKibben 1990). A 1990 study by the Department of Health and Human Services predicted an increasingly profound shortage of nurses, possibly exceeding 800,000 by the year 2020 ("RN Population Seen Declining" 1990).

An idea that surfaces in almost any discussion of nursing shortages is that large numbers of nurses are not working and that if those could be attracted back into active practice, the shortage would be solved. The fact is that in 1987 almost 80 percent of American nurses were employed, as compared with about 50 percent of all women ("Breaking the Shortage Cycle" 1987). It is true that many nurses, unlike most professional employees, work part-time. In 1988, more than 25 percent of all employed registered nurses worked part-time. This represents over a half million part-time nurses. If more nurses worked full-time, it could significantly reduce nursing shortages.

Salary compression, which will be discussed in Chapter 5, results when experienced nurses' salaries peak early in their careers and level off. A related problem in hospitals is the small differential paid to nurses with baccalaureate degrees compared with the cost of obtaining the degree. Both of these issues are at least partly responsible for nurses working part-time and leaving hospitals for other nursing positions.

There are no clear-cut answers to the problem of nursing shortages. Short-term solutions such as creating new workers and importing nurses from abroad only increase the difficulty of addressing the real sources of the shortage. The profession of nursing and employers of nurses must address basic problems of autonomy, salaries, benefits, levels of practice, scheduling flexibility, child care, and other issues that affect the desirability of nursing as a lifelong career in order to break the shortage cycle.

CHAPTER SUMMARY

Women have traditionally been socialized to seek security, avoid risk, and avoid conflict. Since nursing is a female-dominated profession, the development of nursing has been affected by the traditional socialization of women. Social trends that have affected nursing include the women's movement, the consumer movement, the "graying of America," multiculturalism, men in nursing, and technological advances in medicine. A powerful social influence, the media, projects an image of nursing that is often distorted. This has led the public to have misconceptions about nursing and nurses themselves. Shortages in nursing have arisen periodically since World War II. Only by addressing basic issues such as salaries, benefits, and working conditions can the shortage cycle be broken.

REVIEW/DISCUSSION QUESTIONS

1. Explain how being a female-dominated profession has affected the development of the nursing profession.
2. Analyze the social influences that affected your decision to enter the nursing profession. Did the media image of nursing and nurses play a positive role or a negative role?
3. Describe your ideal nurse. What social stereotypes does your description reveal? Does your "ideal nurse" belong to a particular gender, race, or ethnic group?
4. What positive and negative impacts has the consumer movement had on health care in the United States?
5. List three social factors that have the potential to stimulate interest in nursing as a profession.
6. Describe three actions you can personally take to improve the public's image of nursing in your community.

REFERENCES

Boylston, H. D. (1945). *Sue Barton*. Boston: Little, Brown.

Breaking the shortage cycle. (1987). *American Journal of Nursing*, 87(12), 1616–1620.

Dean, P. G. (1978). Toward androgyny. *Image: Journal of Nursing Scholarship*, 10(1), 10.

Dentzer, S. (1989). How we will live. *U.S. News & World Report*, December 25, 1989, 62–65.

Friedman, E. (1990). Troubled past of an invisible profession. *Journal of the American Medical Association*, 264(24), 2851.

Glynn, N. J., and Bishop, G. R. (1986). Multiculturalism in nursing. *Journal of Nursing Education*, 25(1), 39–41.

Hart, P. (1990). *A nationwide survey of attitudes toward health care and nurses*. Washington, D.C.: Peter D. Hart Research Associates.

Kalisch, P. A., and Kalisch, B. J. (1982). Nurses on prime time television. *American Journal of Nursing*, 82(2), 264.

Mangum, S., et al. (1991). Perceptions of nurses' uniforms. *Image: Journal of Nursing Scholarship*, 23(2), 127–130.

McKibben, R. (1990). *The nursing shortage and the 1990s: Realities and remedies*. Kansas City, MO: American Nurses Association.

Muff, J. (1988). *Women's issues in nursing: Socialization, sexism, and stereotyping.* Prospect Heights, IL: Waveland Press.

Murphy, J., Belinger, J. E., and Johnson, B. (1988). Charting by exception: Meeting the challenge of cost containment. *Nursing Management,* 19(2), 56, 72.

Phelps, S., and Austin, N. (1975). *The assertive woman.* San Luis Obispo, CA: Impact Publishers.

RN population seen declining after the year 2000. (1990). *American Journal of Nursing,* 90(9), 97–98.

RN shortage suddenly surfaces in many states. (1986). *American Journal of Nursing,* 86(7), 851–861.

Smith, B. (1986). Recognizing image is power. *Imprint,* 33(1), 26–30.

Stewart, T. A. (1989). The resurrection of Ralph Nader. *Fortune,* May 22, 1989, 106.

Tatham, J. (1952). *Cherry Ames: Clinic nurse.* New York: Grosset & Dunlap.

U.S. Department of Commerce, Bureau of the Census. (1989). *Statistical Abstract of the United States.* Washington, D.C.: Author.

Wells, H. (1945). *Cherry Ames: Flight nurse.* New York: Grosset & Dunlap.

Chapter

4

*Professional Associations**

Barbara K. Redman

CHAPTER OBJECTIVES

What students should be able to do after studying this chapter:

1. Explain why professions have associations.

2. Describe basic functions that nursing associations perform, both as individual organizations and in coalitions with other organizations.

3. Describe a professional development program for yourself that incorporates membership in a professional association.

4. Analyze organized nursing's management of select issues, according to the values they depict, and the political stances/strategies used.

VOCABULARY BUILDING

Terms to know:

certification

coalition

Code for Nurses

collective action

economic and general welfare

issues management

lobby

professional association

professional boundary

---

* This chapter is written in the author's private capacity. The views expressed herein do not necessarily represent those of the American Nurses Association, except as noted.

*A*ssociations are organizations of persons with common interests. Merton (1958, p. 50) defined a **professional association** as: "An organization of practitioners who judge one another as professionally competent and have banded together to perform social functions which they cannot perform in their separate capacity as individuals." Associations exist in all professions and in all parts of the world. While state governments have legal control of nursing licensure, associations' voluntary control of their members serves to assure the public of the availability and quality of services from that profession. Associations also serve their individual members through a variety of services.

Major nursing associations in Great Britain, Canada, and the United States all formed at about the same time at the turn of the century. Chapter 1 described the instrumental role played by Isabel Hampton Robb in establishing the forerunners of the American Nurses Association (ANA) and the National League for Nursing (NLN). Also mentioned was Lillian Wald's role in establishing the National Organization of Public Health Nurses.

The Work of Nursing Associations

As mentioned in Chapter 1, the initial concerns of nursing association founders were twofold: the need for laws to protect the public from poorly prepared nurses, and lack of standardization in nursing preparation. The newly formed associations won those battles first by successfully lobbying for the establishment of state licensure laws and later by promoting accreditation of schools of nursing.

As society changes, the nursing profession must also change so that it can continue to meet its responsibilities to the public. Professional associations provide a vehicle for nurses to meet present and future challenges and work toward positive, professionwide changes.

Who Do Professional Associations Serve?

Nursing associations have three major constituents: society (the public), the profession of nursing, and individual practitioners of nursing. They serve the public in three major ways:

1. By establishing codes of ethics and standards of practice.
2. By socializing new members to these codes and standards.
3. By enforcing codes and standards in practice.

Associations serve the profession by being the mechanism by which the collective interests of its members are pressed collectively and focused politically (Aydelotte 1990). **Collective action** is a frequently misunderstood term. It simply means that activities are undertaken on behalf of a group of people who have common interests. Professional associations help nurses use collective action to push for political responses that will benefit consumers of health care and members of the profession.

Associations serve individual members by providing continuing education, recognizing skill in practice through credentialing, and ensuring mechanisms for a professional workplace. They serve all of these interests by working for adequate numbers of practitioners to serve the public; by forming relationships with the public and other professions; and by ensuring that the profession's work is properly understood and supported by the public, government officials, and other health care professionals.

Examples of Professional Association Activities

One of the most important activities of professional associations is communicating information to members. Most nursing associations have either newsletters or journals, and some have both. These publications carry news stories of interest to nurses, information about pending legislation and political issues affecting nursing and health care, and editorials and articles on issues of interest to members.

The official newspaper of the ANA is *The American Nurse*, published ten times each year. The ANA's professional journal is the *American Journal of Nursing*, which is published monthly. Other associations' publications include *Nursing and Health Care*, published monthly by the NLN; *Imprint*, published quarterly by the National Student Nurses Association; and *Image, Journal of Nursing Scholarship*, published quarterly by Sigma Theta Tau. There are many others. Some journal subscriptions are included in the association's dues, and others must be subscribed separately.

In addition to communicating with members, there are many other activities of professional associations. Let us now look at the specific activities of the ANA. These activities will serve as examples of the range of issues with which professional associations deal and demonstrate how there is sometimes a delicate balance between serving the public and the profession.

1. *Example A*. A hospital is threatened with closure for financial reasons. Although the hospital is in a city that is "overbedded" (has many unoccupied hospital beds that cost the community money even though unfilled), this institution serves a low-income, primarily minority community. If the hospital were closed, the individuals it serves would have to travel farther in order to obtain health care.

Secure employment for the nurses who work at the hospital is also at stake. The hospital provides jobs for a number of nurses who are represented by the state nurses association (SNA), a constituent of the ANA, for purposes of collective bargaining. The nurses therefore would benefit personally if the hospital remained open.

The difficulty is that the resolution of this problem must serve both the public's and the nurses' needs. Through their SNA, the nurses can form a **coalition,** that is, a temporary alliance of distinct parties, with other providers of health care and consumer groups. The coalition can consider options of obtaining a buyer for the hospital or obtaining care for patients and jobs for providers at other facilities in the city. In this process, they may work with the office of the mayor and the city council and with the corporation that owns the hospital.

Box 4–1 The Code for Nurses

1. The nurse provides services with respect for human dignity and the uniqueness of the client unrestricted by considerations of social or economic status, personal attributes, or the nature of health problems.
2. The nurse safeguards the client's right to privacy by judiciously protecting information of a confidential nature.
3. The nurse acts to safeguard the client and the public when health care and safety are affected by the incompetent, unethical, or illegal practice of any person.
4. The nurse assumes responsibility and accountability for individual nursing judgments and actions.
5. The nurse maintains competence in nursing.
6. The nurse exercises informed judgment and uses individual competence and qualifications as criteria in seeking consultation, accepting responsibilities, and delegating nursing activities to others.

7. The nurse participates in activities that contribute to the ongoing development of the profession's body of knowledge.
8. The nurse participates in the profession's efforts to implement and improve standards of nursing.
9. The nurse participates in the profession's efforts to establish and maintain conditions of employment conducive to high quality nursing care.
10. The nurse participates in the profession's effort to protect the public from misinformation and misrepresentation and to maintain the integrity of nursing.
11. The nurse collaborates with members of the health professions and other citizens in promoting community and national efforts to meet the health needs of the public.

(From American Nurses Association. (1985). *Code for nurses with interpretive statements.* Kansas City, MO: Author. Used by permission.)

2. *Example B.* As the acquired immunodeficiency syndrome (AIDS) has become a full-blown epidemic, there have been concerns about protecting both health care workers and patients. Various health professions disagree about whether infected health care workers should voluntarily restrict their practices in situations where patients could be infected. They also disagree about whether mandatory reporting of HIV-positive health care workers should be instituted.

While the profession's ethics require protection of patients, as of 1992 there is very scanty evidence about the degree of risk to patients posed by human immunodeficiency virus (HIV)–positive workers. Meantime, cases are being tried, and resolution of the issue may come through the courts. The ANA has been asked to take a public position on this issue, including supporting various bills before Congress.

American Nurses Association Position Statement on Promotion of Comfort and Relief of Pain in Dying Patients

"Summary: Nurses should not hesitate to use full and effective doses of pain medication for the proper management of pain in the dying patient. The increasing titration of medication to achieve symptom control, even at the expense of life, thus hastening death secondarily, is ethically justified."

(From American Nurses Association. (1992). *Position statement on promotion of comfort and relief of pain in dying patients.* Kansas City, MO: Author.)

3. *Example C.* New technologies, such as ventilators, now keep people in comas alive even though the quality of life is no longer what they would have desired. Lifetime savings of families may be wiped out by maintaining a family member in a persistent vegetative state.

Nurses are frequently caught in situations in which patients or their families no longer want to continue this kind of existence and yet the health care system has not developed adequate legal and decision mechanisms to deal with patients' desires. In response to the need for guidance on ethical issues, a special task force of the ANA (1985) created a document entitled the **Code for Nurses** to help nurses clarify their responsibilities. Box 4–1 contains an abbreviated form.

While the *Code for Nurses* provides broad direction, the ANA also provides more specific direction on particular ethical issues. In addition to the code, the ANA has published a number of position statements on specific issues, including one on promotion of comfort and relief of pain in dying patients.

These three examples of real, yet very diverse problems demonstrate several common elements related to the work of associations:

1. They are all issues in which there is no clearly right or wrong answer.
2. All the examples involve balancing the interests of individual practitioners and patients with the common good of the public nurses serve.
3. All the issues are political in that significant stakeholder groups do not agree on the right course to take.
4. From its position as a voice for experts within the area of concern, the professional association provides guidance on resolution of issues, guidance that is frequently adopted by institutions or jurisdictions.

This is the nature of the work of associations.

Joining and Using Professional Associations in Nursing

Nurses have a responsibility to belong to one or more nursing associations both as an extension of their interest in nursing and to support their fellow nurses. In Chapter 6 you will see that having a strong professional organization is a characteristic of mature professions. Let us now discuss how nurses can make effective decisions about which nursing association(s) to join and learn how to use these groups to meet their needs for professional growth and stimulate activities on behalf of the members of the group (otherwise known as collective action).

TYPES OF ASSOCIATIONS

A list (not comprehensive) of nursing associations in the United States appears in Box 4–2. This list dramatically demonstrates the number and variety of associations that nurses may choose to join. Understandably, individual nurses often express confusion about which association(s) to join.

In general, the associations listed can be classified as one of three main types:

1. Broad purpose professional associations.
2. Specialty practice associations.
3. Special interest associations.

The American Nurses Association is the broad purpose association in nursing. Individual nurses belong to SNAs, and SNAs compose the ANA. The ANA is a federation made up of 53 state and territorial nurses associations. Its purposes are threefold:

1. To work for the improvement of health standards and the availability of health care services for all people.
2. To foster high standards for nursing.
3. To stimulate and promote the professional development of nurses and advance their **economic and general welfare.**

As the nursing profession has grown and diversified, many nurses have limited their practice to a specialty area such as maternal/infant health, school health, community health, critical care, perioperative nursing, or emergency/trauma nursing. Members of specialty nursing associations frequently choose to belong to an SNA also, since specialty associations focus on standards of practice in that specialty only and on the particular professional needs of that group of nurses only.

Examples of special purpose organizations include Sigma Theta Tau, the international nursing honor society, which one must be invited to join, and the Transcultural Nursing Society, which focuses on a particular area of study in nursing. A comprehensive updated list of nursing organizations is published annually in the April issue of the *American Journal of Nursing.*

Box 4-2 Nursing Organizations in the United States

American Nurses Association
American Academy of Ambulatory Nursing Administration
American Academy of Nurse Practitioners
American Assembly for Men in Nursing
American Association for Continuity of Care
American Association for the History of Nursing
American Association of Colleges of Nursing
American Association of Critical-Care Nurses
American Association of Neuroscience Nurses
American Association of Nurse Anesthetists
American Association of Nurse Attorneys
American Association of Occupational Health Nurses
American Association of Office Nurses
American Association of Spinal Cord Injury Nurses
American College of Nurse-Midwives
American Holistic Nurses' Association
American Nephrology Nurses' Association
American Organization of Nurse Executives
American Psychiatric Nurses' Association
American Radiological Nurses Association
American Society of Plastic and Reconstructive Surgical Nurses
American Society of Post Anesthesia Nurses
Association of Black Nursing Faculty in Higher Education
Association of Community Health Nursing Educators

Association of Nurses in AIDS Care
Association of Operating Room Nurses
Association of Pediatric Oncology Nurses
Association of Rehabilitation Nurses
Chi Eta Phi
Dermatology Nurses Association
Drug and Alcohol Nursing Association
Emergency Nurses Association
Hospice Nurses Association
Intravenous Nurses Society
National Alliance of Nurse Practitioners
National Association of Hispanic Nurses
National Association of Neonatal Nurses
National Association of Orthopedic Nurses
National Association of Pediatric Nurse Practitioners and Associates
National Association of School Nurses
National Black Nurses Association
National Flight Nurses Association
National Gerontological Nurses Association
National League for Nursing
National Nurses Society on Addictions
National Organization for the Advancement of Associate Degree Nursing
National Student Nurses Association
Nurses Association of the American College of Obstetricians and Gynecologists
Nurses Organization of the Veterans Administration
Oncology Nursing Society
Sigma Theta Tau
Society for Peripheral Vascular Nursing
Society of Nursing History
Transcultural Nursing Society

(From *American Journal of Nursing*, Vol. 92, 1992 Directory of Nursing Organizations, April 1992.)

BENEFITS OF BELONGING TO PROFESSIONAL ASSOCIATIONS

A variety of benefits result from membership in professional associations. Most nurses were drawn to their profession because it exemplifies caring for others; because it makes a difference in others' lives; and because it demands full use of their intellectual, interpersonal, and emotional talents. Once in nursing, however, both students and practicing nurses have many needs.

Students usually want to socialize with, and learn from, other nursing students on both state and national levels. They need to develop leadership and organizational skills that will help them in many phases of their professional and personal lives. They need to learn how associations function and how to participate as active, effective members. The National Student Nurses Association (NSNA), which has local and state chapters in addition to the national organization, provides all these opportunities and more.

Practicing nurses want to be recognized, both by salary and by position, for their level of professional expertise. They may seek recognition for their expertise through certification in a specialty area, which is granted by professional associations. **Certification** is a formal but voluntary process of demonstrating expertise in a particular area of nursing. Certified nurses often receive salary supplements and special opportunities.

As their careers develop, nurses may obtain master's level preparation or become nurse practitioners and practice independently outside an institution. These nurses desire and deserve direct reimbursement for their work. They need state laws that mandate direct reimbursement of nurses. Others work in nursing homes and may be concerned that there aren't enough registered nurses (R.N.s) available to provide the quality of care the residents need. They need states to regulate nurse:patient ratios and control educational requirements for nurse aides.

Some nurses work in settings where they have little voice in the quality of care in that institution, are paid poorly, and are required to "float" to cover specialized units for which they have not been trained. These nurses may wish to be represented for purposes of collective bargaining so they can negotiate for improved salary and work conditions.

In each of these instances, nursing's general purpose association, the ANA, is involved in vital work supporting nurses as they fulfill their roles as professionals. State nurses associations **lobby** the government to influence laws affecting nursing, such as those that mandate that insurance companies reimburse nurse practitioners for the services they provide. They also influence laws determining how many R.N.s are required to staff nursing homes and educational requirements for nurse aides, for whom nurses are legally responsible. And if invited to do so, many state nurses associations will assist nurses in dealing with workplace issues such as salaries, working conditions, and patient care issues such as staffing ratios.

These examples represent major benefits of membership. There are many others, such as publications; eligibility for group health and life insurance; continuing education offerings; and discounts on travel, eyeglasses, and other goods and services.

DECIDING WHICH ASSOCIATION(S) TO JOIN

In making a decision about joining an association nurses should ask several questions:

1. What are the purposes of this association?
2. Are the association's purposes compatible with my own?
3. How many members are there nationally, statewide, and locally?
4. What activities does the association undertake?
5. How active is the local chapter?
6. What are the benefits of membership?
7. Does this organization lobby for improved health care legislation? How successful is it?
8. Is membership in this association cost-effective?

Answering these questions should provide nurses with adequate information to make reasoned membership decisions.

BECOMING A PRODUCTIVE ASSOCIATION MEMBER

How do nurses get involved with a nursing association? They join as members, attend meetings, volunteer for committees, and participate in the association's

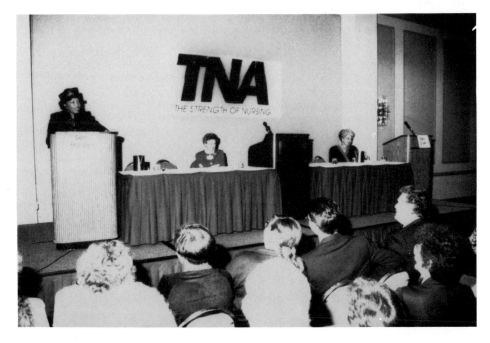

Figure 4–1 Nurses who are active participants in their professional associations can make a difference in nursing and health care. (Courtesy of *Tennessee Nurse*. Photo by Chip Powell.)

activities. Members directly influence the association's priorities, and they provide the volunteer labor that makes the association function. By becoming active participants in professional associations, nurses become part of something bigger than their present work situation, something central to their professional role, and something through which they can make a difference throughout their professional lives (Fig. 4–1).

Perspectives of Nursing Leaders About Professional Associations

In order to present the readers of this chapter a personal view of what organizations do and mean to nurses, the presidents of three major nursing organizations were asked to describe the benefits members receive from belonging to their organizations and what they personally have attained by involvement with their organizations.

Dr. Billye Brown, President, Sigma Theta Tau International

(The society exists to recognize superior achievements in nursing, encourage leadership development, foster high nursing standards, stimulate creative work, and strengthen the commitment to the ideals of the profession. Chapters exist at colleges and universities with accredited programs granting baccalaureate and higher degrees in nursing. There are currently 301 chapters.)

> There are many benefits extending to individual members of Sigma Theta Tau. Members are able to access the latest scientific information through the unique international nursing library maintained by the association. They receive publications and have access to conference and networking opportunities. Members have the chance to participate in activities which enhance their professional credentials, and a structure through which they are able to give back to the profession.
>
> This is an organization into which students in baccalaureate and higher degree programs may be inducted, by invitation, and may continue membership throughout their professional careers. Students need to get directly and actively involved in organizations because I believe it helps them develop their leadership potential, and provides opportunities to observe, and thus learn from, leaders in the organization.
>
> I think the most important issues that are being addressed in the nursing profession at this time are the health care agenda, and increasing standards of nursing practice. (Brown 1991)

Carol A. Fetters, President, National Student Nurses Association

(At the time of this communication, Miss Fetters was a nursing student at Grand View College in Iowa.)

> The purpose of NSNA is to contribute to nursing education in order to provide for the highest quality health care; . . . to aid in development of the whole person, his/her professional role, and his/her responsibility for the health care of people in all walks of life.

This year NSNA will be offering leadership development sessions throughout the year. We are working in collaboration with deans and faculty from nursing programs across the country to develop independent study guidelines for members to use and seek college credit for their active involvement in NSNA. The association also does conferences and conventions, and at these events offers licensing exam review classes free to members, opportunities to meet and hear nursing leaders speak about issues that affect our profession, and to interact with hundreds of recruiters from health care employers from all over the country. Through local and state chapters and on a national level, students have the opportunity to develop important contact networks with many of the future leaders in nursing.

My involvement with organized nursing has helped me complete an integral part of my nursing education, and to develop my own leadership abilities. I was honored to be inducted into Sigma Theta Tau Honor Society on the same day that I was installed as NSNA president. That will be a tough day to follow in my career, as both of the honors are very important to me.

I would tell students to get involved in NSNA. Studies can seem overwhelming at times, but it helps to avoid tunnel vision. As students we have made a commitment to ourselves to leave nursing better than we found it. Get involved early. The profession belongs to all of us. As students we are proud to work alongside organized nursing to bring about positive changes in access to health care. (Fetters 1991)

Dr. Patty Hawken, President, National League for Nursing

(The league is a coalition of nurses, other health professionals, and consumers working to improve the quality of health care through accreditation, continuing education programs, test services, research, publications, videos, and lobbying efforts.)

Benefits of NLN membership include: a free subscription to *Nursing and Health Care*; discounts on all NLN programs, conventions, and publications; and networking, which is so important to professional development. Membership also provides direct involvement in policies affecting nurses, patients, and the profession. It gives you an opportunity to see nursing's and nurses' efforts accomplished. And, you interact with tremendous people and exchange ideas and work on solutions.

Among the most important issues nursing is presently addressing are: Nursing's National Health Agenda; the shortage of nurses, faculty, and space; concerns that wages are too low and too compressed; and further availability of third party reimbursement for nurses.

My advice to students is to learn about your profession and be involved. Get to know other professionals early to learn what their contributions are to the health delivery system. Network, network, network! Share your talents with others. (Hawken 1991)

Analysis of Selected Issues Nursing Associations Address

Several issues are of critical importance to the future of the nursing profession and the purposes it serves. Each of these issues required collective action by organized nursing in coalition with other stakeholders. One involves a threat from organized medicine to nursing's **professional boundary** (dividing line between two professions), and the other involves constructing a new boundary made necessary because of predicted massive change in the health care system. Neither initiative would have been possible without associations, and each issue directly impacts nurses working in all settings.

Registered Care Technologists and Other Assistive Personnel

For some time, nursing has been plagued with periodic shortages. These shortages impact health care settings, particularly hospitals, which sometimes have to close beds because there aren't enough nurses to staff them. Shortages also impact physicians who may not be able to admit nonemergency patients because staffed beds are not available. Closing hospital beds and restricting admissions create adverse economic conditions for both hospitals and physicians.

From time to time when the pressure from this kind of economic impact has been strong, various groups have suggested that nurse substitutes be trained. In the midst of a nursing shortage that peaked in 1988, the American Medical Association (AMA) introduced a proposal for a new health care worker they called the "registered care technologist"(R.C.T.). A series of proposals from the AMA offered different options for supervision of this worker, sometimes suggesting that R.C.T.s would report to nurses and other times suggesting that they would be responsible only to physicians. Proposals also varied widely concerning the number of months of preparation to become R.C.T.s.

Nurses were furious! Instead of supporting appropriate changes in the workplace to alleviate the nursing shortage, such as improving nurses' working conditions and salaries, the AMA appeared to be taking advantage of the shortage to infringe on a boundary nursing had already established as its own. It appeared that the AMA was suggesting that although R.C.T.s would be doing nursing work, and both their supervision and resulting legal liabilities would be the responsibility of nurses, physicians would educate them. This was unacceptable to organized nursing and most individual nurses.

In spite of nursing's opposition, the AMA attempted to find hospitals in which the R.C.T. proposal could be pilot tested. In each potential site, nurses protested so loudly that plans were dropped. Next, the AMA attempted to find test sites in nursing homes, but the same thing occurred. At state and local levels, nurses formed coalitions with sympathetic physicians and medical societies to persuade these colleagues, with whom they frequently worked very closely, that this was not a good idea. Two years after the original proposal, the AMA's House of Delegates essentially barred further active promotion of the R.C.T. The curriculum plan for training such workers, however, remains available to those who wish to purchase it.

It is important to note that this external threat brought all of organized nursing together, not only to fight the R.C.T. proposal but also to deal more proactively with the causes of recurrent shortages. The Tri Council for Nursing, which is a coalition of four major nursing associations, issued a statement on assistive personnel to the registered nurse, which is reprinted in Box 4–3. This statement is meant to guide the profession as it struggles with the long-term resolution of issues involved in using assistive personnel.

Box 4–3 Tri Council for Nursing Statement on Assistive Personnel to the Registered Nurse

Nursing is an essential component of health care, and the consumer of health care needs to be assured of the availability, accessibility, and quality of nursing care. It is in the spirit of this responsibility that this statement related to the use of assistive personnel has been developed.

Historically, unlicensed personnel have assisted registered nurses in the delivery of patient care. However, in recent years, with economic demands driving the delivery system, there have been increasing concerns about the role of assistive personnel. It is extremely important to use assistants in a manner that assures appropriate delegation or assignment of nursing functions and adequate direction and supervision of individuals to whom nursing activities are delegated.

Patient care is delivered today by a staff mix of Registered Nurses (RN), Licensed Practical Vocational Nurses (LPN or LVN), and unlicensed personnel in assistive roles. The term "assistive personnel" is used to recognize the trained/unlicensed health care worker who is employed within the continuum of acute hospital care to home health, ambulatory and long term care. Two categories of assistive personnel are generally recognized: the patient care assistant to whom the RN delegates or assigns aspects of nursing care and who functions under the supervision of the Registered Nurse, and the unit assistant who supports the nursing care system through a variety of nonnursing activities.

Many clinical settings are revising the staff mix needed for the delivery of patient care because of changing patient needs, the economics of reimburse-ment, and demand driven shortages of nursing personnel. A variety of manpower models is being explored and refined as the industry strives to balance quality and cost issues. The ultimate aim is to reallocate nursing and nonnursing activities to enable the registered nurse to focus on the patient. Specific models are best crafted at the point of delivery of care.

The nursing profession is accountable for the quality of the service it provides to the consumer. This includes the responsibility for developing nursing policies and procedures and setting the standards of practice for the nursing care of populations being served. It is further incumbent on the nursing profession to define the appropriate educational preparation and role of any group providing services within the scope of nursing practice. The State Board of Nursing is responsible for the legal regulation of nursing practice for the RN and LPN and should be responsible for the regulation of any other category of personnel who assists in the provision of direct nursing care. Professional and statutory provisions require that when the RN delegates and assigns direct nursing care activities to LPNs and assistive personnel, appropriate reporting relationships are established and the RN supervises all personnel to whom these activities have been delegated. In all situations, registered nurses and licensed practical nurses are responsible and accountable for their respective individual nursing activities. These relationships should be made explicit in workplace policies.

(Courtesy of American Nurses Association.)

Development of Nursing's Agenda for Health Care Reform

There are many indicators that America's health care system is not working as well as it should and needs reform. While we have the most technologically sophisticated system in the world, millions of Americans must overcome enormous obstacles to get even the most elementary services. For example, increasing numbers of children are not receiving immunizations, and there is a resulting resurgence of diseases, such as measles, that are preventable.

Nurses see people daily who are denied or delayed in obtaining appropriate care because of inability to pay or lack of adequate health insurance. These people often delay seeking help until they appear in hospital emergency rooms in advanced stages of illness. Often they have problems that could have been treated in less costly settings or prevented altogether with earlier treatment or prevention services.

Organized nursing felt a professional responsibility to contribute its expertise to the national debate about how health care will be financed and how people, especially those who cannot pay, can gain access to practitioners. In essence, the problems are:

1. Inequitable and limited access to health care providers.
2. Soaring costs.
3. Inconsistencies in quality of care.

Since the *Code for Nurses* (Box 4–1), in points 1 and 11, directs nurses to be advocates for their clients, it is clearly nursing's responsibility to participate actively in seeking solutions for the nation's health care problems.

Realizing that public demand for changes in the health care system was building, the American Nurses Association and the National League for Nursing each began to design a reformed health care system. In spring 1991, their efforts were merged into a single plan, and 65 other nursing organizations have since endorsed the resulting document, now known as *Nursing's Agenda for Health Care Reform* (1991).

Many of the elements of nursing's plan reflect the profession's values. Examples of nursing's values expressed in the agenda include:

1. Special attention to the unique needs of population groups whose health care needs have been neglected—vulnerable groups such as the poor, minorities, and persons with AIDS.
2. A core of federally defined essential health services available to all citizens and residents, regardless of income level or existing health conditions.
3. A major change in the focus of health care—from current practice, which emphasizes acute care only after a patient becomes ill, to a balance of illness and wellness care.
4. Expanded direct consumer access to a range of qualified health care providers, including nurses, in familiar, accessible, and convenient community settings such as schools, the workplace, the home, and community clinics.

It is worth noting that health reform proposals put forth by other individuals and groups are much more focused on financing and downplay the need to reform the system for delivery of care. Organized nursing believes that total reform, not just tinkering, is crucial to ensure access to care for all the nation's citizens.

Developing such a comprehensive proposal and following through on it requires a considerable commitment of time, money, and political clout. This kind of effort is uniquely appropriate for associations and is impossible without them. What was developed in the process of generating *Nursing's Agenda* was a coalition of more than 65 nursing professional associations representing a total of 700,000 nurses. There is tremendous strength in numbers of this magnitude. Many of these nurses are now organized into grass roots political networks, which means they can educate their senators and representatives and urge them to adopt particular legislative proposals to address the problem. In addition, this coalition of associations will:

1. Try to influence other coalitions to support nursing's solutions to health care problems.
2. Hold public hearings to focus debate on the recommendations included in the agenda.

Nursing's Agenda for Health Care Reform and the activities designed to promote it are examples of **issues management** by professional associations. Issues management involves assisting a group to resolve a particular question on which there are significant differences of opinion. Through its agenda, organized nursing is attempting to assist the nation to resolve its health care crisis. This process offers many opportunities for nurses to be involved in reforming the system that impacts the welfare of their patients and their own professional practices.

CHAPTER SUMMARY

Professional associations are the vehicle through which nursing takes collective action to improve health care and nursing. There are many nursing associations from which to choose, and they offer a variety of benefits to the public, to the nursing profession as a whole, and to individual members. Membership in professional associations is considered essential for true professionals, but selecting which association(s) to join can be a challenge. Prospective members can ask several key questions that will help them select wisely. The American Nurses Association, which represents all nurses, is at the forefront in addressing issues of importance to all nurses including the use of assistive personnel and development of *Nursing's Agenda for Health Care Reform*.

REVIEW/DISCUSSION QUESTIONS

1. Look in the local newspaper for articles about the health care system, especially its costs and problems with lack of access for the poor. How does

Nursing's Agenda for Health Care Reform address these problems? Could you sell this plan to a group of consumers, other students, or health professionals?

2. Find out if there is a student nurses association on your campus. If there is, learn all you can about it and consider joining. If there isn't one, consider establishing one.

3. Based on what you now know about associations, how will you personally be involved with them? Establish goals for participation while you are a student, for the first two years after graduation, and for five years after that. Share your goals with a classmate.

4. From the list of associations, contact one that interests you. Ask how one becomes a member and what the association offers its members. Would you want to join? Why or why not? At what stage of your career? Does the cost seem to equal the benefits? What three major issues is that association now addressing, and what has been its effectiveness?

5. In 1991, a program called *The Nightingales* was aired on network television. Most nurses believed it represented a very inaccurate and derogatory image of nurses. Nursing organizations worked together to get the program off the air. Was their action justified? Why or why not?

6. Interview a nurse who is active in a professional association. Ask what he or she sees as the benefits of membership.

REFERENCES

American Nurses Association. (1985). *Code for nurses with interpretive statements.* Kansas City, MO: Author.

American Nurses Association. (1992). *Position statement on promotion of comfort and relief of pain in dying patients.* St. Louis, MO: Author.

Aydelotte, M. K. (1990). The evolving profession: The role of the professional organization. In N. L. Chaska (Ed.), *The nursing profession: Turning points.* St. Louis: C.V. Mosby.

Brown, B. (1991). Personal communication.

Fetters, C. A. (1991). Personal communication.

Hawken, P. (1991). Personal communication.

Merton, R. K. (1958). The functions of the professional association. *American Journal of Nursing,* 58(1), 50–54.

Nursing's agenda for health care reform. (1991). Kansas City, MO: American Nurses Association.

SUGGESTED READINGS

Barnum, B. J. (1990). An interview with Kay Clark. *Nursing and Health Care,* 11, 536–538.

Gunning, C. S., and Hawken, P. L. (1990). Identifying nursing's future leaders. *Nursing Outlook,* 38(1), 78-80.

ıking ICN a catalyst of change. *International Nursing Review*, 36, 171–

9). Nursing code of ethics: An international comparison. *International* , 145–148.

S., and Wakefield, M. (1991). Public policy: New opportunities for *d Health Care*, 12, 16–22.

ts 90th birthday. *International Nursing Review*, 36, 167–170.

Chapter

Nursing Today

Leslie B. Himot

CHAPTER OBJECTIVES

What students should be able to do after studying this chapter:

1. Describe the "typical" registered nurse of today.

2. Identify settings other than hospitals in which registered nurses practice.

3. Differentiate between traditional and nontraditional practice settings.

4. Cite examples of nursing roles in hospital settings.

5. Explain advanced or expanded roles and how nurses prepare to assume them.

6. Analyze the impact of salary compression on the nursing profession.

VOCABULARY BUILDING

Terms to know:

advanced practice
ambulatory care
autonomy
clinical ladder
clinical specialist
entrepreneur
extended care

flexible staffing
home health nursing
moonlighting
nontraditional practice
    settings
nurse anesthetists
nurse managers

nurse midwives
nurse practitioner
private practice
salary compression
traditional settings

A merica's far-reaching economic and social changes have profoundly changed the way health care is delivered. Many of the changes outlined in Chapter 3 have opened avenues to new and exciting employment for nurses. This chapter provides an overview of the registered nurse population in the United States and briefly presents a selection of employment opportunities available to nurses today both within and outside of hospitals. Integrated into the chapter are interviews with several nurses who describe their work and tell what they find are the rewards and challenges of their positions.

Current Status of Nursing in the United States

Nurses today have a wide array of career choices open to them. They may commit their lives to direct patient care in **traditional settings** such as hospitals or practice in nontraditional roles such as owning a health-related business. Nurses should be encouraged to choose freely from the vast number of opportunities open to them; to claim ownership of these roles for nurses and nursing; and to use their positions, whether traditional or nontraditional, as platforms to serve as advocates for their patients and nursing colleagues.

First, let us profile the nurses of today. Is there a "typical" registered nurse (R.N.) of the 1990s? Where do nurses work? What incomes do they earn in today's market? Are there enough jobs to provide employment for all nurses? These are interesting questions and worth exploring.

Every few years since 1977 the federal government has conducted a national survey of registered nurses in the United States. The most recent survey was conducted in 1988. These data were published by the U.S. Department of Health and Human Services in a document entitled *The Registered Nurse Population: 1988* (1990). It describes many of the characteristics of registered nurses today.

Characteristics of Registered Nurses

More than 2 million individuals held licenses as registered nurses in 1988, with nearly 80 percent of that number actively working in nursing. The remaining 20 percent of the registered nurse population were either not working or working in fields other than nursing.

According to the 1988 survey, almost one third (32.4 percent) of employed R.N.s worked part-time. Hospitals were the primary work site reported. More than 67.9 percent of R.N.s reported working in hospital settings. In addition, 7.7 percent worked in **ambulatory care** settings such as clinics; 6.8 percent worked in community health settings such as home health nurses; and 6.6 percent worked in nursing homes or **extended care** facilities. Figure 5–1 shows the percentages of nurses working in settings other than hospitals in 1988.

According to McKibben's 1990 report of the nursing shortage, about two thirds of all employed R.N.s surveyed held staff nurse positions. Staff nurses are

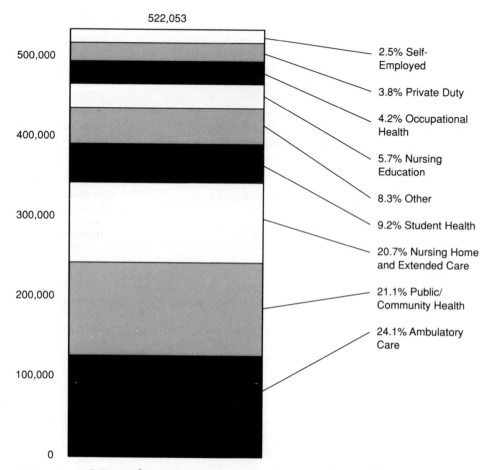

Figure 5–1 R.N. employment in settings other than hospitals, 1988. (From McKibben, R. (1990). *The nursing shortage and the 1990s: Realities and remedies.* Kansas City, MO: American Nurses Association. Used by permission.)

first-line direct patient care providers and work in many settings both in and out of hospitals.

Registered nurses who worked for temporary employment services as their primary work source constituted 3 percent (51,000) of all employed R.N.s. Another 37,000 reportedly worked for temporary employers in addition to holding another nursing position (McKibben 1990). "**Moonlighting,**" or holding more than one position, is a fairly common practice in nursing.

The 1988 figures also showed that most registered nurses were white females. Among employed R.N.s, 3.3 percent were males, and 7.6 percent were from ethnic/racial minority backgrounds. The proportion of minority nurses reported in 1988 represented a decline from 1984, when 11.5 percent of the employed R.N. population were members of minority groups (McKibben 1990).

Like the rest of American society, the R.N. population is getting older. In 1988 more than one third of R.N.s were between the ages of 30 and 39. Their average age was 39. Seventy percent were married, and the majority of married nurses (55 percent) had children at home (McKibben 1990).

Newly Licensed Nurses

The National League for Nursing (NLN) conducted a survey of 28,000 newly licensed nurses in 1990. This survey showed that the average new R.N. was 31 years old. Almost 50 percent had at least one dependent child living at home. Other findings:

> New RNs are attracted to and stay in positions that enable them to practice in their desired nursing specialty. About half of the new RNs cited the ability to practice their specialty as the primary source of their satisfaction, and almost one-third cited it as the reason for selecting their current position. (National League for Nursing 1990)

The survey also found that despite reports that nurses are leaving the profession, 98 percent of new nurses surveyed in 1990 were employed in nursing after nine months in the field. Eighty-five percent were working full-time. Of the 2 percent not employed in nursing, the majority were voluntarily unemployed because they were continuing their education or because of family obligations (National League for Nursing 1990).

According to the American Nurses Association (ANA) publication *Nursing and the American Nurses Association* (1991), nurses are the backbone of the health care system. They are present around the clock, 7 days a week, for 365 days a year. Nurses are responsible for developing and carrying out a personalized care plan for each patient that is consistent with and coordinated with the physician's plan of treatment. Using the nursing process allows nurses to monitor responses to treatment and to modify the care plan as the patient's needs change.

Employment Opportunities for Nurses

Today's 2 million registered nurses serve in hospitals, military service, community clinics, and patient's homes, and some even "hang out their own shingle" in private practice.

Not all nurses provide direct patient care as a primary part of their roles. Nurses conduct research, teach undergraduate and graduate students, are chief executives of companies, and practice in rural clinics. Nurses who have advanced education, such as master's and doctoral degrees, are prepared to become researchers, nurse practitioners, clinical specialists, educators, and administrators.

In deciding which of the many available options to select, nurses should consider their special talents, likes and dislikes, and whether their talents and preferences are a good match with the employment opportunity under consideration.

Nontraditional Employment Opportunities for Nurses

Although two thirds of nurses are employed in hospitals, many others are pursuing challenges elsewhere. Numerous new opportunities and roles are being developed that use nurses' skills in different and exciting ways. Figure 5–1 shows where nurses in nontraditional settings can be found.

What follows are descriptions of a sampling of nontraditional settings in which nurses now practice. In some instances, nurses actually practicing in these settings are interviewed. It must be stressed that these represent only a few of the opportunities available.

RURAL NURSING

Are you independent, intolerant of red tape, and dedicated to the needs of others? Are you from or interested in living far from the maddening crowd? If so, rural nursing may be for you. Today, rural Americans are increasingly elderly and poor. These are the two populations frequently characterized by chronic illness and frailty.

A complicating factor in providing health care to people in rural areas is the scarcity of physicians. The fact that many rural hospitals are closing means even fewer doctors will choose rural areas. Since 1980 there have been 160 closures of rural community hospitals. Of the remaining 2700 rural hospitals, 600 report they are in financial jeopardy. Yet the predominantly elderly, poor rural population remains to be served.

In South Dakota, it is common for patients to drive 100 miles each way for routine health care. South Dakota nurses, like rural nurses in other states, believe that registered nurses are prepared to meet the rural health care challenge. South Dakota senator Tom Daschle agrees.

A recent development expected to improve health care in rural areas is the Rural Nursing Incentive Act, introduced by Senator Daschle. This act requires Medicare, a federally funded insurance program for the elderly, to reimburse nurse practitioners directly for services they provide in rural areas. This act was strongly supported by the ANA and is an example of the power of collective action through professional associations.

Nurses are experts at assessing the whole person. Nurses are also experts in illness prevention and patient education, both of which can greatly improve the quality of health care and keep health care costs low. Since nurses are often the only health professionals in remote rural areas, this expertise is critical in assisting rural patients to develop their personal self-care abilities and independence.

A South Dakota R.N. had this to say about her job in a rural hospital: "A smaller hospital offers nurses the opportunity to be more autonomous and to use all their nursing education and interpersonal skills. We do it all here."

For many nurses, the advantages of living in a rural area outweigh the benefits of working in a big-city facility. On the personal side, they prefer to raise their families away from cities and enjoy the atmosphere of country living. In a professional sense, having a lot of **autonomy**, or freedom from the influence of others, is a plus. The ability to form close relationships with their patients, who

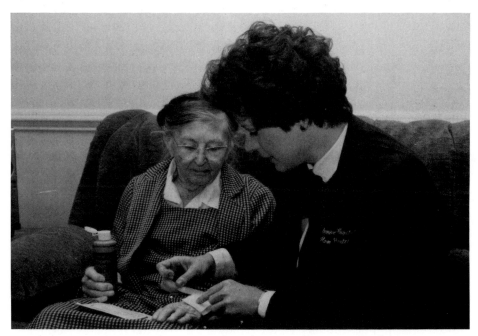

A growing area of nursing practice is home health nursing. (Courtesy of Memorial Hospital, Chattanooga, TN.)

are also their neighbors and friends, is a major reason nurses like working in rural areas.

HOME HEALTH NURSING

Are you creative? Can you improvise? Do you like to deal with people in the context of the family, rather than strictly as individuals? If so, you may find your niche in **home health nursing**.

Lillian Wald is credited with initiating public health nursing when she established the Henry Street Settlement in New York City. Home health care, which includes visiting nurses and hospice nurses, is an outgrowth of public health nursing. Today nurses employed by health departments work in clinics, where patients come to them, and also go into patients' homes to deliver care.

Since 1980 there has been a tremendous increase in the number of private agencies providing home health services. In fact, home health care is one of the fast-growing segments of the entire health care industry. Expenditures for home health care nationwide in 1990 totaled about $16 billion. That figure is expected to reach about $23 billion by 1993. Many home health nurses predict that most health care services in the future will be provided in the home.

Home health care has traditionally been, and will continue to be, nursing's "turf." Home health nurses across the country provide quality care in the most cost-effective and, for patients, the most comfortable setting possible—the home. Patients cared for at home today are sicker than ever. Therefore, more and more high-technology equipment is being used in the home. Equipment formerly unheard of outside of hospital settings, such as pumps that deliver pain medication and treatment for cancer through tubes implanted directly into patients' veins, is routinely encountered in home care today.

Home health nurses must possess up-to-date nursing knowledge and be secure in their own nursing skills. They do not have the backup of a physician or a more experienced nurse as they might in a hospital. They must have good assessment skills, make independent judgments, recognize patients' and families' teaching needs, and have good communication skills. They must also know what their limits are and seek help when the patient's needs are beyond the scope of their abilities.

A registered nurse working in home health in Atlanta, Georgia, relates:

> I have always found a tremendous reward in working with the terminally ill and the elderly, and I get a great deal of contact with this particular population working in home health. One patient I cared for developed a pressure ulcer while at home. I was able to assess the patient's physiological needs as well as teach the family how to care for their loved one to prevent future skin breakdown. Within a few weeks the skin looked good, and the family felt important and involved. To me this is real nursing.

NURSE ENTREPRENEURS

Are you a self-starter? Are you a risk taker? Can you make independent decisions? Can you lead others? If you answer yes to all of these questions, you may want the challenge of being a nurse entrepreneur. A nurse **entrepreneur** identifies a need and creates a service to meet the identified need. Some nurses are creative and energetic people who like the idea of new forms of expression. They are good candidates for entrepreneurship.

Nurse entrepreneurs enjoy the autonomy that is derived from owning and operating their own health-related businesses. Groups of nurses, some of whom are faculty in schools of nursing, have opened nurse-managed centers to provide direct care to clients. Nurses are self-employed as consultants to hospitals, nursing homes, and schools of nursing. Others have started private practices and carry their own caseload of patients with physical or emotional needs. They are sometimes involved in presenting educational workshops and seminars. Some nurses establish their own creative apparel businesses, which provide articles of clothing for premature babies or handicapped people. Others own and operate their own health equipment companies and home health agencies.

Here are a few comments from one such entrepreneur, the chief executive officer of a privately owned home health agency:

> I like working for myself. I know that my success or failure in my business is up to me. Having your own home health agency is a lot of work. You have to be very organized and have excellent communication skills. You cannot be afraid to say no to people. There is nothing better than the feeling you get from a family calling to say our nurses have made a difference in their loved one's life, but I also have to take the calls of complaint about my agency. Those are tough.

A number of nurses are taking the business of health care into their own hands. They seem to agree that the opportunity to create their own businesses has never been better. One such business, based in Columbus, Ohio, offers nursing care for mothers, babies, and children. The emphasis is the care of women whose pregnancies may be complicated by diabetes, hypertension, or multiple births. "Our main specialty is managing high-risk pregnancies and high-risk newborns," reports the R.N. founder. She continued:

> Home care for these individuals is a boon not only to the patients themselves but also to hospitals, insurance companies, and doctors. With the trend toward shorter hospital stays, risks are minimized if skilled maternity nurses are on hand to provide patients with specialty care in their homes.

As with almost any endeavor, there are disadvantages that come with owning a small business. There is the risk of losing your investment if the business is unsuccessful. Fluctuations in income are common, especially in the early months, and regular paychecks may become a memory, at least at first. A certain amount of pressure is created due to the total responsibility for meeting deadlines and paying bills, salaries, and taxes. But there is great opportunity, too.

Aspiring entrepreneurs can eliminate much of the risk involved in small business ownership by completing four steps:

1. Conduct a thorough needs assessment to determine if the service or product is really needed and wanted by consumers.
2. Develop a detailed business plan complete with short- and long-term goals, marketing plans, and schedules for business development.
3. Have enough capital (money) to carry the business for at least a year, even if there is no profit, and keep overhead (expenses) low.
4. Prepare appropriately by learning about effective business practices, for example, budgeting, accounting, personnel policies, and legal aspects of small business.

Beginning entrepreneurs may find value in obtaining the guidance of the Small Business Bureau, which can be found in most cities, prior to starting business. The Service Corps of Retired Executives (SCORE), an arm of the Small Business Bureau, is heavily involved in assisting people to start small businesses with the potential for success. They can help identify the pitfalls and help plan how to avoid them.

In addition to financial incentives, there are also intangible rewards in entrepreneurship. For some people, the autonomy and freedom to control one's own practice are more than enough to compensate them for increased pressure and initial uncertainty.

With rapid changes occurring daily in our health care system, there are always new and exciting horizons. Alert nurses who possess creativity, initiative, and business savvy have tremendous opportunities as entrepreneurs.

NURSES IN OFFICE SETTINGS

Nurses who are employed in office settings work directly with physicians and their patients. Nursing activities include performing health assessments, drawing blood, giving immunizations, administering medications, and providing health education. Nurses in office settings also act as liaisons between patients and physicians. They amplify and clarify orders for patients as well as provide emotional support to anxious patients. They may visit hospitalized patients, and some assist the employing physician in surgery. Often they supervise other office workers such as practical nurses, nurse aides, scheduling clerks, and record clerks. Educational requirements, hours of work, and specific responsibilities differ, depending on the preferences of the employer.

A registered nurse who works for a group of three nephrologists (kidney specialists) in Atlanta, Georgia, describes a typical day:

> I first make rounds independently on patients in the dialysis center, making sure that they are tolerating the dialysis procedure and answering questions regarding their treatments and diets. I then make rounds with one of the physicians in the hospital as he visits patients and orders new treatments. The afternoon is spent in the office assessing patients as they come for their physician's visit. I may draw blood for a diagnostic test on one patient and do patient teaching regarding diet to another. No two days are alike, and that is what I love about this position. I have a sense of independence but still have daily patient contact.

Registered nurses considering employment in office settings need good communication skills, since a large part of their responsibilities includes communicating with patients, families, physicians, pharmacists, and hospital admitting clerks. They should inquire about the specifics of the role since office nursing ranges from very routine tasks to the multifaceted functions described by the nurse interviewed above.

CAMP NURSING

If you enjoy the outdoors, love children, and like to work independently, camp nursing may be your choice. Often used as additional employment in the summer or as a refreshing alternative to work in traditional settings, camp nursing can be both challenging and enjoyable.

Most camp nursing jobs are for a specific span of time such as a summer, although there are year-round camps. The hours are often long, and salaries tend to be modest, but housing and meals are provided and uniforms are usually not required.

Unless the camp is very large, the camp nurse is usually the only health professional on the premises and provides care for counselors as well as children. Nursing activities range from treating minor injuries such as splinters to severe ones such as broken bones. Camp nurses are involved in every phase of camp life and often are sought out for their counseling skills when children are homesick or having difficulty in relationships with other campers.

Some camps are designed for children with specific health problems such as asthma, diabetes mellitus, cancer, or various physical and emotional handicaps. A nurse in a camp for blind children shared her perspective of the role:

> This is a nice change from my usual position of ICU [intensive care unit] nurse. Every summer I take three weeks off from my regular job and work here as a

camp nurse. It has a way of keeping things in perspective for me and lets me use my nursing skills in a different setting and with children.

Requirements for camp nurses, except in highly specialized camps, are usually limited to licensure in the state in which the camp is located. Skills required for camp nurses include knowledge of normal growth and development of children, physical assessment skills, understanding of childhood communicable diseases, first-aid skills, and emergency/CPR (cardiopulmonary resuscitation) competency. For those nurses in camps for children with health problems, an in-depth understanding of the specific illness or disability, its treatment, expected outcomes, and teaching needs of children affected are necessary. A baccalaureate degree or speciality certification may be required in these instances.

Owing to its seasonal nature, camp nursing is unlikely to be a long-term career. It is a pleasant and stimulating form of professional renewal enjoyed by many nurses and demonstrates the range of options open to today's nurses.

NURSES IN OCCUPATIONAL HEALTH SETTINGS

Would you enjoy working in a large company or manufacturing plant with adults? Are you wellness oriented? Do you enjoy teaching people how to live healthy life-styles? These are some of the characteristics of occupational health nursing.

Many large companies today employ nurses to deliver basic health care services, health education, screenings, and emergency treatment to company employees. Corporate executives have long known that good employee health reduces absenteeism, insurance costs, and worker errors, thereby improving company profitability.

Occupational health nurses represent an important investment by companies. They are often asked to serve as consultants on health matters within the company. They may participate in health-related policy development, such as policies governing employee smoking or family leaves (formerly known as maternity leaves). Depending on the size of the company, the nurse may be the only health professional employed and therefore could have a good deal of autonomy.

The usual educational requirement for nurses in occupational health roles is licensure. Some positions call for a baccalaureate degree in nursing. These nurses must possess knowledge and skills that enable them to perform routine physical assessments, including vision and hearing screening for all employees. Good interpersonal skills in order to provide counseling and referrals for life-style problems, such as stress or substance abuse, are a plus for these nurses. They must also have first-aid and CPR skills. If employed in a heavy manufacturing setting where burns or severe injuries are a risk, they must have special training in those medical emergencies.

The responsibilities of occupational health nurses extend to the entire work environment. They must be able to assess the environment for potential safety hazards and work with management to eliminate or reduce them. They need a working knowledge of governmental regulations, such as the requirements of the Occupational Safety and Health Administration (OSHA), and ensure that the company is complying with them. They also need to understand Worker's Compensation regulations and coordinate the care of injured workers with the treating physician.

Nurses in occupational settings have to be confident in their nursing skills, be effective communicators with both employees and management, motivate employees to adopt healthier habits, and be able to function independently in delivering care.

SCHOOL NURSING

Nurses choosing school nursing must love to work with children, their families, and teachers. School nurses make up 7 percent of the nursing work force in the United States. While some states have well-developed school health programs, others do not. Health care futurists (people who study trends) believe that school nursing is the wave of the future (Moccia 1992). Some even believe that in the future the role of school nurse will expand to include members of the school child's immediate family.

Most school systems require nurses to have a minimum of a baccalaureate degree in nursing, whereas some school districts have higher educational requirements. Prior experience working with children is also usually required. School health is becoming a specialty in its own right, and in states where school health is a priority, graduate programs in school health nursing have been established.

Like camp nurses, school nurses need a working knowledge of growth and development in order to detect developmental problems early. First aid for minor injuries and emergency care for more severe ones are additional skills school nurses use. Counseling skills are important since many children turn to the school nurse as counselor. School nurses keep records of children's immunizations and are responsible for seeing that immunizations are current. When an outbreak of a childhood communicable disease occurs, school nurses educate parents, teachers, and students about treatment and prevention of transmission.

Legislation requiring mainstreaming of children has brought many physically challenged children into regular school classrooms. School nurses must work closely with parents and teachers to provide these children with the special care they need while at school.

School nurses work closely with teachers to incorporate health concepts into the curriculum. They conduct vision and hearing screenings. Parents expect school nurses to make referrals to qualified physicians and other health care providers when routine screenings identify problems outside the nurses' scope of practice.

School nurses must be prepared to handle both routine illnesses of children and adolescents and emergencies. One of their major concerns is safety. Accidents are the leading cause of death in children of all ages, yet accidents are preventable. Preventive aspects of child health are a major focus of school health nurses. In terms of safety, prevention requires both protection from obvious hazards and education of teachers, parents, and students about how to avoid accidents. School nurses practice safety, are alert to safety needs in the school and surrounding environment, and recognize the need for safety education in contributing to accident reduction.

School nursing is a complex and multifaceted field which is constantly expanding. It represents a challenge for those nurses who choose it as a career.

Traditional Employment Opportunities for Nurses

As reviewed in Chapter 1, nursing care originated in the home setting and moved into hospitals only within the last century. For most of nursing's history, therefore, nursing care was delivered outside hospitals. Given that history, it would seem that out-of-hospital nursing settings would be called traditional ones, but that is not the case. In this context, **traditional settings** means employment in hospitals, clinics, and nursing homes. The discussion of employment opportunities in this chapter is limited to those available in hospitals.

THE HOSPITAL SETTING

Most nurses (two thirds) work in hospital settings. Hospitals vary widely in size, services offered, and geographic location. In general, nurses in hospitals work with patients who have medical or surgical conditions, with children, with women and their newborns, with cancer patients, with people who have had severe traumas (injuries) or burns, in operating rooms or emergency rooms, and in many other capacities. In addition to direct patient care roles, nurses in hospitals serve as educators, managers, and administrators who teach or supervise others and establish the direction of nursing hospitalwide. There is perhaps no other setting that offers so much variety within the same organization as do hospitals.

The educational credentials required of registered nurses practicing in hospitals can range from associate degrees and diplomas to doctoral degrees. Generally, entry-level positions require only a license. Many hospitals require nurses to hold baccalaureate degrees to move up the clinical ladder or to move into management. Clinical coordinators, who are responsible for the management of more than one unit, are generally expected to hold master's degrees, as are clinical specialists, whose role is described below.

Most new nurses choose to work in acute care hospitals initially in order to gain experience in organizing and delivering patient care. For some, staff nursing is extremely enjoyable, and they continue in this role for their entire careers.

Others pursue additional education, often provided by the hospital, and move into specialty units such as coronary care. Although specialty units usually require experience and advanced training, some hospitals do allow exceptional new graduates to work in these units.

Still others find that management is their strength. Head nurses, often called **nurse managers**, are in charge of all activities on their units, including patient care, continuous quality improvement, personnel selection and evaluation, and resource (supplies and money) management. Being a head nurse in a hospital today is somewhat like running a business, and head nurses need a somewhat entrepreneurial spirit to be effective.

Most nurses in hospitals provide direct patient care. In the past, it was necessary for nurses to move into administrative or management roles in order to be promoted or receive salary increases. This took them away from the bedside. Today clinical ladder programs allow nurses to progress while staying in direct patient care roles.

A **clinical ladder** is a multiple-step program that begins with entry-level staff nurse positions. As nurses gain experience, participate in continuing education, demonstrate clinical competence, pursue formal education, and become certified, they are eligible to move up the rungs of the ladder.

At the top of most clinical ladders are clinical specialists. **Clinical specialists** are nurses with master's degrees in specialized areas of nursing such as oncology. The role varies but generally includes responsibility for serving as a clinical mentor and role model for other nurses as well as setting standards for nursing care on the particular unit. The oncology clinical specialist, for example, works with the nursing staff on the oncology unit to help them stay abreast of the latest research in the care of cancer patients. The clinical specialist is a resource person for the unit and often provides direct care to patients or families with particularly difficult or complex problems. He or she establishes nursing protocols and is responsible for seeing that nurses adhere to high standards of care.

Salaries and responsibilities increase at the higher levels of clinical ladders. The clinical ladder concept benefits nurses by allowing them to advance while still working directly with patients. Hospitals also benefit by retaining experienced clinical nurses in direct care roles, thus improving the quality of nursing care throughout the hospital.

Each hospital nursing role has its own unique characteristics. In the following profile, an R.N. discusses his role as a bedside nurse in a burn unit:

> A burn nurse has to be gentle, strong, and patient enough to go slow. You must be confident enough to work alone; you must believe that what you're doing is in the patient's best interest because some of the procedures hurt far worse than anyone can imagine. Every burn is unique and a challenge. Fifteen years ago, the prognosis for surviving an intensive burn was not good, but with today's techniques for fluid replacement and the development of effective antibiotics, many patients are surviving the first few critical days. During the long hours of one-on-one care you really get to know your patient. There is nothing more rewarding.

When the "fit" between nurses and their role requirements are good, nursing is a gratifying profession. An oncology nurse demonstrated that gratification as she discussed her role:

> Being an oncology nurse and working with people with potentially terminal illnesses brings you close to patients and their families. The family room for our patients and their families is very homelike. Families bring food in and have dinner with their loved one right here. Working with dying patients is a tall order. You must be able to support the family and the patient through many stages of the dying process including anger and depression. Experiencing cancer is always

traumatic with the diagnosis, the treatment, and the struggle to cope. But today's statistics show that more people experience cancer and live. Because of research and early detection, being diagnosed with cancer is no longer the automatic death sentence it used to be. I love getting involved with patients and their families and feel that I can contribute to their positive mental attitude, which can impact their disease process, or hold their hand and help them to die with dignity. They cry, I cry—it is part of my nursing, and I would have it no other way.

These are only two of the many possible roles nurses in hospital settings may choose. Though brief, these descriptions convey a flavor of the responsibility, complexity, and fulfillment to be found in hospital-based nursing today.

SALARIES OF NURSES PRACTICING IN HOSPITAL SETTINGS

The latest survey of the National Association for Healthcare Recruitment (*NAHCR Survey* 1989) shows positive signs in terms of salaries for registered nurses. Salaries are up nationwide.

Discussing salaries from a national perspective is often misleading. Salary figures in San Francisco and Chicago are much higher than those in smaller communities. Readers should bear this in mind when reviewing these pages.

In 1989, average minimum salaries for staff nurses went up 6 to 8 percent, whereas average maximum salaries for staff nurses went up 10 percent. "Other" nurse salaries, that is, salaries of nurses who are not staff nurses, rose only 6 to 7 percent (*NAHCR Survey* 1989). While figures can be misleading, this may mean that the work of staff nurses is valued more highly than it was in the past.

In 1989, more facilities (31 percent) paid salary supplements for nurses holding baccalaureate degrees. Nonsalary benefits were also positive in the 1989 survey. Nonsalary benefits include such things as favorable work schedules, tuition reimbursement, and salary differentials for advanced education or undesirable shifts.

One of the greatest drawbacks to hospital nursing in the past was the necessity for nurses to work rigid schedules, which usually included evenings, nights, and weekends. While nurses still must work a fair share of undesirable times, **flexible staffing** is becoming the norm. Some hospitals go so far as to encourage the nurses on a particular unit to negotiate with each other and establish their own schedules. In the 1989 survey, flexible staffing showed significant gains, with 87 percent of surveyed nurses reporting a greater degree of flexibility in staffing patterns. This represents an increase from 63 percent in 1987.

In keeping with the trend in nursing for continuing formal education, many hospitals now offer tuition reimbursement to nurses pursuing baccalaureate and master's degrees. Once offered as an enticement to get nurses to work at hospitals offering reimbursement, the 1989 survey revealed that 98 percent of hospitals reported offering some tuition reimbursement. There was a modest increase of 1 to 3 percent in the dollar amount of tuition reimbursement reported over the previous year. Offering a salary differential to nurses working evening and night hours is a nearly universal practice. In 1989, 97 percent of institutions offered a differential, with little regional variation. Weekend differential pay-

	AVERAGE MINIMUM	AVERAGE MAXIMUM	RANGE
LPN/LVN			
Northeastern	$18,035	$23,962	$12,000-35,000
Southern	14,561	20,700	9,800-28,000
North Central	15,405	20,660	10,200-25,300
Western	17,119	22,891	13,300-28,600
National	16,263	22,013	9,800-35,000
RN			
Northeastern	25,977	36,104	20,600-56,000
Southern	22,342	32,904	19,500-45,000
North Central	22,733	31,808	17,600-43,800
Western	25,702	37,667	17,500-52,000
National	24,150	34,376	17,500-56,000
Head Nurse			
Northeastern	31,448	42,216	22,700-67,000
Southern	27,998	39,880	22,100-53,900
North Central	28,392	40,157	19,400-56,000
Western	32,895	45,891	25,300-64,700
National	29,972	41,682	19,400-67,000
Supervisor			
Northeastern	32,222	44,090	24,500-73,200
Southern	28,945	41,052	20,800-55,700
North Central	29,507	41,733	22,000-70,300
Western	34,151	47,469	24,500-68,300
National	31,000	43,255	20,800-73,200
Director of Nursing			
Northeastern	44,495	61,755	28,400-100,000
Southern	38,704	54,771	27,800- 85,000
North Central	39,842	56,814	25,400-105,100
Western	47,223	68,386	30,000-125,000
National	42,360	59,972	25,400-125,000

Figure 5–2 Nurses' salaries across the country, 1989. (Reprinted with permission from the September issue of *Nursing '89.* Copyright 1989 Springhouse Corporation, 1111 Bethlehem Pike, Springhouse, PA 19477-0908. All rights reserved.)

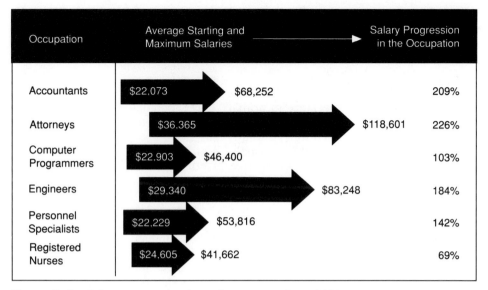

Occupation	Average Starting and Maximum Salaries ———→	Salary Progression in the Occupation
Accountants	$22,073 → $68,252	209%
Attorneys	$36,365 → $118,601	226%
Computer Programmers	$22,903 → $46,400	103%
Engineers	$29,340 → $83,248	184%
Personnel Specialists	$22,229 → $53,816	142%
Registered Nurses	$24,605 → $41,662	69%

Figure 5–3   Salary progression in various occupations, 1989. (From U.S. Department of Labor, Bureau of Labor Statistics. (1990). *White-collar pay: Private service–producing industries* (Bulletin 2347). Washington, D.C.: Author.)

ment also occurs nationwide. Figure 5–2 shows salaries for nurses across the country.

Other benefits reported by hospitals include paid time off for continuing education, offered by 85 percent; critical care internships, offered by 52 percent; and clinical ladder programs, offered by 49 percent.

An important issue to R.N.s is the problem of salary compression. **Salary compression** is a term meaning that pay increases are limited during a typical career. This means that nurses "top out" early in their careers and nurses with years of experience sometime make little, if any, more than their younger counterparts.

Salary progression in other fields is much greater than in nursing. Attorneys, for example, can expect a 226 percent salary progression, whereas nurses average only a 69 percent salary progression in the typical career span. This issue is certainly one of concern to nurses. Figure 5–3 depicts salary progression in various occupations including nursing.

Nursing Opportunities Requiring Higher Degrees

Many registered nurses choose to pursue roles that require either a master's degree or specialized education in a specific area. These are known as **advanced practice** or expanded roles. Already mentioned in this chapter are clinical specialists, nurse managers, and nurse executives in hospital settings. Nursing educators, whether in clinical or academic settings, also are required to hold advanced degrees. The scope of this chapter does not allow a complete listing of all specialty areas requiring master's degrees, but a few will be mentioned.

Nurse Practitioners

Nurse practitioners specialize in primary (basic ambulatory) health care of a particular group, such as children (pediatric nurse practitioner) or the elderly (gerontological nurse practitioner). In any episode of illness, primary care providers are the first people patients usually contact when they enter the health care system. Nurses prepare for the role of nurse practitioner in master's or certificate programs that emphasize health assessment and deviations from normal. This education enables them to detect common health problems and prescribe treatments and medications from a limited range specified by state law.

A Tennessee geriatric nurse practitioner is the medical manager for the intermediate medicine service, which is a 20-bed inpatient unit in a Veterans Administration hospital. She coordinates a multidisciplinary team that includes a clinical nurse specialist, a social worker, a pharmacist, and other health professionals to provide care for the patients on her service. She has liberal clinical privileges, including writing medication orders, performing certain procedures, and ordering diagnostic tests. Her competence has made it unnecessary for the hospital to hire a medical resident for the unit. This nurse has a master's degree in nursing and a bachelor of science in nutrition (Oliver 1992).

Nurse Midwives

Nurse midwives assist women and couples during uncomplicated pregnancies, deliveries, and postdelivery periods. They work in groups affiliated with maternity hospitals and birthing centers or under the direction of physicians. Nurse midwives are educated for their expanded responsibilities through either master's degree or specialty certification programs.

Nurse Anesthetists

Nurse anesthetists administer anesthetic agents to patients undergoing operative procedures. Specialized education in master's or certification programs is required. The accrediting body for the nation's schools of anesthesia is requiring that by 1998 all accredited programs in nurse anesthesia will offer master's preparation.

Private Practice Nursing

Private practice nursing was mentioned in the section on nurse entrepreneurs. It is important to point out that nurses in private practice—whether they are consultants or counselors or are providing hands-on care—must have advanced degrees or specialized education, training, and certification. The specific requirements differ according to state law. A careful reading of the state's nurse practice

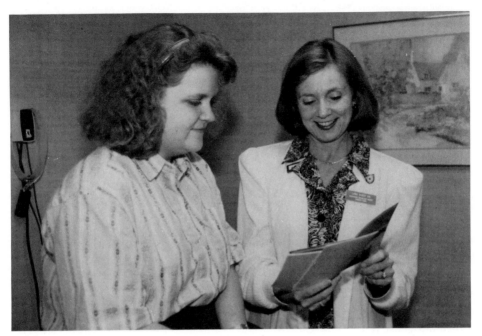

A private practice nurse educates her patient. (Courtesy of Memorial Hospital, Chattanooga, TN.)

act is important for all nurses but particularly for those nurses in advanced practice, such as nurse midwives, nurse practitioners, nurse anesthetists, and private practice nurses.

CHAPTER SUMMARY

There are more than 2 million registered nurses in the United States, and nearly 80 percent are actively practicing. Two thirds of working nurses are employed in hospitals, a traditional setting for nursing practice. An exciting trend is toward **nontraditional practice settings** such as home health, school nursing, and small health-related businesses. As nurses make more opportunities for themselves in nontraditional settings, competition to keep nurses in hospitals will increase. Resolving the issue of salary compression in hospitals will help in the retention of nurses, as will continued innovations in flexible scheduling and other benefits.

REVIEW/DISCUSSION QUESTIONS

1. What characteristics do nurses of today have in common and how do they differ?
2. Think of the areas of nursing that interest you most. Are they traditional

settings or nontraditional settings? How do your personal and professional qualifications compare with the characteristics needed in the roles discussed in this chapter?

3. Interview nurses in traditional and nontraditional settings. Find out how they prepared for their positions, what their daily activities are, and what they enjoy most and least about their work.

4. Call the nurse recruiter or personnel office of a nearby hospital and inquire about salaries and other benefits for entry-level and advanced nursing positions. How do they compare with those listed in this chapter?

REFERENCES

American Nurses Association. (1991). *Nursing and the American Nurses Association.* Kansas City, MO: Author.

McKibben, R. (1990). *The nursing shortage and the 1990s: Realities and remedies.* Kansas City, MO: American Nurses Association.

Moccia, P. (1992). In 1992: A nurse in every school. *Nursing & Health Care,* 13(1), 14–18.

National Association for Healthcare Recruitment survey, Nursing '89. (1989). Springhouse, PA: Springhouse Corporation.

National League for Nursing. (1990). *Nursing datasource 1990: A research report.* New York: Author.

Oliver, G. (1992). Nurse in the news: Sarah Senn. *R.N. Communiqué,* 23(3), 4.

U.S. Department of Health and Human Services. (1990). *The registered nurse population: 1988.* Washington, D.C.: Author.

U.S. Department of Labor, Bureau of Labor Statistics. (1990). *White-collar pay: Private service–producing industries* (Bulletin 2347). Washington, D.C.: Author.

Chapter

Defining Profession

Kay K. Chitty

CHAPTER OBJECTIVES

What students should be able to do after studying this chapter:

1. Identify the characteristics of a profession.
2. Distinguish between the characteristics of professions and occupations.
3. Evaluate nursing's current status as a profession.
4. Recognize characteristic behaviors of professional nurses.

VOCABULARY BUILDING

Terms to know:

accountability	cognitive	profession
altruism	Flexner Report	professional
autonomy	nursing process	professionalism
code of ethics	occupation	

What is a **profession** and who can be called a **professional**? These terms are used loosely in everyday conversation. Historically, only medicine, law, and the ministry were accepted as professions. Today, however, *professional* is a term commonly used to identify many types of people ranging from wrestlers and rock stars to college professors and archaeologists. Are all these individuals professionals? The answer to that question depends on how profession is defined.

In sports, a professional is distinguished from an amateur by being paid. Amateur golfers, for example, cannot accept money; professional golfers compete for it. So in sports, making money is one characteristic of being a professional. Professionals are generally better at what they do than are others. Therefore, in most fields, expertise is also a part of being a professional. But being paid and having expertise are not the only criteria for being professional.

Characteristics of a Profession

Over the years many thoughtful people have grappled with the meaning of **professionalism**. In the early 1900s the Carnegie Foundation issued a series of papers about professional schools. The first of these reports was based on Abraham Flexner's 1910 study of medical education (Flexner 1910). The **Flexner Report**, as it became known, is a classic piece of educational literature that provided the impetus for the much-needed reform of medical education.

Flexner went on to study other disciplines and later, in a paper about social work, published a list of criteria that he felt were characteristic of all true professions (Flexner 1915). Since Flexner's original criteria were published, they have been widely used as a benchmark for determining the status of various occupations in terms of professionalism.

Flexner's Criteria

Flexner believed that professional work:

1. Is basically intellectual (as opposed to physical).
2. Is based on a body of knowledge that can be learned.
3. Is practical, rather than theoretical.
4. Can be taught through a process of professional education.
5. Has a strong internal organization of members.
6. Has practitioners who are motivated by **altruism** (the desire to help others).

Since 1915 a number of other authorities have also identified criteria for professions, which vary slightly from Flexner's.

Bixler and Bixler's Criteria

Genevieve and Roy Bixler, a husband and wife team of nonnurses who were nevertheless advocates and supporters of nursing, first wrote about the status of nursing as a profession in 1945. In 1959 they again appraised nursing according to their original seven criteria, noting the progress made (Bixler and Bixler 1959). Their criteria included the following:

1. "A profession utilizes in its practice a well-defined and well-organized body of specialized knowledge which is on the intellectual level of the higher learning" (p. 1142).
2. "A profession constantly enlarges the body of knowledge it uses and improves its techniques of education and service by the use of the scientific method" (p. 1143).
3. "A profession entrusts the education of its practitioners to institutions of higher education" (p. 1144).
4. "A profession applies its body of knowledge in practical services which are vital to human and social welfare" (p. 1145).
5. "A profession functions autonomously in the formulation of professional policy and in the control of professional activity thereby" (p. 1145).
6. "A profession attracts individuals of intellectual and personal qualities who exalt service above personal gain and who recognize their chosen occupation as a life work" (p. 1146).
7. "A profession strives to compensate its practitioners by providing freedom of action, opportunity for continuous professional growth, and economic security" (p. 1146).

A comparison of Flexner's and Bixler and Bixler's criteria reveal many similarities. General agreement exists about what constitutes a profession, but not all people agree about which occupations are professional. How contemporary nursing stacks up as a profession is discussed later.

Differences in "Profession" and "Occupation"

Occupation is often used interchangeably with *profession*, but their definitions differ. Webster defines **occupation** as "what occupies, or engages, one's time; business; employment." *Profession* is defined as "a vocation requiring advanced training . . . , and usually involving mental rather than manual work, as teaching, engineering, etc.; especially, medicine, law, or theology (formerly called the learned professions)" (*Webster's* 1989). There is widespread overall agreement that a profession is different from an occupation in at least two major ways— preparation and commitment.

Preparation

Professional preparation usually takes place in a college or university setting. Preparation is prolonged in order to include instruction in the specialized body of knowledge and techniques of the profession. Professional preparation includes more than knowledge and skills, however. It also includes orientation to the beliefs, values, and attitudes expected of the members of the profession. Standards of practice and ethical considerations are also included. These components of professional education are part of the process of socialization into a profession. They will be discussed in Chapter 8.

Table 6–1 Characteristics of Occupations and Professions

Occupation	Profession
Training may occur on the job	Education takes place in a college or university
Length of training varies	Education is prolonged
Values, beliefs, and ethics are not prominent features of preparation	Values, beliefs, and ethics are an integral part of preparation
Commitment and personal identification vary	Commitment and personal identification are strong
Workers are supervised	Workers are autonomous
People often change jobs	People unlikely to change professions
Accountability rests with employer	Accountability rests with individual

Commitment

Professionals' commitment to their profession is strong. They derive much of their personal identification from their work and consider it an integral part of their lives. People engaging in a profession often consider it their "calling." Whereas people may readily change occupations, it is uncommon for people to change professions.

Several critical differences between occupation and profession are summarized in Table 6–1.

Nursing as a Profession

An ongoing subject for discussion in nursing circles has been the question, Is nursing a profession? Much has been written on both sides of this issue over the years. Nursing sociologists do not all agree that nursing *is* a profession. Some believe that it is, at best, an "emerging profession." Others cite the progress nursing has made toward meeting the commonly accepted criteria for full-fledged professional status.

Kelly's Criteria

Kelly (1981, p. 157) reiterated and expanded Flexner's criteria in her 1981 listing of characteristics of a profession:

1. The services provided are vital to humanity and the welfare of society.
2. There is a special body of knowledge which is continually enlarged through research.
3. The services involve intellectual activities; individual responsibility (**accountability**) is a strong feature.

4. Practitioners are educated in institutions of higher learning.
5. Practitioners are relatively independent and control their own policies and activities (**autonomy**).
6. Practitioners are motivated by service (**altruism**) and consider their work an important component of their lives.
7. There is a **code of ethics** to guide the decisions and conduct of practitioners.
8. There is an organization (association) which encourages and supports high standards of practice.

Let us examine how well contemporary nursing fulfills these criteria.

1. *"The services provided are vital to humanity and the welfare of society."* If ten students were asked why they chose nursing, most would reply, "To help people." Certainly nursing is a service that is essential to the well-being of people and to society as a whole. Nursing promotes the maintenance and restoration of health of individuals, groups, and communities. Assisting others to attain the highest level of wellness of which they are capable is the goal of nursing. Caring, meaning nurturing and helping others, is a basic component of professional nursing.

2. *"There is a special body of knowledge which is continually enlarged through research."* In the past, nursing was based on principles borrowed from the physical and social sciences and other disciplines. Today, however, there is a body of knowledge that is uniquely nursing's. While this was not always so, the amount of investigation and analysis of nursing care has expanded rapidly in the past 20 years. Nursing theory development is also proceeding swiftly. Nursing is no longer based on task orientation, intuition, or trial and error but increasingly relies on research as a basis for practice. Several theoretical models of nursing will be discussed in Chapter 11, and issues in research will be discussed in Chapter 12.

3. *"The services involve intellectual activities; individual responsibility (accountability) is a strong feature."* Nursing has developed and refined its own unique approach to practice, called the **nursing process**. The nursing process is essentially a **cognitive** (mental) activity that requires both critical and creative thinking and serves as the basis for providing nursing care. There is more about the nursing process in Chapter 17.

Individual accountability in nursing has become the hallmark of practice. **Accountability**, according to the American Nurses Association's (ANA) *Code for Nurses* (1985, p. 10), is "being answerable to someone for something one has done. It means providing an explanation to self, to the client, to the employing agency, and to the nursing profession." Organized nursing has also demonstrated a commitment to accountability in the ANA's *Standards of Nursing Practice* (1973). Through legal opinions and court cases, society has demonstrated that it, too, holds nurses individually responsible for their actions as well as for those of personnel under their supervision.

4. *"Practitioners are educated in institutions of higher learning."* As presented in Chapter 2, the first university-based nursing program began in 1909 at the University of Minnesota. Several studies, including Esther Lucille Brown's 1948 report *Nursing for the Future,* called for nursing education to be based in universities and colleges. Recall that another milestone was the 1965 position paper of

the ANA, which called for all nursing education to take place in institutions of higher education (American Nurses Association 1965).

The majority of programs offering basic nursing education are now associate degree and baccalaureate programs located in colleges and universities. There are master's and doctoral programs in nursing, although the number of graduates is small compared with other health professions. Since professional status and power increase with postgraduate education, a legitimate question is, "How can nursing take its place as a peer among the professions when most nurses currently in practice hold less than a baccalaureate degree?" The differentiation between professional nursing and technical nursing is a challenging issue that nursing has not yet resolved. Diversity within the ranks of nursing has slowed the progress toward acceptance of the baccalaureate or higher degree as the prerequisite for professional practice. Lack of resolution of these differences threatens to undermine nursing's development as a profession.

5. *"Practitioners are relatively independent and control their own policies and activities (autonomy)."* Autonomy, or control over one's practice, is another controversial area for nursing. While many nursing actions are independent, most nurses are employed in organizations where authority resides in one's position. One's place in the hierarchy, rather than expertise, confers or denies power and status. Physicians are widely regarded as gatekeepers, and their authorization or supervision is required before many activities can occur. Nurse practice acts in most states reinforce nursing's lack of self-determination by requiring that nurses perform certain actions only when authorized by supervising physicians or hospital protocols.

There are at least three groups who wish to control nursing practice: organized medicine, health service administration, and organized nursing. Both the medical profession and health service administration are attempting to maintain control of nursing because they believe it is in their best interest to keep nurses dependent on them. Both are well organized and have powerful lobbies at state and national levels. Organized nursing, on the other hand, promotes independence and autonomy, but its power is fragmented by subgroups and dissension. Rivalry between diploma-educated, associate degree–educated, and baccalaureate-educated nurses saps the energy of the profession. The proliferation of nursing organizations (see Box 4–2 for a partial list of nursing organizations) and competition among them also diminish nursing's potential. Only 10 percent of the nation's registered nurses are members of the American Nurses Association (Little 1992). The fact that most nurses are not members of any professional organization impairs nursing's ability to lobby effectively. These are major challenges for nursing if it is to realize its potential collective professional power and autonomy.

6. *"Practitioners are motivated by service (altruism) and consider their work an important component of their lives."* As a group, nurses are dedicated to the ideal of service to others, which is also known as altruism. This ideal has sometimes become intertwined with economic issues and historically has been exploited by employers of nurses. No one questions the right of other professionals to charge reasonable fees for the services they render; when nurses want higher salaries, however, others sometimes call their altruism into question. Nurses must take

Box 6–1   The Florence Nightingale Pledge

I solemnly pledge myself before God and in the presence of this assembly to pass my life in purity and to practice my profession faithfully.

I will abstain from whatever is deleterious and mischievous, and will not take or knowingly administer any harmful drug. I will do all in my power to maintain and elevate the standard of my profession, and will hold in confidence all personal matters committed to my keeping and all family affairs coming to my knowledge in the practice of my calling.

With loyalty will I endeavor to aid the physician in his work and devote myself to the welfare of those committed to my care.

(From Pillitteri, A. (1991). Documenting Lystra Gretter's Student Experiences in Nursing. *Nursing Outlook,* 39(6), pp. 273–279. Reprinted by permission.)

responsibility for their own financial well-being and for the health of the profession. This will, in turn, assure its continued attractiveness to those who might choose nursing as a career. If there are to be adequate numbers of nurses to meet society's needs, salaries must be comparable with those in competing occupations. Being concerned with salary issues does nothing to diminish a nurse's altruism.

Another issue, consideration of work as a primary component of life, has been a thornier problem for nurses. Commitment to a career is not a value equally shared by all nurses. Some still regard nursing as a job and drop in and out of practice depending on economic and family needs. This approach, while appealing to many nurses and conducive to traditional family management, has retarded the development of professional attitudes and behaviors for the profession as a whole.

7. *"There is a code of ethics to guide the decisions and conduct of practitioners."* An ethical code does not stipulate how an individual should act in a specific situation; rather, it provides professional standards and a framework for decision making. The trust placed in the nursing profession by the public requires that nurses act with integrity. To aid them in doing so, both the International Council of Nurses (ICN) and the ANA have established codes of nursing ethics through which standards of practice are established, promoted, and refined. Chapter 4 contains the ANA's *Code for Nurses,* and Chapter 20 contains the *International Council of Nurses Code for Nurses.*

In 1893, long before these codes were written, "The Florence Nightingale Pledge" was created by a committee headed by Mrs. Lystra Eggert Gretter and presented to the Farrand Training School for Nurses located at Harper Hospital in Detroit, Michigan (Pillitteri 1991). The Nightingale pledge can be considered nursing's first code of ethics. The pledge is reprinted in Box 6–1.

8. *"There is an organization (association) which encourages and supports high standards of practice."* As shown in Chapter 4, nursing has a number of professional associations that were formed to promote the improvement of the profession. Foremost among these is the ANA, the purposes of which are to foster high standards of nursing practice, promote professional and educational advancement of nurses, and promote the welfare of nurses to the end that all people have better nursing care (American Nurses Association 1970). The ANA is also the official voice of nursing and therefore is the primary advocate for nursing interests in general. Unfortunately, fewer than one out of ten nurses belong to the official professional organization. The political power that could be derived from the unified efforts of 2 million registered nurses nationwide would be impressive; that goal has not yet been realized.

Characteristic Behaviors of Professional Nurses

If being a professional nurse is different from practicing the occupation of nursing, there must be certain behaviors that differentiate the two. As students develop their ideas of how they want to function as nursing professionals, it may help to have an ideal in mind. Many students already know a nurse they consider to be a role model of professionalism. If not, there may be interest in hearing about Joan.

Joan: A Case Study

Professional Behavior Demonstrated

Joan is a 32-year-old married mother of two. She graduated from River City College of Nursing at the age of 26 and has been practicing since her graduation. Her first position was as a staff nurse at Providence Hospital, a 300-bed private hospital. Nursing administration at Providence encourages nurses to provide individualized nursing care while protecting the dignity and autonomy of each patient and family. She chose Providence because the philosophy of nursing there paralleled her own. Another reason for selecting this hospital was that Joan wanted to practice oncology (cancer) nursing, and there is an oncology unit at Providence.

Has developed own philosophy of nursing

Self-determination

Each day Joan uses the nursing process in caring for her patients and in dealing with their families. That means she assesses their condition, plans and implements their care, and evaluates the care she has given. Then she writes what she has done in each patient's chart in the accepted format. She communicates clearly to the other members of the nursing staff and to the other health care professionals involved in the care of the patients on her unit.

Uses critical thinking

Collaborates and communicates with other health professionals

After two years as a staff nurse, Joan accepted a position as a team leader. This means that now she takes responsibility not only for her own practice but for supervising licensed practical nurses and nursing assistants on her team. In order

Demonstrates accountability for self and others

to do this effectively, she stays abreast of changes in her state's nurse practice act and Providence Hospital's policies and procedures. In addition, she updates her knowledge by reading current journals and research periodicals. She makes it a policy to attend at least two nursing conferences each year to stay on top of trends. She belongs to her professional organization and participates as an active member. She finds that this is another source of the latest information on professional issues.

Committed to lifelong learning

Active in professional organization

Joan looks forward to working with the nursing students who are learners at Providence Hospital. She remembers when she was a student and how a word from a practicing nurse could make or break her day. Of course, students do mean extra work, but she sees this as a part of her role and patiently provides the guidance they need, even when she is busy.

Mentors aspiring professionals

In the course of her daily work, Joan sometimes has a question about certain procedures. She is not embarrassed to seek help from more experienced nurses, from textbooks, or from other health professionals. Sometimes she offers suggestions to the head nurse and the oncology clinical nurse specialist about possible research questions and participates in gathering data when the unit takes on a research study.

Recognizes own limits; seeks help when needed

Contributes to expansion of nursing's body of knowledge

Providence Hospital uses a shared governance model, which means nurses serve on committees that develop and interpret nursing policies and procedures. Joan serves on two committees and chairs another. Right now the hospital is preparing a self-study for an upcoming accreditation, so the meetings are frequent. Instead of complaining about the meetings, Joan prepares and organizes her portion of the meeting so everyone's time is used most effectively. She has to delegate some of her patient care responsibilities to others while she is attending meetings. Because she has taken the time to know the other workers' skills and abilities, she does not worry about what happens while she is gone.

Provides leadership

Uses principles of time management

Delegates responsibility wisely

At the end of the day when Joan goes home, she occasionally gets a call from a friend with a health-related question or a request to give a neighbor's child an allergy injection. Although she is tired, she recognizes that in the eyes of others, she represents the nursing profession. She is proud to be trusted and respected for her knowledge, skills, and dedication. Helping others through nursing care is something Joan has wanted to do since she was small, and she finds it very fulfilling.

Represents profession to the public

Models altruism

Lately Joan has recognized in herself some troubling signs: She has been irritable, impatient with family and co-workers, and generally out of sorts. She has gained weight and is exercising less than usual. She wonders if working

Possesses self-awareness

with terminally ill patients and their families is the source of
her stress. Joan's husband suggested that she take "a break"
from nursing and stay home with the children, but after   *Demonstrates*
talking it over with her head nurse, she decided to ask for   *commitment to*
assignment to different nursing responsibilities for a while.   *nursing*
She knows that she needs to be her own advocate and take
care of herself. Next week she will begin a three-month stint   *Models healthy*
in outpatient surgery, where the emotional intensity will be a   *coping behavior*
bit less.

This brief description illustrates more than 18 characteristic behaviors exhibited by professional nurses. Nursing is clearly much more than an occupation to
Joan and to many others like her.

CHAPTER SUMMARY

Commitment to a profession is very different from commitment to a job or an
occupation. People who have studied professions agree that there are several
characteristics that all true professions have in common. A body of knowledge,
specialized education, service to society, accountability, autonomy, and ethical
standards are a few of the hallmarks of professions. Although nursing has a
briefer history than some traditional professions and is still dealing with autonomy, preparation, and commitment issues, great progress has been made in
moving nursing toward full professional status. An awareness of the characteristics of professions and professional behavior will help nurses assume leadership
in continuing that progress.

It is important to remember that being a professional is a dynamic process,
not a condition or state of being. Professional growth evolves throughout the
different stages of nurses' careers.

REVIEW/DISCUSSION QUESTIONS

1. How might nursing be different today if all its practitioners viewed it as their
   profession rather than a job?
2. What is the relationship between training and education?
3. On a scale of 1 to 10, rate nursing on each of Flexner's, Bixler and Bixler's,
   and Kelly's criteria for professions.
4. Discuss technical versus professional education.
5. Describe at least five characteristic behaviors of professional nurses.

REFERENCES

American Nurses Association. (1965). *Educational preparation for nurse practitioners and
assistants to nurses: A position paper.* Kansas City, MO: Author.

American Nurses Association. (1970). *Association bylaws.* Kansas City, MO: Author.

American Nurses Association. (1985). *Code for nurses with interpretive statements*. Kansas City, MO: Author.

Bixler, G. K., and Bixler, R. W. (1959). The professional status of nursing. *American Journal of Nursing*, 59(8), 1142–1147.

Brown, E. L. (1948). *Nursing for the future*. New York: Russell Sage Foundation.

Flexner, A. (1910). *Medical education in the United States and Canada: A report to the Carnegie Foundation for the advancement of teaching*. Bethesda, MD: Science and Health Publications.

Flexner, A. (1915). Is social work a profession? *School Society*, 1(26), 901.

Kelly, L. (1981). *Dimensions of professional nursing* (4th ed.). New York: Macmillan.

Little, M. (1992). Sprout growers unite! *Tennessee Nursing Matters*, 1(3), 7.

Pillitteri, A. (1991). Documenting Lystra Gretter's student experiences in nursing. *Nursing Outlook*, 39(6), 273–279.

Webster's new collegiate dictionary. (1989). 9th edition. Springfield, MA: Merriam-Webster.

SUGGESTED READINGS

Diers, D. (1986). To profess—to be a professional. *Journal of Nursing Administration*, 16(3), 25–30.

Hegyvary, S. T. (1991). Freedom and responsibility. *Journal of Professional Nursing*, 7(1), 8.

Kluge, E. H. (1982). Nursing: Vocation or profession? *Canadian Nurse*, 78(2), 34–36.

Larson, M. S. (1977). *The rise of professionalism*. Los Angeles: California Press.

Sarafian, L. B. (1990). Limited view of the profession of nursing. *Clinical Nurse Specialist*, 4(4), 171.

Schutzenhofer, K. K. (1991). Scholarly pursuit in the clinical setting: An obligation of professional nursing. *Journal of Professional Nursing*, 7(1), 10–15.

Segal, E. T. (1985). Is nursing a profession? Yes/no. *Nursing '85*, 15, 40–43.

Stuart, G. W. (1981). How professionalized is nursing? *Image: The Journal of Nursing Scholarship*, 13, 18–23.

Styles, M. M. (1983). The anatomy of a profession. *Heart and Lung*, 12, 570–575.

Chapter

Defining Nursing

Kay K. Chitty

CHAPTER OBJECTIVES

What students should be able to do after studying this chapter:

1. Recognize the evolutionary nature of definitions.
2. Compare early definitions of nursing with contemporary ones.
3. Identify themes in existing definitions of nursing.
4. Develop personal definitions of nursing.

VOCABULARY BUILDING

Terms to know:

active collaborator	high-tech nursing	maximum health
caring	high-touch nursing	potential
educative instrument	holism	milieu
health maintenance	humanistic nursing	nursing practice act
health promotion	care	scientific discipline

*I*t may be surprising to learn that finding a universally acceptable definition of nursing has been an elusive goal. It seems that even nurses themselves have been unable to agree on one definition. Individuals, including the venerable

Nightingale, and organizations, such as the International Council of Nurses (ICN) and the American Nurses Association (ANA), have made attempts to achieve consensus, some more successful than others. In spite of the inability of those in the profession to agree on one definition, most of the definitions reviewed in this chapter have similar themes. Considering the variations in knowledge and technology during the different points in history when these definitions were written, the similarities are remarkable. All the definitions were impacted by significant political and social events of the day that shaped the form of nursing as it is now known.

Why Define Nursing?

Why is it important for people to spend time trying to define nursing? Having an accepted definition of nursing is helpful in a variety of ways and provides a framework for nursing practice. It establishes the parameters, or boundaries, of the profession; identifies the purposes and functions of the work; and guides the educational preparation of aspiring practitioners.

To illustrate the importance of defining human activity, suppose a person was told that he had been selected to play on a major league baseball team, but he didn't know how to play. So he asked the team owner, "What is important for me to know about baseball?" And she said, "Just win games!" Then he went to a pitcher, who showed him a fast ball, a curve ball, and a slider. From there he went to a batting coach, who showed him how to hit fast balls, slow balls, and sliders. When he went to a fielding coach, he was told how to cover the bases and catch balls. Next, he consulted a trainer who showed him how to condition his body to avoid injuries. He has spent a great deal of time and still does not have an overall picture of baseball. Now, suppose he had been told initially, "Baseball is a game played with a ball and a bat on a large field on which there are three bases and a home plate. There are two nine-member teams, one at bat and one in the field. The object of the game is for a member of the batting team to hit a pitched ball and to run around the bases to home plate without being called out. The team with the most runs at the end of nine turns at bat wins." Although this description leaves out a lot of detail, it succinctly states the boundaries of the game, the purpose of the game, and gives guidance on how to play the game. Therefore, it would be more useful as a first step in an attempt to master baseball than the unorganized approach of talking to owners, players, and coaches.

So it is with definitions. They are a good place to begin in attempting to understand any complex entity.

Nightingale Defines Nursing

Considering how relatively undeveloped nursing was during her time, Florence Nightingale's definitions contain very contemporary concepts. Remember that during Nightingale's day, formal schooling in nursing was just beginning. In writing *Notes on Nursing: What It Is and What It Is Not* in 1859, she became the first person to attempt a definition of nursing. She wrote, "And what nursing has to do . . . is put the patient in the best condition for nature to act upon him" (Nightingale 1946, p. 75). She also wrote:

> I use the word nursing for want of a better. It has been limited to signify little more than the administration of medicines and the application of poultices. It ought to signify the proper use of fresh air, light, warmth, cleanliness, quiet, and the proper selection and administration of diet—all at the least expense of vital power to the patient. (p. 6)

Although Nightingale lived in a time when little was known about disease processes and available treatments were extremely limited, these definitions foreshadowed contemporary nursing's focus on the therapeutic **milieu** (environment) as well as the modern emphasis on **health promotion** and **health maintenance**. Nightingale was also the first person to differentiate between nursing provided by a professional nurse using a unique body of knowledge and nursing care such as a mother would perform for an ill child.

The Evolution of Definitions of Nursing

In the decades since Nightingale thought about, practiced, wrote about, and transformed nursing, many others have attempted to distill into one definition the essence of nursing. This section will review a number of definitions that evolved over the years.

Early Twentieth-Century Definitions

Fifty years after Nightingale, the search for a definition began in earnest. Following the English model, many schools of nursing had been established in the United States, and numbers of "trained nurses" were in practice. They sought to develop a professional identity for their rapidly expanding discipline. Shaw's *Textbook of Nursing* (1907, pp. 1–2) defined nursing as an art: "It properly includes as well as the execution of specific orders, the administration of food and medicine, the personal care of the patient." Harmer's *Textbook of the Principles and Practice of Nursing*, published in 1922, elaborated on Shaw's bare-bones definition: "The object of nursing is not only to cure the sick . . . but to bring health and ease, rest and comfort to mind and body. Its object is to prevent disease and to preserve health" (p. 3). The fourth edition of the Harmer text, which showed the influence of coauthor and nursing notable Virginia Henderson, redefined nursing: "Nursing may be defined as that service to an individual that helps him to attain or maintain a healthy state of mind or body" (Harmer and Henderson 1939, p. 2).

Post–World War II Definitions

World War II, like all wars, helped advance the technologies available to treat people, which in turn influenced nursing. The war also made nurses aware of the influential role emotions play in health, illness, and nursing care. Hildegard Peplau (1952), widely regarded as a pioneer among contemporary nursing theorists and herself a psychiatric nurse, defined nursing in interpersonal terms: "Nursing is a significant, therapeutic, interpersonal process. . . . Nursing is an **educative instrument** . . . that aims to promote forward movement of personality in the direction of creative, constructive, productive, personal and community living" (p. 16). She reinforced the idea of the patient as an **active collaborator** in his own care.

During the late 1950s and early 1960s the number of master's programs in nursing increased. As more nurses were educated at the graduate level and learned about the research process, they were anxious to test new ideas about nursing. Nursing theory was born. (See Chapter 11 for a fuller discussion of nursing theory.)

One of the theorists who began work during this period was Dorothea Orem. Her 1959 definition of nursing captures the flavor of her later, more completely elaborated self-care theory of nursing: "Nursing is perhaps best described as the giving of direct assistance to a person, as required, because of the person's specific inabilities in self-care resulting from a situation of personal health" (Orem 1959, p. 5). Orem's belief, that nurses should do for a person only those things the person cannot do without assistance, also emphasized the patient's active role.

By 1960, Henderson's earlier definition had evolved into a statement that had such universal appeal that it was adopted by the ICN:

> The unique function of the nurse is to assist the individual, sick or well, in the performance of those activities contributing to health or its recovery (or to a peaceful death) that he would perform unaided if he had the necessary strength, will or knowledge. And to do this in such a way as to help him gain independence as rapidly as possible. (Henderson 1960, p. 3)

Never before or since has one definition of nursing been so widely accepted both in this country and worldwide. Many feel it is still the most comprehensive and appropriate definition of nursing in existence.

Another pioneer nursing theorist, Martha Rogers, included the concept of the nursing process in her definition: "Nursing aims to assist people in achieving their **maximum health potential**. Maintenance and promotion of health, prevention of disease, nursing diagnosis, intervention, and rehabilitation encompass the scope of nursing's goals" (Rogers 1961, p. 86).

A Controversial Definition Emerges

Definitions are not usually considered controversial, but in 1980 the ANA issued a statement of beliefs called *Nursing: A Social Policy Statement* that contained perhaps the most controversial definition of nursing to date. It states: "Nursing is the diagnosis and treatment of human responses to actual and potential health problems" (p. 9). This definition has been criticized for a number of reasons, a chief one being that it fails to identify health as a goal of nursing. The emphasis on diagnosis and treatment ignores the health promotion and maintenance

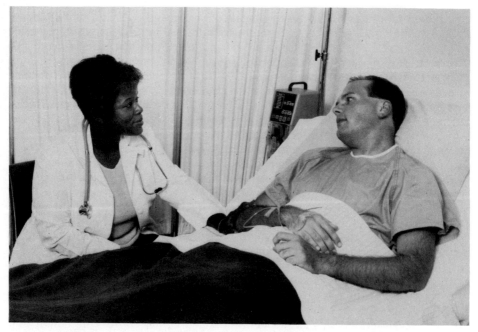

Holistic nursing practice takes the whole person into consideration.

aspects that others define as the essence of nursing. Terming the ANA definition "incomplete and in part illogical," prominent nurse educator Rozella Schlotfeldt (1987) went so far as to assert that the definition, by its incompleteness, "may delay or deter progress in theory development" (p. 6). She suggested that a more accurate and appropriate definition, and one that can inform and guide current and future practitioners would be: "Nursing is the appraisal and the enhancement of the health status, health assets, and health potentials of human beings" (p. 67).

A Focus on Caring, Humanism, and Holism

After a period of intense interest in "**high-tech**" **nursing** during the late 1960s and 1970s, modern nursing returned to its "**high-touch**" roots, so to speak, in the late 1970s with a renewed interest and public recognition as the health discipline that "cares." That trend has continued to the present.

A **caring** professional is one who watches over, attends to, and provides for the needs of others. Contemporary nursing stresses **humanistic nursing care**, that is, viewing professional relationships as human to human rather than nurse to patient. The meaning of the patient's experience is a very important aspect of humanistic nursing. Holism is also receiving emphasis in modern definitions of nursing. **Holism** is a system of comprehensive care that takes the physical, emotional, social, economic, and spiritual needs of the person into consideration.

Jean Watson, a nursing theorist, illustrated the return to caring and humanism in 1979 when she wrote, "Nursing is both scientific and artistic. I seek to combine science with humanism. . . . Nursing is a therapeutic interpersonal process. . . . Nursing is a **scientific discipline** that derives . . . its practice base from scientific research" (p. pxvii). Nurses can expect to hear more about the caring aspects of nursing as a counterbalance to the dizzying array of technologies anticipated in the future.

This brief review of selected definitions of nursing in vogue during the past 150 years is summarized in Table 7–1.

Developing Personal Definitions of Nursing

Students may not realize that faculties of accredited schools of nursing are encouraged to develop definitions of nursing as part of the school's statement of philosophy. Some of the most spirited discussions during faculty meetings center around what one or another faculty member believes nursing really is. A description of nursing that combines humanistic and holistic values can be found in the University of Rochester School of Nursing's thoughtful and comprehensive philosophy statement:

> We believe that the profession of nursing has as its essence, assisting people to attain and maintain optimal health and to cope with illness and disability. Nursing derives its rights and responsibilities from society and is, therefore, accountable to society as well as to the individuals who comprise it. The nurse functions as a caring professional in both autonomous and collaborative professional roles, using critical thinking, ethical principles, effective communication, and deliberative action to render holistic care, facilitate access to health care, and aid consumers in making decisions about their health. (Radke et al. 1991, p. 12)

All nursing students and practicing nurses, whether or not they realize it, are in the process of developing and refining their own definitions of nursing. From time to time it is helpful to write down just what your personal definition is and compare it with those developed by nursing scholars over the years.

On a practical note, it is important to keep in mind that the most significant definition of nursing for every nurse is contained in the **nursing practice act** of the state in which that nurse practices. Regardless of how restrictive or permissive it may be, this definition constitutes the legal definition of nursing in that state, and the wise nurse maintains familiarity with the latest version of the act. The current nurse practice act in each state can be obtained by calling or writing the state board of nursing. The addresses of the boards of nursing are found in Table 7–2.

Table 7–1 Themes in the Evolution of Definitions of Nursing, 1859–1987

	Definition	Theme
Nightingale 1859 (1946)	". . . nursing. . . . ought to signify the proper use of fresh air, light, warmth, cleanliness, quiet, and the proper selection and administration of diet—all at the least expense of vital power to the patient" (p. 6).	The nurse's center of concern is the patient. Nature and a healthful, restful environment are the nurse's allies.
	"And what nursing has to do . . . is put the patient in the best condition for nature to act upon him" (p. 75).	Health maintenance and restoration are the nurse's goals.
Shaw 1907	"Nursing is an art. . . . It properly includes as well as the execution of specific orders, the administration of food and medicine, the personal care of the patient. . . . To fill such a position requires certain physical and mental attributes as well as special training" (pp. 1–2).	More than knowledge and skills are needed by nurses. The attribute of personal caring is also required.
Harmer 1922	"Nursing is rooted in the needs of humanity. . . . Its object is not only to cure the sick . . . but to bring health and ease, rest and comfort to mind and body. Its object is to prevent disease and to preserve health" (p. 3).	Disease prevention and health promotion are the focus. Nursing is based on human needs.
Harmer and Henderson 1939	"Nursing may be defined as that service to an individual that helps him to attain or maintain a healthy state of mind or body" (p. 2).	Nursing deals with the health of both psyche (mind) and soma (body).
Peplau 1952	"Nursing is a significant, therapeutic, interpersonal process. . . . Nursing is an educative instrument . . . that aims to promote forward movement of personality in the direction of creative, constructive, productive, personal and community living" (p. 16).	Effective nursing results from a therapeutic relationship between nurse and patient.

Source	Definition	Focus/Goal
Orem 1959	"Nursing is . . . described as the giving of direct assistance to a person, as required, because of the person's specific inabilities in self-care resulting from a situation of personal health" (p. 5).	Nursing is doing for a person what he cannot do at this time due to health-related limitations. Return to self-care is the goal.
Henderson 1960	"The unique function of the nurse is to assist the individual, sick or well, in the performance of those activities contributing to health or its recovery (or to a peaceful death) that he would perform unaided if he had the necessary strength, will or knowledge. And to do this in such a way as to help him gain independence as rapidly as possible" (p. 3).	Both well and ill people are the focus of nursing. Responsibility for care is shared by nurse and patient. The goal is independence of the patient.
Rogers 1961	"Nursing aims to assist people in achieving their maximum health potential. Maintenance and promotion of health, prevention of disease, nursing diagnosis, intervention, and rehabilitation encompass the scope of nursing's goals" (p. 86).	Each person has a personal maximum health potential. Nursing seeks to strengthen each human being's capacity to achieve that potential.
American Nurses Association 1980	"Nursing is the diagnosis and treatment of human responses to actual and potential health problems" (p. 9).	Nursing focuses on human responses to illness or the threat of illness.
Watson 1979	"Nursing is both scientific and artistic. I seek to combine science with humanism. . . . Nursing is a therapeutic interpersonal process. . . . Nursing is a scientific discipline that derives . . . its practice base from scientific research" (p. pxvii).	Nursing represents a balance between science and humanism. The interpersonal features of nursing are paramount. Nurses care for people with a holistic approach even while using the scientific approach.
Schlotfeldt 1987	"Nursing is the appraisal and the enhancement of the health status, health assets, and health potentials of human beings" (p. 67).	Regardless of where a person is on the continuum of wellness to illness, nursing focuses on enhancing that person's health care status.

Table 7–2   State Boards of Nursing

Board of Nursing
One/East Building
Suite 203
500 East Blvd.
Montgomery, AL 36117

Board of Nursing
Dept. of Commerce and Economic
   Development
Division of Occupational Licensing
PO Box D-LIC
Juneau, AK 99811–0800

Board of Nursing
1123 S. University Avenue
Suite 800
Little Rock, AR 72204

State Board of Nursing
2001 W. Camelback Rd.
Suite 350
Phoenix, AZ 85015

Board of Registered Nursing
1030 13th St.
Suite 200
Sacramento, CA 94244–2100

Board of Nursing
1560 Broadway
Suite 670
Denver, CO 80202

Department of Health Services, Nurse
   Licensure
150 Washington St.
Hartford, CT 06106

Board of Nursing
PO Box 1401
Dover, DE 19901

Nurses' Examining Board
614 H St. NW
Room 904
Washington, D.C. 20001

Board of Nursing
111 E. Coastline Drive
Suite 504
Jacksonville, FL 32202

Board of Nursing
166 Pryor St. SW
Suite 400
Atlanta, GA 30303

Board of Nursing
PO Box 3469
Honolulu, HI 96801

Board of Nursing
500 S. 10th St.
Suite 102
Boise, ID 83720

Nursing Committee
Dept. of Registration and Education
320 W. Washington St.
Springfield, IL 62786

State Board of Nursing
One American Square
Suite 1020
Indianapolis, IN 46282-0001

Board of Nursing
State Office Bldg.
1223 E. Court
Des Moines, IA 50319

Board of Nursing
900 S.W. Jackson
Suite 551-S
Topeka, KS 66612–1256

Board of Nursing
4010 Dupont Circle
Suite 430
Louisville, KY 40207

State Board of Nursing
150 Baronne St.
Room 907
New Orleans, LA 70112

Board of Nursing
295 Water St.
Augusta, ME 04330–2240

Board of Examiners of Nurses
4201 Patterson Ave.
Baltimore, MD 21215–2299

Board of Registration in Nursing
100 Cambridge St.
Room 1519
Boston, MA 02202

Board of Nursing
611 N. Otiana
Lansing, MI 48909

Table 7–2 (Continued)

Board of Nursing
2700 University Ave. W
Suite 108
St. Paul, MN 55114

Board of Nursing
239 N. Lamar St.
Suite 401
Jackson, MS 39201

Board of Nursing
3524 N. Ten Mile Dr.
Jefferson City, MO 65102

Board of Nurses
Dept. of Commerce
1424 Ninth Ave.
Helena, MT 59620–0407

Board of Nursing
Dept. of Health, Bureau of Examining Boards
PO Box 95007
Lincoln, NE 68509

Board of Nursing
1281 Terminal Way
Suite 116
Reno, NV 89502

Board of Nursing
Education and Registration
6 Hazen Dr.
Concord, NH 03301

New Jersey Board of Nursing
1101 Raymond Blvd.
Room 508
Newark, NJ 07102

Board of Nursing
4253 Montgomery NE
Suite 130
Albuquerque, NM 87109

Board of Nursing
State Education Department
Cultural Education Center
Albany, NY 12230

Board of Nursing
PO Box 2129
Raleigh, NC 27602

Board of Nursing
Kirkwood Office Tower
7th and Arbor Ave.
Suite 504
Bismarck, ND 58504

Board of Nursing
Education and Registration
77 S. High St.
Columbus, OH 43266-0316

Board of Nurse Registration and Nursing
  Education
2915 N. Classen Blvd.
Suite 524
Oklahoma City, OK 73106

Board of Nursing
1400 S.W. 5th Ave.
Suite 904
Portland, OR 97201

Board of Nurse Examiners
PO Box 2649
Harrisburg, PA 17105–2649

Board of Nurse Education and Registration
Cannon Health Bldg.
75 Davis St.
Suite 104
Providence, RI 02908

Board of Nursing
1777 St. Julian Pl.
Suite 102
Columbia, SC 29204

Board of Nursing
304 S. Phillips Ave.
Suite 205
Sioux Falls, SD 57102

Board of Nursing
283 Plus Park Blvd.
Nashville, TN 37219–5407

Board of Nurse Examiners
9101 Burnet Rd.
Suite 104
Austin, TX 78758

Board of Nursing
160 E. 300 South
Salt Lake City, UT 84145

Board of Nursing
26 Terrace St.
Montpelier, VT 05602

Board of Nursing
1601 Rolling Hills Drive
Richmond, VA 23229

(continued)

Table 7–2 (Continued)

Board of Nursing	Board of Nursing
Division of Professional Licensing	PO Box 8935
PO Box 9649	Room 174
Olympia, WA 98504	Madison, WI 53708
Board of Examiners	Board of Nursing
922 Quarrier St.	Barrett Bldg., 3rd Floor
Suite 309	2301 Central Ave.
Charleston, WV 25301	Cheyenne, WY 82002

(From Mattera, M. D. (Ed.). (1992). *RN presents: Nursing opportunities for 1992* (23rd ed.). Montvale, NJ: Medical Economics. Used by permission.).

CHAPTER SUMMARY

Although attempting to define nursing has been an interesting activity since the days of Nightingale, all attempts have fallen short of capturing the scope, diversity, and richness that is nursing. Storlie struck a chord of truth when she wrote, "The glorious thing about nursing is that it cannot be defined. The irony is that we never give up trying. . . . Nursing will resist being reduced to so-called facts no matter how precise the researcher" (Storlie 1970, pp. 254–255).

Note that the definitions reviewed in this chapter have more similarities than differences. Review some of their major themes highlighted in Table 7–1. Notice how the definitions have evolved over time even though many themes are constant. It is possible to find definitions by some of the same authors that are different from the ones given in this chapter. This is because definitions evolve over time as nursing changes and each individual's perceptions about, and experiences in, nursing change. Although nursing may wish for one, succinct definition, the dynamic nature of the nursing profession, society, and health care will likely prevent us from ever developing one eternal, universally accepted definition of nursing.

REVIEW/DISCUSSION QUESTIONS

1. From the definitions of nursing presented in this chapter, select the one you most prefer and explain your choice.
2. Using your thoughts as well as elements of others' definitions, write your own definition of nursing. Explain it to a classmate, giving your rationale for what you included and excluded.
3. How might new developments and practice options for nurses affect future definitions of nursing?
4. How has your personal definition of nursing changed over time?
5. Using the appropriate address from Table 7–2, obtain a copy of the nurse practice act for your state. Find the legal definition of nursing and compare it with other definitions found in this chapter. How are they alike, and how are they different?

REFERENCES

American Nurses Association. (1980). *Nursing: A social policy statement*. Kansas City, MO: Author.

Harmer, B. (1922). *Textbook of the principles and practice of nursing*. New York: Macmillan.

Harmer, B., and Henderson, V. (1939). *Textbook of the principles and practice of nursing* (4th ed.). New York: Macmillan.

Henderson, V. (1960). *Basic principles of nursing care*. London: International Council of Nurses.

Mattera, M. D. (1992). *RN presents: Nursing opportunities for 1992* (23rd ed.). Montvale, NJ: Medical Economics.

Nightingale, F. (1946 facsimile of 1859 edition). *Notes on nursing: What it is and what it is not*. Philadelphia: J.B. Lippincott.

Orem, D. (1959). *Guidelines for developing curricula for the education of practical nurses*. Washington, D.C.: Government Printing Office.

Peplau, H. (1952). *Interpersonal relations in nursing: A conceptual frame of reference for psychodynamic nursing*. New York: G.P. Putnam's Sons.

Radke, K. J., et al. (1991). Curriculum blueprints for the future: The process of blending beliefs. *Nurse Educator* 16(2), 9–13.

Rogers, M. (1961). *Educational revolution in nursing*. New York: Macmillan.

Schlotfeldt, R. M. (1987). Defining nursing: A historic controversy. *Nursing Research*, 36(1), 64–67.

Shaw, C. W. (1907). *Textbook of nursing* (3rd ed.). New York: Appleton.

Storlie, F. (1970). Nursing need never be defined. *International Nursing Review*, 70(17), 255–258.

Watson, J. (1979). *The philosophy and science of caring*. Boston: Little, Brown.

SUGGESTED READING

Brooks, J. A., and Kleine-Kracht, A. E. (1983). Evolution of a definition of nursing. *Advances in Nursing Science*, 5(4), 51–85.

Chapter

8

Professional Socialization

Kay K. Chitty

CHAPTER OBJECTIVES

What students should be able to do after studying this chapter:

1. Discuss how students' initial images of nursing are modified by professional education.

2. Differentiate between formal and informal socialization.

3. Identify internal and external factors that influence an individual's professional socialization.

4. Describe developmental models of professional socialization and how they can be used.

5. Differentiate between the elements of professional socialization that are the responsibility of nursing programs and those that are the individual's responsibility.

6. Discuss Kramer's model for minimizing reality shock.

7. Describe practical steps to ease the transition from student to professional nurse.

8. Discuss employer expectations.

VOCABULARY BUILDING

Words to know:

biculturalism
cognitive rebellion
culture of nursing
dissonance
external factors
formal socialization
inertia

informal socialization
internal factors
internalize
internship
job hopping
mentor
modeling

mutuality
preceptor
professional
  socialization
reality shock
resocialization
work ethic

*I*n Chapter 3, societal influences that have affected the development of nursing were discussed, and the media's impact on nursing's image was explored. It is clear that the image of nursing held by the public over the years has been influenced in large measure by books, television, and motion pictures. Nursing students, too, are affected by the images portrayed by these media as well as by contact with nurses they know. They bring an outsider's view of the nursing profession to school with them.

During formal schooling, the complex process of exchanging an outsider's perception for an insider's understanding of what nursing really is begins. This process requires that students **internalize**, or take in, the knowledge, skills, attitudes, beliefs, norms, values, and ethical standards of nursing and make them a part of their own self-image and behavior (Jacox 1973).

The process of internalization and development of an occupational identity is known as **professional socialization**. Professional socialization in nursing is believed to occur largely, but not entirely, during the period students are in basic nursing programs. It continues after graduation when they enter nursing practice. In this chapter the effects of both school and work settings on nurses' professional socialization will be examined.

Education's Effect on Professional Socialization

What kinds of educational experiences are needed to make the transition from student to professional nurse? Learning any new role is derived from a mixture of formal and informal socialization. Little boys, for example, learn how to assume the father role by what their own fathers purposely teach them (formal socialization) and by how they observe their own and other fathers behaving (informal socialization). In nursing, **formal socialization** includes lessons the faculty intend to teach—such as how to plan nursing care, how to perform a physical examination on a healthy child, or how to communicate with a psychiatric patient. **Informal socialization** includes lessons that occur incidentally, such as overhearing a nurse teach a young mother how to care for her premature infant, participating in the student nurse association, or sitting in on a nursing ethics committee meeting. Part of professional socialization is simply absorbing the **culture of nursing**, that is, the rites, rituals, and valued behaviors of the profession. This requires that students spend enough time with nurses in work settings for adequate exposure to the nursing culture to occur. Most nurses agree that informal socialization is more powerful and memorable than formal socialization.

Learning a new vocabulary is also part of professional socialization. Each profession has its own "jargon," which is not generally understood by outsiders. Professional students usually enjoy acquiring the new vocabulary and practicing it among themselves.

Learning any new role creates some degree of anxiety (Wooley 1978). Disappointment and frustration sometimes occur when students' learning expectations come into conflict with educational realities. Students' ideas of what they need to learn, when they need to learn it, and what might be the best way to learn it may differ from what actually occurs. They sometimes become disillusioned when they observe nurses behaving in ways that differ from their ideas about how nurses *should* behave. Knowing in advance that these things may happen can help students accurately assess the sources of their anxiety and manage it more effectively.

Internal Influencing Factors

As students progress through nursing programs, a variety of internal and external factors challenge their customary ways of thinking. **Internal factors** include personal feelings and beliefs they bring with them. Some of these may conflict with professional values. For example, if they believe in a higher power (God), they may be uncomfortable working with patients who have no such belief. Yet nursing's code of ethics requires that nurses work with all patients regardless of their beliefs (American Nurses Association 1976). Other areas that sometimes challenge students' thinking are substance abuse, self-destructive behaviors, abortion, and issues related to sexuality, such as sexual preference.

External Influencing Factors

External factors also influence professional development. Growing children are first influenced by the values, beliefs, and behaviors of the significant adults around them and later by peers. Ideas about health, health care, and nursing are also shaped through this process. If a nurse's family valued fitness, for example, it may be difficult for that nurse to empathize with an overweight patient who refuses to exercise. In this example, a family value (fitness) comes into conflict with a professional value (empathy toward all patients without judging them).

Nurses need to be aware of their biases and discuss them with peers, instructors, and professional role models. Failure to do so may adversely affect the nursing care provided to certain patients. Professional nurses make every effort to avoid imposing their beliefs on others. See Chapter 18 for further discussion of self-awareness and nonjudgmentalism as necessary attributes of professional nurses.

As seen from this brief discussion, socialization is the key to keeping a profession vital and dynamic. It is not surprising, therefore, that a good deal of attention has been paid to this important process.

Models of Professional Socialization

In thinking about professional socialization, it is helpful to have theoretical models to consider. Cohen (1981) and Hinshaw (1976) described developmental models appropriate for beginning nursing students. Bandura (1977) described an informal type of socialization he called "modeling," which is useful when learning any new behavior. Throwe and Fought (1987) described a developmental model of professional socialization specifically designed to meet the needs of registered nurse students. Let us consider each of these models briefly.

Cohen's Model

Cohen (1981) proposed a model of professional socialization consisting of four stages. Basing her work on developmental theories and studies of students' attitudes toward nursing, she asserted, "Students must experience each stage in sequence to feel comfortable in the professional role" (p. 16). She believed that a positive outcome in all of the four stages is necessary for satisfactory socialization to occur.

Cohen called the first stage in her model "stage I, unilateral dependence." Owing to inexperience and lack of knowledge, students at this stage rely on external limits and controls established by authority figures such as teachers. During stage I, students are unlikely to question or critically analyze the concepts teachers present because they lack the necessary background to do so.

In "stage II, negativity/independence," students' critical thinking abilities and knowledge bases expand. They begin to question authority figures. Cohen called this "**cognitive rebellion.**" Much as a young child learns that he can say "No!", students at this level begin to free themselves from external controls and to rely more on their own judgment.

In "stage III, dependence/mutuality," Cohen described students' more reasoned evaluation of other's ideas. They develop an increasingly realistic appraisal process and learn to test concepts, facts, ideas, and models objectively. Students at this stage are more impartial; they accept some ideas and reject others.

In "stage IV, interdependence," students' needs for both independence and **mutuality** (sharing jointly with others) come together. They develop the capacity to make decisions in collaboration with others. The successfully socialized student completes stage IV with a self-concept that includes a professional role identity that is personally and professionally acceptable and compatible with other life roles (Cohen 1981). Table 8–1 summarizes the key behaviors associated with each stage.

Research Note

Does knowledge have the ability to change people's attitudes? This was the question three Canadian nurse researchers wanted to answer. They were specifically interested in knowing whether having more knowledge about AIDS would change nursing students' attitudes toward people with AIDS. They designed a study that involved 319 undergraduate students in a baccalaureate nursing program in western Canada. The research subjects were given a pre-test to determine their knowledge about the attitudes toward caring for patients with AIDS. They then attended a day-long workshop consisting of presentations by speakers experienced in the care of people with AIDS. These experts included a physician who was involved in infection control at a large hospital, a faculty member in a college of nursing who also practiced in an intensive care unit, an infection control nurse, an epidemiologist, and a social worker. They presented both physiological and psychosocial apects of care. A post-test was given two and one-half weeks later. The researchers found that there were significant changes in both knowledge and attitudes following the workshop, but cautioned that paper and pencil tests are not always true indicators of what people believe. They suggested adding more AIDS content in nursing curricula and recommended that influential people lead the way in changing attitudes toward people with AIDS.

From Brown, Y., Calder, B., and Rae, D. (1990). The effect of knowledge on nursing students' attitudes toward individuals with AIDS. *Journal of Nursing Education,* 29(8), 367–372.

Table 8–1   Cohen's Stages of Professional Socialization

Stage	Key Behaviors
Stage I, unilateral dependence	Reliant on external authority; limited questioning or critical analysis
Stage II, negativity/independence	Cognitive rebellion; diminished reliance on external authority
Stage III, dependence/mutuality	Reasoned appraisal; begins integration of facts and opinions following objective testing
Stage IV, interdependence	Collaborative decision making; commitment to professional role; self-concept now includes professional role identity

(From Cohen, H. A. (1981). *The nurse's quest for professional identity.* Menlo Park, CA: Addison-Wesley. Used by permission.)

Readers may wish to compare themselves and nursing classmates to these four stages. A word of caution, however: Although it is interesting and useful, this is a model that has not been scientifically tested and validated (confirmed). At least one researcher, McCain (1985), concluded that her study "did not support the Cohen (1981) model . . . " because students in McCain's sample of 422 B.S.N. (bachelor of science in nursing) student volunteers in a large southern state university did not show evidence of progression through Cohen's developmental stages (p. 185). McCain recommended further testing of Cohen's model.

Hinshaw's Model

Another potentially useful model describing the educational aspect of professional socialization was proposed by Hinshaw in a 1976 publication for the National League for Nursing (NLN).

In this model, stage I, "initial innocence," is characterized by idealized images and expectations of nursing. Students have gained these images from the media and from their own experiences with nurses. For example, they may expect that as nursing students they will immediately begin to work with sick patients, or that nurses are always treated with the utmost respect by other health care workers, or that they will always be able to make things better for their patients.

In stage II, "incongruities," students realize that their innocent images of nursing differ from reality. For example, they discover that they must complete anatomy, physiology, nutrition, and a host of other courses before working with patients, or they discover that students are expected to defer to more experienced nurses and physicians, or they encounter patients with chronic, intractable pain. This **dissonance** (lack of harmony) between their expectations and reality produces tension and frustration. During the dissonant stage, differences are sufficiently well formulated to discuss with others. Students at this stage may overtly question whether or not they should continue in the program and may choose not to do so (Hinshaw 1976).

In stage III, "identification," students select and carefully observe role models. Role models may be particularly admired instructors or nurses seen in clinical settings. This stage is closely followed by stage IV, "role simulation," in which they practice the role behaviors they observed. At first the new behaviors may feel strange or "phony," which sometimes causes confusion and self-doubt (Hinshaw 1976). Students learning therapeutic communication techniques, for example, often feel awkward and obvious when they first try out these techniques in conversation.

In stage V, "vacillation," there is a desire to cling to the old ideas and images about nursing while recognizing that new ideas and images are based on reality (Hinshaw 1976). Evidence of this stage can be seen in new graduates who feel guilty when they are unable to provide intense, individualized care for every patient in spite of patient load and time constraints.

The last stage, "internalization," occurs when there is stable and reliable use of the internalized professional model (Hinshaw 1976). This can be seen in

Table 8–2   Hinshaw's Stages of Professional Socialization

Stage	Key Behaviors
Stage I. Initial innocence	Initial image of nursing unaffected by reality
Stage II. Incongruities	Initial expectations and reality collide; questions career choice; may drop out
Stage III. Identification	Observes behaviors of experienced nurses
Stage IV. Role simulation	Practices observed behaviors; may feel unnatural in role
Stage V. Vacillation	Old images emerge and conflict with new professional image
Stage VI. Internalization	Acceptance and comfort with new role

(Adapted from Hinshaw, A. S. (1976). *Socialization and resocialization of nurses for professional nursing practice*. New York: National League for Nursing. Used by permission.)

nurses who, after practicing for some time, have developed a balance between their expectations of themselves as professionals, employers' expectations, and their other life role expectations. Table 8–2 contains the stages of socialization described in the Hinshaw model.

Bandura's Concept of Modeling

Another method of professional socialization is **modeling**, discussed by Bandura (1977). In modeling, students learn by observing role models. Bandura believed that there are two requirements for successful modeling: Models must be seen as competent, and students must have an opportunity to practice the behaviors they see modeled. This is different from the informal socialization process described earlier because modeling involves a conscious decision on the part of the learner.

Students who wish to try modeling should identify nurses or instructors who share their values and attitudes and observe them closely. The next step is to "try out" the behaviors they most admire. Since people are not equally talented in all areas, students may choose to observe several models, each of whom excels in a different area. The basis of modeling as a method of professional socialization is careful observation and intentional simulation of the admired behaviors or characteristics. This is a legitimate method of acquiring desirable professional behaviors that can be useful to students interested in being more active in their own socialization.

Throwe and Fought's Model for Socialization of Registered Nurse Students

When registered nurses (R.N.s) return to school to work on their baccalaureate degrees, their needs are different from those of basic nursing students. They may experience feelings of frustration and anger caused by returning to the student role. Often, these nurses have practiced for years and wonder what anyone can

Table 8–3 Assessment Tool for Socialization to the Professional Nurse Role

Developmental Task	Role-Resisting Behaviors Observed	Role-Accepting Behaviors Observed
Trust/mistrust	Learns to trust the worlds of education and work through consistency and repetitive experiences	Physically isolated from peers both in class, clinical Does not initiate interactions with others Responds only if called upon	Involved with classmates Readily and quickly forms/joins groups when directed Initiates discussions with others Asks for clarification
Autonomy/doubt	Begins to develop independence while under supervision	Delays joining groups for unstructured activities Does not contribute equally Forgets or suppresses assignment dates Does not meet target dates Self-conscious about being evaluated by others	Joins groups for unstructured activities (study groups) Shares information with group; prepares for activities Meets target dates Able to interact in the teaching/learning environment Begins to develop independence with guidance
Initiative/guilt	Can independently identify, plan, and implement skills/assignments	Perceives objectives and assignments as not worthwhile Stress-related symptoms increase Has difficulty setting priorities Waits for instructor to initiate priority setting Lacks initiative to deal with conflicts Unaware of available resources	Objectives and assignments take on meaning Applies new skills, content to other work settings Effective in time management Renegotiates deadline extensions when appropriate Takes initiative in resolving conflict situations Aware of and uses available resources
Industry/inferiority	Behavior is dominated by performance of tasks and curiosity—individuals need encouragement to attempt and master skills	Elicits performance rewards and feedback from others Needs direct encouragement especially when performing affective and cognitive skills	Able to reward self Confidence thrives Eager to try out new skills; takes risks

(continued)

Table 8–3 (Continued)

Developmental Task	Role-Resisting Behaviors Observed	Role-Accepting Behaviors Observed
	Last to volunteer to demonstrate new behaviors	Volunteers to demonstrate new behaviors
	Seeks rewards by performing old familiar skills rather than those in new dimensions	Profits from guidance and direction of others
	Demonstrates disengaging behaviors (late, uninterested, resistive to learning opportunities)	Applies self beyond family/work settings
		Curiosity channeled through educational system
Identity/role confusion	The individual searches for continuity and structure, is concerned with how he/she is accepted by others; how he/she is accepted by self; each individual struggles to shape or formulate own identity	Needs a structured clinical setting to further develop ego identity	Searches for continuity and structure but can adapt to unstructured clinical settings
	Sees old job as ideal and denies need for change	Identifies role models in clinical setting
	Serious about learning (content and clinical practice)	Articulates need for change or for modification of job-related roles and procedures
	Frustrated with nursing as a career choice	Appears to enjoy learning and performing in clinical settings
	Too ideological or overly critical of others	Realistic about own achievements and progress in educational system
Intimacy/isolation	Seeks to combine his/her identity with other self-selected individuals	Participates as a member but resists group leader role	Volunteers to lead work/study groups
	Does not participate in professional meetings	Participates in professional organizations
	Unsupportive of others' educational advancement	Recruits others and represents school
	Feels no increased esteem in performing new role behaviors	Demonstrates pride in new role behaviors and shares with others in work settings
	Meets minimal requirements and sees instructor only in evaluative role	Seeks out instructor for additional learning, information, and professional growth opportunities
		Values symbols of profession (using assessment tools, R.N. name tags)

144

Stage	Description	Negative behaviors	Positive behaviors
		Resists using newly developed; Resists using newly developed skills; more comfortable with previous level of performance; Avoids giving feedback to agency personnel	Evaluates ability of clinical agencies to facilitate meeting learner objectives; Provides feedback to agency personnel
Generativity/stagnation	Efforts are made to guide and direct incoming students; assists others	Avoids social interaction and information sharing with incoming students; Provides minimal care; unconcerned about continuity of patient care; Selects patients with common, familiar clinical disorders; No increase ease of learning or improved test-taking abilities; Does not elect to test out of course requirements; Stagnates in same job setting	Guides and directs incoming students; Provides quality nursing care to patient, family, and community; Takes calculated risks (questions level of care, seeks multiple learning opportunities, shares level of expertise, elects to test out of required/elective courses); Demonstrates critical problem-solving skills; Attains mastery of test-taking skills; Self-directed learner; Demonstrates clinical problem solving in own work setting; Uses holistic approach to delivery of health care.
Ego integrity/despair	Acceptance of one's own progress, achievement, and goals through realistic self-appraisal	Frustrated with progress and achievement; stagnated in developing new goals; Crisis prone when changing roles; Self-appraisal unrealistic; Does not participate in structured educational opportunities; Returns to old job and does not modify role performance; See no reward in risk taking; High risk for dissatisfaction with profession	Accepts progress, achievement, and goal attainment; Realistic in self-appraisal; Resets professional goals (graduate school, participation in CE, certification); Joins new perspectives on old job by use of critical thinking; Takes risks (new jobs, different clinical setting, and leadership roles)

CE = Continuing education.

(From Throwe, A. N., and Fought, S. G. (1987). Landmarks in the Socialization Process from RN to BSN. *Nurse Educator*, 12(6), 15–18. Used by permission.)

teach them about nursing. It may seem almost insulting when they are placed in classes with students who are just beginning in nursing education. These registered nurses are not being socialized into nursing; if anything, they are in the process of **resocialization**, a process that often creates uncomfortable tension.

Throwe and Fought (1987) believed that the stages R.N.s must master during resocialization could be assessed using Erikson's theory. Erikson's (1950) theory described eight developmental stages individuals master as they progress from infancy to old age. Throwe and Fought designed a framework for R.N.s in B.S.N. programs to assess their own growth as they progress through school. The framework can also be used by faculty and non–R.N. students to help them appreciate R.N.s' experiences. Table 8–3 contains Throwe and Fought's assessment tool.

Actively Participating in One's Own Professional Socialization

So far in this discussion, professional socialization has sounded like something that happens *to* students. While much is out of their control, students don't have to be passive recipients of socialization. As active participants, they can influence the socialization process. For some ideas about how to become an active participant in the socialization process, use the checklist in Box 8–1.

As consumers of educational services, students need to know what to expect of their nursing programs in terms of professional socialization. Schools are responsible for some activities, whereas the individual is responsible for others. The checklist in Box 8–2 provides ideas about what takes place in nursing programs around the country to enhance students' professional socialization. Students can compare their experiences with those in this guide.

Socialization to the Work Setting

When nurses graduate, is their professional socialization over? Most authorities believe that socialization, like learning, is a lifelong activity. The transition from student to professional is just another of life's challenges and, like most transitions, is one that helps people grow. Most new nursing graduates feel somewhat unprepared and overwhelmed with the responsibilities of their first positions. Although agencies that employ new graduates realize that the orientation period will take time, graduates may have unrealistic expectations of themselves and others.

During the early days of practice, most graduate nurses quickly realize that the ideals taught in school are not always possible to achieve in everyday practice. This is largely due to time constraints and produces feelings of conflict and even guilt. In school, students are taught to spend time with patients and to consider their emotional as well as their physical needs. In practice, the emphasis seems to be on getting things done, and spending time talking with patients may be viewed as unproductive. Comprehensive, individualized nursing care planning, such a staple of life for nursing students, may become an unrealistic luxury. New nurses also must adapt to depending on other nursing care person-

Box 8–1   A Do-It-Yourself Guide to Professional Socialization

Listed below are 20 possible behaviors demonstrated by students who take responsibility for their own professional socialization. Place a check next to the behaviors you regularly exhibit. Be honest with yourself.

_____ 1.   I interact with other students in and out of class.

_____ 2.   I participate in class by asking intelligent questions and initiating discussion occasionally.

_____ 3.   I have formed or joined a study group.

_____ 4.   I use the library, labs, and teachers as resources.

_____ 5.   I organize my work so I can meet deadlines.

_____ 6.   If I have a conflict with another student or a teacher, I take the initiative to resolve it.

_____ 7.   I don't let minor personality problems distract me from my goals.

_____ 8.   I seek out new learning experiences and sometimes volunteer to demonstrate new skills to others.

_____ 9.   I have chosen professional role models.

_____ 10. I am realistic about my performance.

_____ 11. I try to accept constructive criticism undefensively.

_____ 12. I recognize that *trying* to do good work is not the same as *doing* good work.

_____ 13. I recognize that each teacher has different expectations, and it is my responsibility to learn what is expected by each.

_____ 14. I demonstrate respect for my teachers' time by making appointments whenever possible.

_____ 15. I demonstrate respect for my classmates and patients by never coming to class or clinical unprepared.

_____ 16. I recognize my responsibility to help create a dynamic learning environment and am not satisfied to be merely an academic spectator.

_____ 17. I participate in the student nurse association and encourage others to do the same.

_____ 18. I represent my school with pride.

_____ 19. I project a professional appearance.

_____ 20. One of my goals is to become a self-directed, lifelong learner.

Scoring: 1 to 10 checks: You need to examine your behavior and think about taking more responsibility for your own socialization.

11 to 15 checks: You are active in your own behalf. See if you can begin using some of the remaining behaviors on the list or come up with your own.

More than 15 checks: You are a role model of positive action in your own professional socialization process.

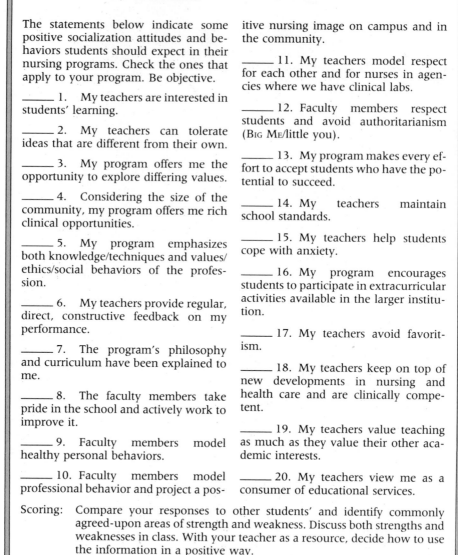

Box 8–2   A Consumer's Guide to Professional Socialization

The statements below indicate some positive socialization attitudes and behaviors students should expect in their nursing programs. Check the ones that apply to your program. Be objective.

_____ 1.   My teachers are interested in students' learning.

_____ 2.   My teachers can tolerate ideas that are different from their own.

_____ 3.   My program offers me the opportunity to explore differing values.

_____ 4.   Considering the size of the community, my program offers me rich clinical opportunities.

_____ 5.   My program emphasizes both knowledge/techniques and values/ethics/social behaviors of the profession.

_____ 6.   My teachers provide regular, direct, constructive feedback on my performance.

_____ 7.   The program's philosophy and curriculum have been explained to me.

_____ 8.   The faculty members take pride in the school and actively work to improve it.

_____ 9.   Faculty members model healthy personal behaviors.

_____ 10. Faculty members model professional behavior and project a positive nursing image on campus and in the community.

_____ 11. My teachers model respect for each other and for nurses in agencies where we have clinical labs.

_____ 12. Faculty members respect students and avoid authoritarianism (BIG ME/little you).

_____ 13. My program makes every effort to accept students who have the potential to succeed.

_____ 14. My teachers maintain school standards.

_____ 15. My teachers help students cope with anxiety.

_____ 16. My program encourages students to participate in extracurricular activities available in the larger institution.

_____ 17. My teachers avoid favoritism.

_____ 18. My teachers keep on top of new developments in nursing and health care and are clinically competent.

_____ 19. My teachers value teaching as much as they value their other academic interests.

_____ 20. My teachers view me as a consumer of educational services.

Scoring: Compare your responses to other students' and identify commonly agreed-upon areas of strength and weakness. Discuss both strengths and weaknesses in class. With your teacher as a resource, decide how to use the information in a positive way.

nel such as nursing assistants, patient technicians, and other unlicensed personnel to assist them in caring for patients. This is a difficult adjustment for some nurses who are unaccustomed to delegating or believe only they can provide quality care.

REALITY SHOCK

Kramer (1974) termed the feelings of powerlessness and ineffectiveness experienced by new graduates **reality shock**. Psychological stresses generated by reality shock decrease the ability of individuals to cope effectively with the demands of the new role. Unfortunately, some new nurses drop out at this point before they take steps to resolve reality shock.

Kramer identified several ways to drop out: dropping out mentally and becoming part of the problem; driving self and others to the breaking point trying to do it all; dropping out by **"job hopping"** (looking for the perfect, nonstressful job that is perfectly compatible with professional values); or dropping out by prematurely returning to school. Sadly, both for themselves and the nursing profession, some even sacrifice all the years of education they have invested in nursing and decide not to work in nursing at all. This is a loss neither nursing nor society can afford.

Being aware that there are stages most new graduates go through before settling comfortably into their professional roles can help reduce anxiety and increase coping. Kramer identified a model for resolving reality shock that consists of four stages.

1. *Mastery of skills and routines.* In busy acute care settings, which most new nurses choose for their first jobs, certain activities must be accomplished each day, and specific behaviors are required in order to accomplish them. During this stage, nurses focus on the mastery of essential skills and routines. They may temporarily lose sight of the bigger picture and may have to be reminded not to get so focused on the technical aspects of care that they fail to see patients' emotional needs.

2. *Social integration.* In this stage, which overlaps with stage 1, new nurses face the challenge of fitting into the work group. Issues of getting along and being accepted surface. Most people have a desire for peer recognition and approval. It is sometimes a challenge to retain the goodwill of coworkers while keeping high ideals and standards. Learning that they may have to sacrifice the esteem of some workers in order to maintain their professional values can be a painful, but necessary, lesson for nurses in this stage.

3. *Moral outrage.* Once they realize that they can't do it all because their commitments to the needs of the organization (hospital), to the profession, and to patients often conflict, frustration and anger result. Is it more important to attend a staff meeting or to talk to Mr. Jameson's daughter who needs to discuss home care versus nursing home placement for her father? Managing these sorts of priorities is a challenge even for experienced nurses.

4. *Conflict resolution.* Kramer identified several possible resolutions of these problems:
   a. Change behavior while retaining values. For example, find a new work setting that is more compatible with beliefs, or, if that is impossible, leave nursing altogether.
   b. Give up professional values (attending to patients' emotional needs) and accept bureaucracy's values (get work done quickly); just try to fit into the system.
   c. Give up both sets of values; for example, adopt a "go-with-the-flow" attitude; survival becomes the goal.
   d. Become a "bicultural nurse" (p. 162) who learns to use the values of both profession and bureaucracy to influence positive change in the system.

According to Kramer, adopting biculturalism is the most effective of these options.

BICULTURALISM

Biculturalism is a term Kramer used to describe nurses who learn to balance both cultures—the ideal nursing culture they learned about in school and the real one they experience in practice—and use the best of both. We can learn about bicultural nurses by examining their behaviors.

How do bicultural nurses behave? First, they are realists. They recognize that there is no perfect work situation. They also recognize that if they are able to establish credibility and gain respect, they can later be leaders in making improvements.

Next, they accept the fact that newcomers have to demonstrate competence before they can become leaders. They know that people will follow only those whom they respect. So they invest time in proving themselves before they start trying to make changes in the system. During that time, they demonstrate, through their own work, the approach to nursing care they value. They do this quietly and without fanfare, however, seeking support from like-minded peers.

Bicultural nurses observe the political system around them. Who are the real opinion makers? Who are the formal and informal leaders? Are they the same? When changes are made, who is involved and how is it done? Who can be counted on to react to new ideas positively, and who is always negative and complaining? Is there anything that "turns on" the complainers? Are there some people who are so chronically underfunctioning that they just can't or won't change? Answering these questions will provide an appraisal of some of the political realities in the system.

Bicultural nurses willingly serve on committees in order to demonstrate their ability to address institutionwide issues and to meet others within the system who may share their values. They limit their committee service, however, to those that they feel are useful and constructive.

Bicultural nurses work at having rewarding personal lives. They realize that when people get most of their emotional needs met at work, they are vulnerable.

They want to fit in so badly that they tend to sacrifice their professional values if they conflict with the system or the values of others.

Bicultural nurses take care of themselves. They negotiate for a position, not just accept what is offered. They expect reasonable compensation and also expect reasonable work hours most of the time, although they work their fair share of undesirable shifts. They do not routinely allow the system to take advantage of them and set them up for physical and emotional exhaustion, or burnout. On the other hand, they are cooperative. They demonstrate commitment and loyalty to the organization and show that nursing is more than just a job to them.

Bicultural nurses demonstrate many of the behaviors discussed in Chapter 6. In the final analysis, biculturalism and professionalism have many of the same attributes.

Minimizing Reality Shock

Much can be done to reduce reality shock in the transition from student to professional. Students must recognize that schools cannot provide enough clinical experience to make graduates comfortable on their first day as new nurses. They can take responsibility for obtaining as much practical experience as possible outside of school. Working in a health care setting during summers, on school breaks, and on weekends is helpful. They should avoid work during the school week, if at all possible, or keep it to an absolute minimum since academic responsibilities take priority during that time and exhausted students make poor learners.

Some schools offer programs in which students are paired with practicing nurses (**preceptors**) and work closely with them to experience life as registered nurses do. If your school offers such a program, take advantage of it. If not, seek out information about similar programs at area hospitals. Many hospitals are now providing excellent opportunities for students nearing graduation to function in expanded roles.

KNOWING EMPLOYERS' EXPECTATIONS

New nurses approaching graduation should realistically appraise their strengths, weaknesses, and preferences. To reduce reality shock, it is important to ensure that there is a good "match" between one's abilities and employers' expectations. Ellis and Hartley (1988, pp. 346–349) suggest that nurses examine themselves in seven areas in which employers of new graduates have expectations.

1. *Theoretical knowledge* should be adequate to provide basic patient care and make clinical judgments. Employers expect new nurses to be able to recognize the early signs and symptoms of patient problems, such as an allergic reaction to a blood transfusion, and take the appropriate nursing action, that is, turn off the transfusion. They are expected to know potential problems related to various patient conditions, such as postoperative status, and what nursing actions to take to prevent complications.

2. The ability to *use the nursing process* systematically as a means of planning nursing care is important. Employers will evaluate nurses' understanding of the

phases of the process: assessment, analysis, nursing diagnosis, planning, intervention, and evaluation. They expect nurses to ensure that all elements of a nursing care plan are used in delivering nursing care and that there is documentation in the patient's record to that effect.

3. *Self-awareness* is critically important. Employers will ask prospective employees to identify their own strengths and weaknesses. They need to know that new nurses are willing to ask for help and recognize their limitations. New graduates who are unable or unwilling to request help pose a risk to patients that employers are unwilling to accept.

4. *Record-keeping ability* is an increasingly important skill that employers value. While patient documentation systems differ from facility to facility, employers expect new graduates to know what patient data should be charted and that all nursing care should be entered in patient documents. Accuracy, legibility, spelling, and use of correct grammar and approved abbreviations are all minimal expectations.

5. *Work ethic* is another area in which employers are vitally interested. **Work ethic** means that prospective employees understand what is expected of them and are committed to providing it. Nursing is not, and never has been, a nine-to-five profession. While work schedules are more flexible today than ever before, patient care still goes on around the clock, on weekends, and on holidays. Employers expect new graduates to recognize that the most desirable positions and work hours do not usually go to entry-level workers in any field. Nursing is no different in this respect from accounting, broadcasting, or investment banking. In nursing, others cannot leave work until they turn patient care responsibilities over to a qualified replacement; therefore, being late to work or "calling in sick" when not genuinely incapacitated are luxuries professional nurses cannot afford. Tardy nurses quickly lose credibility with their peers. In sum, employers expect new nurses to recognize and accept that employment means some sacrifices in personal convenience—as in every other profession.

6. *Skill proficiency* of new graduates varies widely, and employers are aware of this. Most large facilities now provide fairly lengthy orientation periods when each nurse's skills are appraised and opportunities are provided to practice new procedures. In general, smaller and rural facilities have less formalized orientation programs, and earlier independent functioning is expected. It can be very useful to keep a log of nursing procedures learned during school. Many schools provide a skills checklist that is helpful in identifying areas in which students need more practice. Students can then be assertive in seeking specific types of patient assignments.

7. *Speed of functioning* is another area in which new nurses vary widely. By the end of the orientation period, the new graduate should be able to care for the average patient load without too much difficulty. Time management is a skill that is very closely related to speed of functioning. Managing time well means managing yourself well and requires self-discipline. The ability to organize and prioritize nursing care for a group of patients requires time management skills. See Box 8–3 to determine what can be done to keep poor time management from being a problem.

Box 8–3   Time Management Self-Assessment

Good time management is a skill that can be developed. Listed below are principles reflecting good time management. Circle the answer most characteristic of how you manage your time. Be honest.

1. I spend some time each day planning how to accomplish my school and other responsibilities.
   0. Rarely
   1. Sometimes
   2. Frequently
2. I set specific goals and dates for accomplishing them.
   0. Rarely
   1. Sometimes
   2. Frequently
3. Each day I make a "to do" list and prioritize it. I complete the most important tasks first.
   0. Rarely
   1. Sometimes
   2. Frequently
4. I plan time in my schedule for unexpected problems and unanticipated delays.
   0. Rarely
   1. Sometimes
   2. Frequently
5. I ask others for help when possible.
   0. Rarely
   1. Sometimes
   2. Frequently

6. I take advantage of short but regular breaks to refresh myself and stay alert.
   0. Rarely
   1. Sometimes
   2. Frequently
7. When I really need to concentrate, I work in a specific area that is free from distractions and interruptions.
   0. Rarely
   1. Sometimes
   2. Frequently
8. When working, I turn down other people's requests when they would interfere with my completing my priority tasks.
   0. Rarely
   1. Sometimes
   2. Frequently
9. I avoid unproductive and prolonged socializing with fellow students or employees during my workday.
   0. Rarely
   1. Sometimes
   2. Frequently
10. I keep a calendar of important meetings, dates, and deadlines and carry it with me.
    0. Rarely
    1. Sometimes
    2. Frequently

Scoring: Give yourself   2 points for each "Frequently"
                         1 point for each "Sometimes"
                         0 points for each "Rarely"

If your score is:
    0–10   You need to improve your time management skills.
    11–15 You are doing fine and can still improve.
    16–18 You have very good time management skills.
    19–20 Your time management skills are too good to be true!

OTHER MEASURES TO REDUCE REALITY SHOCK

Other measures to reduce reality shock include seeking an employment situation with an **internship** or long orientation period. Inquire about preceptor opportunities, that is, working along side an experienced nurse, and assess the level of professional development activities offered in each facility under consideration.

Recognize that all large systems have a certain amount of **inertia** (disinclination to change), and as good as a new nurse's ideas are, they may not be welcomed. Learning how change is accomplished in the institution is an important first step in becoming a positive influence on the system. Identifying which battles to fight and which to ignore is a learning process for all new professionals.

Talking with other new graduates about feelings is one of the best ways to combat reality shock. Take the initiative to form a group for mutual support—others need it too! Another interpersonal strategy is to seek a professional mentor. A **mentor** is an experienced nurse who is committed to nursing and to sharing knowledge with less experienced nurses to help advance their careers. A mentor can be a great source of all types of knowledge as well as another source of support. Ask an admired nurse to be a mentor and identify what he or she can offer. Some inexperienced nurses are fearful of approaching potential mentors with this request. They should remember that this process is not a one-way street; it complements and validates the mentor's self-esteem as well as providing important information and support to the nurse being mentored.

CHAPTER SUMMARY

Professional socialization is a critical process that turns novices into fully functioning professionals. The two major components of socialization to professional nursing are socialization through education and socialization in the workplace. There are several models of professional socialization that identify stages in the process and key behaviors occurring at each stage. Individuals have significant responsibility for active participation in their own professional socialization. They can identify needed learning experiences and seek opportunities that provide them. Reality shock has been identified as a stressful period new nurses may experience upon entering nursing practice. Understanding the stages and how to resolve them can assist new graduates through this transition. In addition, knowing what employers expect can help students plan more effectively and help them be more assertive in seeking experiences they need.

REVIEW/DISCUSSION QUESTIONS

1. Describe how both formal and informal socialization experiences in school have modified the image of nursing you brought with you.
2. Select one model of socialization discussed in this chapter and place yourself in one of the stages. Give your rationale for that placement. If none of the models fit your experience, design one and share it with the class.

3. List five things you can do to take active responsibility for your own professional socialization.

4. Interview a new nurse and assess his or her reality shock experience. How is this individual handling the transition from student to practicing nurse? What can you learn from his or her experience?

REFERENCES

American Nurses Association. (1976). *Code for nurses with interpretive statements*. Kansas City, MO: Author.

Bandura, A. (1977). *Social learning theory*. Englewood Cliffs, NJ: Prentice-Hall.

Cohen, H. A. (1981). *The nurse's quest for professional identity*. Menlo Park, CA: Addison-Wesley.

Ellis, J. R., and Hartley, C. L. (1988). *Nursing in today's world: Challenges, issues, trends* (3rd ed.). Philadelphia: J.B. Lippincott.

Erikson, E. (1950). *Childhood and society*. New York: W.W. Norton.

Hinshaw, A. S. (1976). *Socialization and resocialization of nurses for professional nursing practice*. New York: National League for Nursing.

Jacox, A. (1973). Professional socialization of nurses. *Journal of the New York State Nurses' Association*, 4(4), 6–15.

Kramer, M. (1974). *Reality shock: Why nurses leave nursing*. St. Louis, MO: C.V. Mosby.

McCain, N. L. (1985). A test of Cohen's developmental model for professional socialization with baccalaureate nursing students. *Journal of Nursing Education*, 24(5), 180–186.

Throwe, A. N., and Fought, S. G. (1987). Landmarks in the socialization process from RN to BSN. *Nurse Educator*, 12(6), 15–18.

Wooley, A. S. (1978). From RN to BSN: Faculty perceptions. *Nursing Outlook*, 26(2), 104–106.

SUGGESTED READINGS

Adams-Ender, C. L. (1991). Mentoring: Nurses helping nurses. *RN*, 91(4), 21–23.

Benner, P. (1984). *From novice to expert: Excellence and power in clinical nursing practice*. Menlo Park, CA: Addison-Wesley.

Bevis, E. O., and Watson, J. (1989). *Toward a caring curriculum*. New York: National League for Nursing.

Hammer, R. M., and Tufts, M. A. (1985). Nursing's self-image: Nursing education's responsibility. *Journal of Nursing Education*, 24(7), 280–284.

Chapter 9

Philosophies of Nursing

Marilynn K. Bodie
and Kay K. Chitty

CHAPTER OBJECTIVES

What students should be able to do after studying this chapter:

1. Define and give an example of a belief.
2. Define and give an example of a value.
3. Cite examples of nursing philosophies.
4. Discuss the impact of beliefs and values on nurses' professional behaviors.
5. Explain why nurses need a philosophy of nursing.
6. Begin to identify personal beliefs, values, and philosophies as they relate to nursing.

VOCABULARY BUILDING

Terms to know:

aesthetics	ethics	philosophy
beliefs	logic	politics
bioethics	metaphysics	values
epistemology	nonjudgmental	

*U*p to now, this book has focused on describing and defining nursing from the outside. The historical milestones of the profession, how its practitioners are educated, the social context in which nursing has evolved, the organizations nurses belong to, how nursing measures up as a profession, how nurses define their profession, and how new nurses are socialized have all been examined. Now the book begins to examine what nurses think, believe, and value and how their care of patients is influenced by these thoughts, beliefs, and values. In other words, nursing will be explored from the inside.

Certain beliefs about what nursing is have evolved during the development of professional nursing. Specific statements of beliefs were generated by the members of the American Nurses Association and published in the *Code for Nurses with Interpretive Statements*. This document can be reviewed in Box 4–1 of this book. Statements such as the code exist to affirm the beliefs of the profession as a whole and to guide the practice of nursing.

This chapter will examine the relationship of beliefs, values, and philosophies to the practice of nursing; review several philosophies of nursing that were developed by an individual, two hospitals, and a school of nursing; and assist readers in beginning to develop their own philosophies of nursing.

Beliefs

A **belief** represents the intellectual acceptance of something as true or correct. Beliefs can also be described as convictions or creeds. Beliefs are opinions that may be, in reality, true or false. They are based on attitudes that have been acquired and verified by experience. Beliefs are generally transmitted from generation to generation.

Although all people have beliefs, few have spent much time examining their beliefs. In nursing, it is important to know and understand one's beliefs because the practice of nursing frequently challenges nurses' beliefs. While this may create temporary discomfort, it is ultimately good because it forces nurses to consider their beliefs carefully. They have to answer the question, Is this something I really believe, or have I accepted it because some influential person [such as a parent or teacher] said it? Issues such as abortion, living wills, the right to die, the right to refuse treatment, alternative life-styles, and similar issues confront all members of contemporary society. Professional nurses must develop and refine their beliefs about these and many other issues.

Beliefs are exhibited through attitudes and behaviors. Simply observing how nurses relate to patients, their families, and nursing peers reveals something about those nurses' beliefs. Every day nurses meet people whose beliefs are very different from, or even diametrically opposed to, their own. Effective nurses recognize that they need to adopt **nonjudgmental** attitudes toward patients' beliefs. A nurse with a nonjudgmental attitude makes every effort to convey neither approval nor disapproval of patients' beliefs and respects each person's right to his or her beliefs.

Box 9–1 Religion and Health Care Beliefs

God's will vs. doctor's orders. Deciding which to follow is an agonizing choice for many parents. Justin Barnhart, a two-and-a-half-year-old youngster who lived in Pennsylvania, suffered from a Wilms' tumor, a form of kidney cancer. As the tumor grew larger it obstructed his intestines and took all the nourishment from his food. Justin died from starvation. His parents, William and Linda Barnhart, had never taken him to a doctor. They were charged with, and eventually convicted of, involuntary manslaughter and endangering the welfare of a child. A state appeals court upheld the conviction in 1985.

The Barnharts loved their son and grieved when he died. But they had been members of the Faith Tabernacle Church all their lives (as had Mr. Barnhart's father before him). Central to that religion are the beliefs that life rests in God's hands and that trust in medicine harms one's spiritual and eternal interests, which are more important than physical well-being.

The Barnhart case illustrates one of the most troubling ethical dilemmas involving children and medical care. Religious freedom and family privacy are cherished values in our society; so too is the concept that the medical profession and the government have an obligation to protect the health and welfare of all children. In the most extreme cases, involving life and death, honoring one value inevitably means violating the other.

(From Levine, C. (1989). God's will versus doctor's orders. *Parents' Magazine*, 64(3), 220, 222, 226–227. Used by permission.)

An example of differences in beliefs that directly affect nursing is the position taken by some religious groups that all healing should be left to a divine power. Seeking medical treatment, even lifesaving ones such as blood transfusions or chemotherapy for cancer, is not condoned. From time to time there have been news reports of parents who are charged with criminal acts because they did not take a sick child to the doctor. Box 9–1 contains such a story. While reading it, think about how your health care beliefs differ from or concur with those of the family described in the article. What feelings might you have if assigned to work with this family? From this brief exercise it can be seen how difficult maintaining a nonjudgmental attitude toward the beliefs of patients can be.

Three Categories of Beliefs

People often use the terms **beliefs** and **values** interchangeably. Even experts disagree about whether they differ or are the same. Although they are related, beliefs and values will be differentiated in this chapter and discussed separately.

Rokeach (1973, pp. 6–7) identified three main categories of beliefs:

1. *Descriptive* or *existential beliefs* are those that can be shown to be true or false. An example of a descriptive belief is: "The sun will come up each morning."
2. *Evaluative beliefs* are those in which there is a judgment about good or bad. The belief "Dancing is immoral" is an example of an evaluative belief.
3. *Prescriptive* (encouraged) and *proscriptive* (prohibited) *beliefs* are those in which certain actions are judged to be desirable or undesirable. The belief "Every citizen of voting age should vote in every election" is a prescriptive belief, whereas the belief "People should not engage in sexual intercourse outside of marriage" is a proscriptive belief. Prescriptive and proscriptive beliefs are closely related to values.

Values

Values are the social principles, ideals, or standards held by an individual, class, or group that give meaning and direction to life. Values reflect what people consider desirable and consist of the subjective assignment of worth to behavior. Although many people are unaware of it, values help them make both small, day-to-day choices and important life decisions. Just as beliefs influence nursing practice, values also influence how nurses practice their profession, often without their conscious awareness. Diann Uustal (1985), a contemporary nurse who has written extensively about values, said, "Everything we do, every decision we make and course of action we take is based on our consciously and unconsciously chosen beliefs, attitudes and values" (p. 100).

The Nature of Human Values

Values evolve as people mature. An individual's values today are undoubtedly different from those of ten, or even five, years ago. Rokeach (1973, p. 3) made several assertions about the nature of human values:

1. Each person has a relatively small number of values.
2. All human beings, regardless of location or culture, possess basically the same values to differing degrees.
3. People organize their values into value systems.
4. People develop values in response to culture, society, and even individual personality traits.
5. Most observable human behaviors are manifestations or consequences of human values.

Authorities agree that values influence behavior and that people with unclear values lack direction, persistence, and decision-making skill (Raths, Harmin, and Simon 1978). Since much of nursing involves having a clear sense of direction, the ability to persevere, and the ability to make sound decisions quickly and frequently, effective nurses must have a strong set of professional nursing values. Uustal (1985) identified a number of professional nursing values. They include such values as "individualized patient care," "providing care regardless of patient's ability to pay," "promotion of patient self-determination," and "support of fellow nurses." Uustal's complete list is found in Table 9–1.

The Process of Valuing

Valuing is the process by which values are determined. Raths, Harmin, and Simon (1978) identified steps in the process of valuing. They divided the process into three main components: choosing, prizing, and acting.

Choosing is the cognitive (intellectual) aspect of valuing. Ideally, people choose their values freely from all alternatives after considering the possible consequences of their choices.

Prizing is the affective (emotional) aspect of valuing. People usually feel good about their values and cherish the choices they make.

Table 9–1 Professional Nursing Values

Nonjudgmental attitude
Honesty with patients
Involvement with families
Listening
Patient advocacy
Cooperative work relationships among staff
Dignity of the patient
Sharing self through nursing interventions
Integrity of profession through each nurse's example
Promotion of health
Providing care regardless of patient's ability to pay
Patient education
Emotional involvement with patients
Quality care (physical, emotional, spiritual, social, intellectual)
Individualized patient care
Knowledge
Competence
Empathy
Flexibility
Openness to learning
Trust
Teamwork
Promotion of patient self-determination
Collaboration between patient and nurse
Dependability
Support of fellow nurses
Accountability

(Adapted from Uustal, D. B. (1985). *Values and ethics in nursing: From theory to practice.* East Greenwich, RI: Educational Resources in Nursing and Wholistic Health. Used by permission.)

Acting is the behavioral aspect of valuing. When people affirm their values publicly by acting on their choices, they make their values part of their behavior. A real value is repeated consistently in behavior.

All three steps must be taken, or the process of valuing is incomplete. For example, a professional nurse might believe that learning is a lifelong process and that nurses have an obligation to keep up with new developments in the profession. This nurse would choose continued learning over other alternatives and appreciate the consequences of the choice. He might even publicly affirm his choice and feel very good about it. But unless he follows through consistently with behaviors such as reading journals, attending conferences, and seeking out other learning opportunities, continued learning is not a true value in his life.

Values Clarification

Nurses, and people in other helping professions, need to understand their values. This is the first step in self-awareness, which is important in maintaining a nonjudgmental approach to patients.

A variety of values clarification exercises have been developed to help people understand their values. Most of them are group exercises, but even without a group, considering your reactions to these statements can help in the beginning identification of values:

1. Patients should always be told the truth about their diagnoses.
2. Nurses, if asked, should assist terminally ill patients to die.
3. Severely impaired infants should be kept alive, regardless of their future quality of life.
4. Nurses should never accept gifts from patients.
5. A college professor should receive a heart transplant before a homeless person does.
6. Nurses should be role models of healthy behavior.

As you react, both emotionally and intellectually to these statements, something about your personal and professional values is revealed. Determining where you stand on these and other nursing issues is an important step in clarifying your values. More about values and their relationship to nursing practice is included in Chapters 19 and 20.

Philosophies

Philosophy is defined as the study of the truths and principles of being, knowledge, or conduct (Flexner 1980). A more literal translation, based on the Greek root words, means "the love of exercising one's curiosity and intelligence" (Edwards 1967, p. 216). Nursing students often learn about philosophers such as Plato, Socrates, Aristotle, Bacon, Kant, Descartes, and others in nonnursing classes. These philosophers were searching for the underlying principles of reality and truth.

Philosophy begins when someone contemplates, or wonders, about something. If a group of friends sometimes sit and discuss the relationship between men and women and ponder the differences in males' and females' natures and approaches to life, one might say that they were developing a philosophy about male and female ways of being. It is important to remember that philosophy is not the exclusive domain of a few erudite individuals; everyone has a personal philosophy of life, for example, which is unique from all others'.

People develop personal philosophies as they mature. These philosophies serve as blueprints or guides and incorporate each individual's value and belief systems. Nurses' personal philosophies interact directly with philosophies of nursing and influence professional behaviors.

Branches of Philosophy

Before examining professional philosophies, let us briefly explore the discipline of philosophy itself. Philosophy has been divided into specific areas of study. This section will review six branches: epistemology, logic, aesthetics, ethics, politics, and metaphysics.

1. **Epistemology** is the branch of philosophy dealing with the theory of knowledge. The epistemologist attempts to answer such questions as, "What can be known?" Epistemology attempts to determine how we can know whether our beliefs about the world are true.

2. **Logic** is the study of correct and incorrect reasoning. In logic, the nature of reasoning itself is the subject. It is logical behavior, for example, for fair-skinned individuals to stay out of the midday sun unless wearing protective clothing. Chapter 17 presents the method of logical thinking that nurses use to plan and implement effective patient care, called "the nursing process."

3. **Aesthetics** is the study of what is beautiful. Painting, sculpture, music, dance, and literature are all associated with beauty. Judgments about what is beautiful, however, differ from individual to individual and culture to culture. For example, Eastern music may sound discordant to the Western ear.

4. **Ethics** is the branch of philosophy that studies the propriety of certain courses of action. Moral principles and values make up a system of ethics. Behavior depends on moral principles and values. Ethics, therefore, underlie the standards of behavior that govern us as individuals and as nurses. **Bioethics** is a term describing the branch of ethics that deals with biological issues. Bioethics and nursing ethics are complex areas of study that will be explored in Chapter 20.

5. **Politics**, in the context of a discussion of philosophy, means the area of philosophy that deals with the regulation and control of people living in society. Political philosophers study the conditions of society and suggest recommendations for improving them.

6. **Metaphysics** is the consideration of the ultimate nature of existence, reality, and experience. Metaphysicians believe that we can gain a more complete understanding of reality than even science can provide.

This brief review of the branches of philosophy is presented as a backdrop for the discussion of philosophies of nursing.

Box 9–2   One Nurse's Philosophy

I believe that the essence of nursing is caring about and caring for human beings who are unable to care for themselves. I believe that the central core of nursing is the nurse-patient relationship and that through that relationship I can make a difference in the lives of others at a time when they are most vulnerable.

Human beings generally do the best they can. When they are uncooperative, critical, or otherwise unpleasant, it is usually because they are frightened; therefore, I will remain pleasant and nondefensive and try to understand the patient's perception of the situation. I pledge to be trustworthy and an advocate for my patients.

I realize that my cultural background affects how I deliver nursing care and that my patients' cultural backgrounds affect how they receive my care. I try to learn as much as I can about each individual's cultural beliefs and individualize care accordingly.

My vision for myself as a nurse is that I will provide the best care I can to all patients, regardless of their financial situation, social status, life-style choices, or spiritual beliefs. I will form partnerships with my patients, their families, and my health care colleagues and work cooperatively with them, valuing and respecting what each brings to the situation.

I am individually accountable for the care I provide, for what I fail to do and to know. Therefore, I pledge to remain a learner all my life and actively seek opportunities to learn how to be a more effective nurse.

I will strive for a balance of personal and professional responsibilities. This means I will take care of myself physically, emotionally, socially, and spiritually so I can continue to be a productive care giver.

Philosophies of Nursing

Philosophies of nursing are statements of beliefs about nursing and expressions of values in nursing that are used as bases for thinking and acting. Most philosophies of nursing are built on a foundation of beliefs about people, environment, health, and nursing. Each of these four foundational concepts of nursing will be discussed in Chapter 10.

INDIVIDUAL PHILOSOPHIES

If asked, most nurses could list their beliefs about nursing, but it is doubtful that many have written a formal philosophy of nursing. They are influenced on a day-to-day basis, however, by their unwritten, informal philosophies. It is useful to go through the process of writing down one's own professional philosophy and revising it from time to time. Comparing recent and earlier versions can reveal professional and personal growth over time. It is also helpful to read one's

Box 9–3   Statement of Philosophy and Purpose of the Division of Nursing, Beth Israel Hospital

INTRODUCTION

This revised statement of philosophy and purpose has drawn on the work and recommendations of the Beth Israel Hospital Nursing Services Administrative Planning Group; on the seminal thinking of Henderson, Wiedenbach, and Orlando; and on multiple documents developed by the Beth Israel Hospital Division of Nursing over a ten-year period, including the Division's Statement of Philosophy first issued in 1974.

Statements such as this are meaningless unless they are translated into action. Our philosophy and purpose are perhaps most succinctly expressed in the words of one of our patients: "My primary nurse was truly a gem in the profession of nursing. She combines not only the highest level of professionalism in nursing, but also the many personal qualities which go beyond that in assisting patients to make a full recovery. She had a knack for getting me to motivate myself. Her concern was genuine, her advice sound, and her willingness to assist in my long-range rehabilitation goals ever present."

PURPOSE

The purpose of the Division of Nursing at Boston's Beth Israel Hospital is to ensure that each patient receives professional nursing care that is patient-centered and goal-directed, while supporting nursing and other health care education and research. Each member of the Division carries out his or her activities with one focus in mind: the patient and his welfare.

PHILOSOPHY

Nursing as a Professional Service

We agree with Virginia Henderson that professional nursing is a complex service that assists ". . . people (sick or well) in the performance of those activities contributing to health, or its recovery (or to a peaceful death) that they would perform unaided if they had the necessary strength, will, or knowledge. It is likewise the unique contribution of nursing to help people to be independent of such assistance as soon as possible." The activities which the nurse helps the patient carry out (or carries out for him) include the therapeutic plans prescribed by his physician, by other health care providers, and by the nurse herself. In carrying out these activities, the nurse practices an art through which scientific knowledge and principles; judgment; and technical, communication, observational, and analytical skills are systematically applied to the health needs of others in a caring manner.

We believe that physical and emotional comfort is a universal health need, the provision of which is an historical and fundamental nursing responsibility. Nursing is further distinguished from other direct health care services by its tradition of *continuity in time* with hospitalized patients: around-the-clock observation, recording, and reporting of the patient's condition, and direct provision of care and comfort. For patients who are not hospitalized, continuity is provided over *time* until care is no longer needed. Continuity of care is valued and provided by all nurses at Beth Israel Hospital, whatever their area of practice.

We believe that care is best provided by professional, registered nurses. We further believe that for each patient, continuity, personalization, and excellence of care is best achieved when it is planned and evaluated by a single professional nurse who has continuous accountability for that care, and when it is provided by her and her designated associates. The desired endpoint of all

nursing activity is to maintain or improve the patient's health status and comfort.

The art of professional nursing is acquired through formal higher education. It becomes refined through continuing education and training, manager and self-evaluation, and experience.

(From Division of Nursing, Beth Israel Hospital. (1991). *Statement of philosophy and purpose.* Boston, MA: Author. Used by permission.)

philosophy of nursing from time to time to make sure daily behaviors are consistent with deeply held beliefs. Box 9–2 contains one nurse's philosophy of nursing.

COLLECTIVE PHILOSOPHIES

Although few individuals write down their nursing philosophies, it is very common for hospitals and schools of nursing to express their collective beliefs about nursing in written philosophies. In fact, both hospitals and schools of nursing are required by their accrediting bodies to develop statements of philosophy. Philosophical statements should be relevant to the setting. They are intended to guide the practice of nurses employed in that setting. Examining some of these statements will clarify what constitutes a collective philosophy of nursing.

Philosophies of Nursing in Two Hospital Settings. First look at the philosophy of the Division of Nursing at Beth Israel Hospital in Boston (Box 9–3). Notice that this philosophy includes statements of belief about nursing services, recipients of nursing care, and professional nurses themselves.

Box 9–4 contains the philosophy of nursing of Memorial Hospital in Chattanooga, Tennessee. It describes a commitment to excellence in nursing service, practice, and leadership.

Notice differences and similarities in the two philosophies as well as statements with which one might agree or disagree. Remember that these are both philosophies of departments of nursing in hospital settings. Before taking a position in a hospital or health care agency, it is a good idea to ask for a copy of the philosophy of nursing in that institution. Read it carefully and make sure you accept the beliefs and values it contains.

A College of Nursing's Philosophy. Now examine a philosophical statement of a college of nursing. The philosophy of the faculty in the College of Nursing at the University of Tennessee, Memphis, is printed in Box 9–5. After reading it, identify the differences between the philosophies of nursing in hospitals and the one in this college of nursing.

Box 9–4   Memorial Hospital Philosophy of Nursing

Memorial Hospital Philosophy of Nursing

The Department of Nursing at Memorial Hospital is committed to upholding the corporate values of the Sisters of Charity of Nazareth Health Corporation and promoting the mission of Memorial Hospital. We affirm that the corporate values of

JUSTICE

QUALITY

COMPASSION

STEWARDSHIP

COLLABORATION

are in congruence with our professional values.

Therefore, we believe that the following principles must characterize the Department of Nursing.

Excellence in Service

We believe . . .

- That each of our patients, regardless of circumstances, possess intrinsic value from God and should be treated with dignity and respect.
- That each encounter with patients and families should portray compassion and concern.
- That each patient should receive quality care that is cost-effective, competitive and based on the latest technology.
- That patient confidentiality and privacy should be preserved.
- That meeting the needs of patients and other customers should always be our number one priority.

Excellence in Practice

We believe . . .

- That our profession is a science and an art, the essence of which is nurturing and caring.
- That our primary duty is to restore and maintain the health of our patients in a spirit of compassion and concern.
- That the nursing process is an integral part of our practice as professional nurses.
- That nurses should collaborate with other health care team members to meet the holistic needs of our patients, which include physical, psychosocial and spiritual aspects of care.
- That we should aggressively promote patient and family education to allow each individual the opportunity to prevent illness and/or achieve optimal health.
- That we are accountable to our patients, patients' families and to each other for our professional practice.
- That monitoring and evaluating nursing practice is our responsibility and is necessary to continuously improve care.
- That we should pursue professional growth and development through education, participation in professional organizations and support of research.

Excellence in Leadership

We believe . . .

- That we should provide a progressive environment, utilizing current technology, guided by responsible stewardship to promote the highest quality patient care and employee satisfaction.
- That we should encourage and support collaborative decision-making by those who are closest to the situation, even at the risk of failure.
- That compassion should be characterized in our day to day personal interactions as well as being a motivating factor in management decisions.
- That we should be sensitive to individual needs and give support, praise, and recognition to encourage professional and personal development.
- That we should possess an energy level and personal style that empowers and inspires enthusiasm in others.
- That we should consider suggestions and criticisms as challenges for improvement and innovation.
- That justice should be applied equitably in all employment practices and personnel policies.

(From Department of Nursing, Memorial Hospital, a division of the Sisters of Charity of Nazareth Health Corporation. (1991). *Philosophy of nursing. Chattanooga, TN: Author. Used by permission.*)

An important point about philosophies of nursing is that they are dynamic and change over time. When a collective philosophy is written, it reflects the existing values and beliefs of the particular group of people who wrote it. When the group members change, the philosophy may change. Therefore, once a collective philosophy is written, it should be "revisited" regularly and modified to accurately reflect the group's current beliefs about nursing practice (Cody 1990).

Developing a Personal Philosophy of Nursing

Developing a philosophy of nursing is not merely an academic exercise required by accrediting bodies. Having a written philosophy can help guide nurses in the daily decisions they must make in nursing practice. Because many nurses have ill-defined, uneasy feelings about committing their philosophies of nursing to paper, few nurses have done so.

Writing a philosophy is not a complex, time-consuming task. It simply involves writing down one's beliefs and values about nursing. It answers the question, Why do you practice nursing the way you do? A philosophy should provide direction and promote effectiveness. If it does not, it is a time-wasting collection of words.

Box 9–6 is designed to help you get started in developing your own personal philosophy of nursing. After you develop a beginning philosophy, save it. As you progress through your educational program, take it out and revise it regularly, saving each version. After you graduate, look back at all the different versions and see how your values and beliefs about nursing have changed over time.

Box 9–5   Philosophy of the College of Nursing, University of Tennessee

The philosophy of the College of Nursing is consistent with the University of Tennessee and with the goals and mission of UT Memphis. The College Philosophy focuses upon the nature of the PERSON, ENVIRONMENT, HEALTH, THE PROFESSION OF NURSING, and THE PROCESS OF EDUCATION.

Faculty believe that the PERSON is a unique and continuously evolving being of dignity and growth. The person's behavior reflects the interaction between personal and environmental influences. Each person has the right to participate in making decisions which affect health and to accept or refuse health care within the context of safety to society.

The faculty view ENVIRONMENT as all external influences affecting the life and development of the person. The health of individuals, families and communities is affected by these influences.

HEALTH is viewed as a dynamic state arising from continuous change in the person and environment. The faculty view the promotion, maintenance, and restoration of health as complex phenomena involving the joint responsibility of the person and the health care providers.

NURSING is the diagnosis and treatment of actual or potential health problems. Nursing involves supportive and therapeutic interventions based on theoretical and scientific knowledge. The goal of nursing is to promote health throughout the life span, prevent illness, restore and/or maintain with dignity essential life functions altered by illness. As health care professionals, nurses exert leadership to achieve a viable system of health care delivery and assure quality nursing care. The nurse's role is that of a health care provider who, both independently and in collaboration with others, assesses, plans, implements, and evaluates nursing care.

Nursing is a synthesis of art and science. The art of nursing requires that the practitioner apply knowledge gained from the humanities, arts, and sciences to understand human needs. This knowledge provides the foundation for acceptance and appreciation of the values of the person which may differ from those of the nurse. The science of nursing is the contemplation, exploration and research of the person, environment, and health.

EDUCATION for professional nursing practice includes a sound theoretical knowledge base to support experiential learning. Faculty believe the educational process facilitates continuing personal and professional growth in which the responsibility for outcomes is mutually shared by students and faculty. The intent of the educational programs is to focus on the learner. Education is a lifelong process, with the commitment of the learner to establish patterns of continued inquiry.

(From College of Nursing, University of Tennessee, Memphis. (1991). *Philosophy of the College of Nursing*. Memphis, TN: Author. Used by permission.)

Box 9–6   Philosophy of Nursing Work Sheet

Purpose: To write a beginning philosophy of nursing that reflects the beliefs and values of _____[Your Name]_____.

Today's date is: _____.

I chose nursing as my profession because nursing is _____
_____
_____
_____.

I believe that the core of nursing is ___
_____
_____.

I believe that the focus of nursing is ___
_____
_____.

My vision for myself as a nurse is that I will _____
_____
_____.

In order to live out my philosophy of nursing, every day I must remember this about:

a. My patients _____
_____.

b. My patients' families _____
_____.

c. My fellow health care professionals
_____.

d. My own health _____
_____.

CHAPTER SUMMARY

People develop beliefs and values that affect their attitudes and behaviors. Beliefs and values influence how nurses practice their profession. Nurses need to be aware of their beliefs and values to prevent the unintentional intrusion of personal values into the nurse-patient relationship. A statement of beliefs can be called a philosophy. There are numerous philosophical statements about nursing. Examples in this chapter demonstrate that philosophies rest on a basis of beliefs and values. As nurses progress professionally, they collect ideas about the practice of nursing that they agree with and support. From these they develop their own personal philosophies of nursing. The purpose of developing a philosophy of nursing is to shape and guide nursing practice. As nurses mature in the profession, they may find that their philosophies about nursing also change even though underlying values may not.

REVIEW/DISCUSSION QUESTIONS

1. Name two of your health-related values. How did these become your values? Describe how you expect these values to influence your nursing practice.
2. Compare the nursing philosophies of Beth Israel and Memorial hospitals. What are three common elements and three differences? If you or a family member needed to be hospitalized, which hospital would you choose, based on these philosophies? Why?

3. Obtain the philosophy statement of the faculty of your school of nursing. What concepts are included? Which beliefs do you agree with and disagree with? Why?

4. Using the work sheet in Box 9–6, write a beginning philosophy of nursing. Share your philosophy with one other person.

5. Discuss how having or not having a philosophy of nursing influences a nurse's practice.

REFERENCES

Beth Israel Hospital Division of Nursing. (1991). Statement of philosophy and purpose. Boston: Author.

Cody, B. (1990). Shaping the future through a philosophy of nursing. *Journal of Nursing Administration,* 20(10), 16–22.

College of Nursing, The University of Tennessee, Memphis. (1991). Philosophy of the College of Nursing. Memphis: Author.

Edwards, P. (Ed.). (1967). *Encyclopedia of philosophy.* New York: Macmillan.

Flexner, S. B. (Ed.). (1980). *The Random House dictionary.* New York: Random House.

Levine, C. (1989). God's will versus doctor's orders. *Parents' Magazine,* 64(3), 220, 222, 226–227.

Memorial Hospital Department of Nursing. (1991). Memorial Hospital philosophy of nursing. Chattanooga, TN: Author.

Raths, L., Harmin, M., and Simon, S. (1978). *Values and teaching* (2nd ed.). Columbus, OH: Charles Merrill.

Rokeach, M. (1973). *The nature of human values.* New York: Free Press.

Uustal, D. B. (1985). *Values and ethics in nursing: From theory to practice.* East Greenwich, RI: Educational Resources in Nursing and Wholistic Health.

SUGGESTED READINGS

Brink, P. J. (1989). A philosophy of nursing (editorial). *Western Journal of Nursing Research,* 11(4), 391–392.

Gates, R. J. (1990). From educational philosophy to educational practice: Fidelity and the curriculum in context. *Nurse Education Today,* 10(6), 420–427.

Woods, S., and Edwards, S. (1989). Philosophy and nursing. *Journal of Advanced Nursing,* 14(8), 33–42.

Chapter

10 Major Concepts in Nursing

Marilynn K. Bodie and Kay K. Chitty

CHAPTER OBJECTIVES

What students should be able to do after studying this chapter:

1. Summarize the concepts basic to professional nursing.
2. Describe the components and processes of general systems theory.
3. Explain human needs theory.
4. Recognize how environmental factors such as family, culture, social support, and community influence health.
5. Explain the significance of a holistic approach to nursing care.
6. Apply Rosenstock's model of health beliefs to personal behaviors and the behaviors of others.
7. Devise a personal plan for achieving high-level wellness.

VOCABULARY BUILDING

Terms to know:

adaptation	extended family	health behaviors
closed system	feedback	health beliefs
culture	general systems	high-level wellness
environment	theory	holism
evaluation	health	homeostasis

input	output	system
Abraham Maslow	person	theory of human
nuclear families	self-actualization	motivation
nursing	subsystems	
open system	suprasystem	

*T*here are certain basic concepts, or ideas, that are essential to an understanding of professional nursing practice. You could say that they are the building blocks of nursing. These concepts are person, environment, and health. Everything professional nurses do is in some way related to one of these basic concepts. These concepts are interrelated, as seen in Figure 10–1.

Prior to addressing each of the concepts, it is important to have an understanding of general systems theory (von Bertalanffy 1968), which helps explain how the concepts relate to each other.

General Systems Theory

Ludwig von Bertalanffy described **general systems theory** in the late 1930s. A **system** is a set of interrelated parts that come together to form a whole. Each part is a necessary or integral component required to make a complete and meaningful whole. These parts are input, output, evaluation, and feedback.

The first component of a system is **input**, which is the information, energy, or matter that enters a system. For a system to work well, input should contribute to achieving the purpose of the system.

A second component of a system is **output**, the end result or product of the system. Outputs vary widely, depending on the type and purpose of the system.

Evaluation is the third component of a system. Evaluation means measuring the success or failure of the output and consequently the effectiveness of the system. For evaluation to be meaningful in any system, outcome criteria, against which performance or product quality is measured, must be identified.

The process of communicating what is found in evaluation of the system is called **feedback**, the final component of a system. Feedback is the information given back into the system to determine whether or not the purpose, or end result, of the system has been achieved. Figure 10–2 shows a pictorial explanation of general systems theory.

It may be helpful to use a simple example to clarify the components of systems. In a college system, *input* consists of students, faculty, ideas, the desire to learn, and knowledge. Since the purpose of the system is to educate, the students need to be ready to learn, the faculty should be prepared to teach, and the ideas and knowledge transmitted must be clear and understandable. The *output*, or product, of the system is educated graduates. For *evaluation* of the output, a standardized examination of reading comprehension, mathematics, and analytical skills may be used. Student scores on the comprehensive exami-

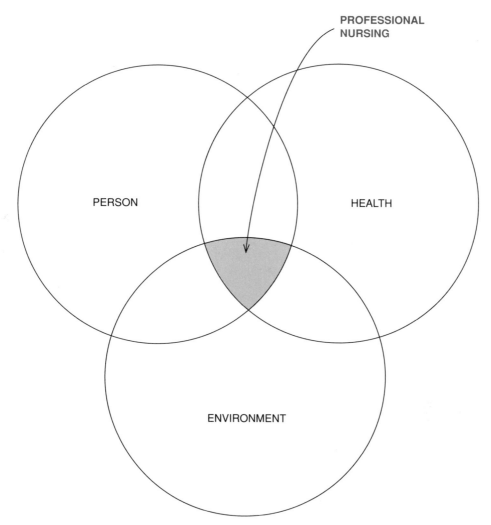

Figure 10–1 Relationship of concepts basic to professional nursing.

nation provide *feedback* to the faculty and administrators. If they score well, the system has achieved its purpose. If not, changes need to be made in the input or in the system itself, for example, to admit brighter students, hire more talented faculty, or design more rigorous courses and curricula.

Systems are usually complex and consist of several parts called **subsystems**. Let us examine a hospital as a system. Technically, it is a system for providing health care, but the success of the system depends on the functioning of many subsystems. The subsystems include the laboratory, radiology, housekeeping, laundry, supply, medical records, dietetics, nursing, pharmacy, and

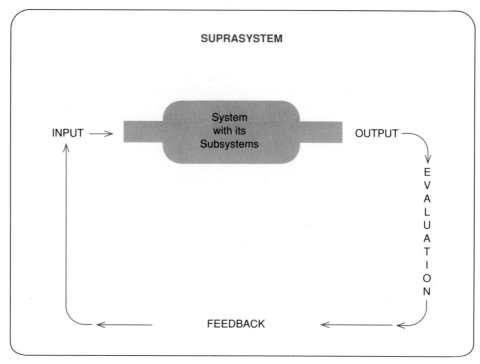

Figure 10–2 General systems model.

medical staff. All these subsystems function collaboratively to make the health care provider system—the hospital—work.

The hospital and all its subsystems are **open systems**. An open system promotes the exchange of matter, energy, and information with other systems and the environment. The larger environment outside the hospital is called the **suprasystem**. A **closed system**, on the other hand, does not interact with other systems or with the surrounding environment. Matter, energy, and information do not flow into or out of a closed system. There are few totally closed systems. A completely balanced aquarium comes very close to being a closed system.

Two more points are essential to a beginning understanding of systems theory. First, the whole is different from and greater than the sum of its parts. Stated another way, the system is different from and greater than the sum of its subsystems. Anyone who has ever been in a hospital, for example, knows that what happens there is different from and more than the sum of the following equation: Laundry + pharmacy + nurses + doctors = hospital. Something additional occurs when all the various subsystems and the people who make them up join forces to work with patients and their families.

The final point to be made about systems is that change in one part of the system creates change in other parts. If the hospital admissions office, for example, decides to admit patients only between the hours of 8:00 A.M. and 10:00 A.M., that decision will create change on the nursing units, in housekeeping, the business office, surgery, the laboratory, and other hospital subsystems. If that change were implemented without prior communication to the other subsystems and coordinated planning, it could create chaos in the system.

The exchange of energy and information *within* open systems and *between* open systems and their suprasystems is continuous. The dynamic balance within and between the subsystems, the system, and the suprasystems helps create and maintain **homeostasis**, or internal stability.

All living systems are open systems. The internal environment is in constant interaction with a changing environment external to the organism. As change occurs in one, the other is affected. For example, walking into a cold room (change in the external environment) affects a variety of physiological and psychological subsystems of the person's internal environment. These in turn change a person's blood flow, ability to concentrate, feeling of comfort, and so on (changes in internal environment).

It is the openness of human systems that makes nursing intervention possible. Understanding systems theory helps nurses assess relationships among all the factors that affect patients, including the influence of nurses themselves. Nurses who understand systems theory view patients holistically, including the subsystems (respiratory system, gastrointestinal system, and so on) and suprasystem (family and community). These nurses appreciate the influence of change in any part of the system. For instance, when a diabetic patient has pneumonia (change in subsystem), the infection increases the blood sugar and may result in hospitalization. Hospitalization may adversely affect the patient's role in the family and community (change in suprasystem). Key concepts of general systems theory are summarized in Table 10–1.

With this beginning understanding of general systems theory as a foundation, the three basic concepts that are fundamental to the practice of professional nursing can now be examined.

Table 10–1 Key Concepts in General Systems Theory

A system is a set of interrelated parts.

The parts form a meaningful whole.

The whole is different from and greater than the sum of its parts.

Systems may be open or closed.

All living systems are open systems.

Systems strive for homeostasis (internal stability).

Change in one part of the system creates change in other parts.

Person

The term "**person**" is used to describe each individual man, woman, or child. There are a number of different approaches to the study of person. This chapter will briefly examine the concept of person according to general systems theory and human needs theory.

As mentioned above, each individual has numerous subsystems that make up the whole person. There are circulatory, musculoskeletal, respiratory, and neurological subsystems that compose the physiological subsystem. There are also psychological, social, and spiritual subsystems that combine with the physiological subsystem to make the whole person. Each person is unique and different from all others. This uniqueness is determined both genetically and environmentally.

Certain personal characteristics are determined before birth by the genes received from parents. Genetically determined characteristics include eye, skin, and hair color; height; gender; and a variety of other features. Other characteristics about persons are determined by the environment. Such environmental factors as the presence or absence of loving parents or parent substitutes, the presence or absence of sufficient nutritious foods, educational opportunities or lack of them, adequate or inadequate housing, the quality and quantity of parental supervision, and safety are all environmental factors that influence how a person develops.

Human Needs Theory

In addition to having personal characteristics, people have needs. A human *need* is something that is a requirement for the person's well-being. In 1954, psychologist **Abraham Maslow** published *Motivation and Personality.* In this book, Maslow discussed his **theory of human motivation** and the relationship of motivation and needs. He suggested that human behavior is motivated by needs. He identified five levels of needs and organized them into a hierarchical order, as shown in Figure 10–3.

The most basic level of needs consists of those necessary for physiological survival: food, oxygen, rest, activity, shelter, and sexual expression. These are needs all human beings, regardless of location or culture, have in common. Maslow identified the second level of needs as safety and security needs. These include both physical safety and security needs as well as psychological safety and security needs. Psychological safety and security include having a fairly predictable environment with which one has some familiarity. The third level of needs consists of love and belonging needs. Each person needs close, intimate relationships, social relationships, and group affiliations. Next in Maslow's hierarchy is the need for self-esteem. This includes the need to feel self-worth, self-respect, and self-reliance. The highest level of needs was termed **self-actualization**. Self-actualized people have realized their maximum potential and use their capabilities to the fullest extent possible. People do not stay in a state of self-actualization but may have "peak experiences" during which they realize self-actualization for some period of time. Maslow believed that many people strive for self-actualization, but few reach that level.

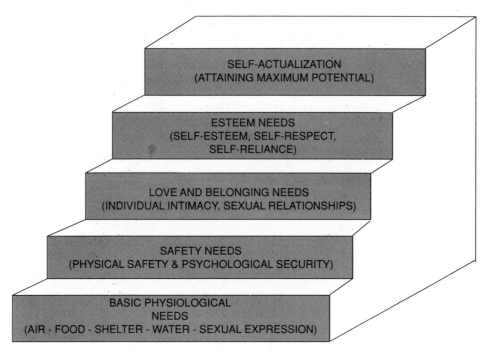

Figure 10–3 Maslow's hierarchy of needs.

Maslow's hierarchy rests on several basic assumptions about human needs. One assumption is that the more basic needs must be at least partially satisfied before higher-order needs can become relevant to the individual. For example, a starving person can hardly be concerned with self-esteem needs until a life-sustaining level of nutrition is established.

A second assumption about human needs is that individuals meet their needs in different ways. One person may need eight or nine hours of sleep to feel rested, whereas another may only require five or six hours. Each individual's sleep needs may vary at different stages of life. Older people usually require less sleep than younger ones. Individuals also eat different diets in differing quantities and at differing intervals. Some prefer to eat only twice a day, whereas others may snack six or eight times a day to meet their nutritional needs. Sexual energy also varies widely from person to person. The frequency with which normal adults desire sexual activity is difficult to determine owing to the broad range of individual interests.

Even though sleep, food, and sex are considered basic human needs, the manner in which these needs are met, as well as the extent to which any one of them is considered a need, varies according to each individual. It is therefore extremely important to determine what a person's needs are in order to provide appropriate, individualized nursing care. If a patient is uncomfortable eating three large meals such as those served in most hospitals, nurses can help that person by saving parts of the large meals in the refrigerator on the nursing unit and serving them to the patient between regularly scheduled meals. This is a simple example of what is meant by the term *individualized nursing care*. Individualized nursing care recognizes each individual's unique needs and tailors the plan of nursing care to take that uniqueness into consideration.

Another aspect of human needs that must be considered is that people change, grow, and develop. Carl Rogers (1961), a well-known psychologist, built a theory of personhood based on the idea that people are constantly adapting and discovering themselves. His book *On Becoming a Person* is considered a classic in psychological literature. Rogers's idea that a person's needs change as the person changes is important for nurses to remember. Nurses can tap into the human potential to grow and develop to assist patients to change unhealthy behaviors and to reach the highest level of wellness possible. The concept of **adaptation** is also helpful in understanding that people admitted to hospitals and removed from their customary, familiar environments frequently become anxious. Even the most confident person can become fearful when in an uncertain, perhaps threatening, situation. Under these circumstances, nurses have learned to expect people to regress slightly and to become more concerned with basic needs and less focused on the higher needs in Maslow's hierarchy. A "take-charge" professional person, for example, may become somewhat demanding and self-absorbed when hospitalized.

Homeostasis

When a person's needs are not met, homeostasis is threatened. Remember that homeostasis is a dynamic balance achieved by effectively functioning open systems. It is a state of equilibrium, a tendency to maintain internal stability. In humans, homeostasis is attained by coordinated responses of organ systems that automatically compensate for environmental changes. When someone goes for a brisk walk, for example, heartbeat and respiratory rates automatically increase to keep vital organs supplied with oxygen. When the individual comes home and sits down to read the newspaper, heart rate and breathing slow down. No conscious decision to speed up or slow down these physiological functions has to be made. Adjustments occur automatically to maintain homeostasis.

Individuals, as open systems, also endeavor to maintain balance between external and internal forces. When that balance is achieved, the person is healthy, or at least is resistant to disease. When environmental factors affect the homeostasis of a person, the person will attempt to adapt to the change. If adaptation is unsuccessful, disequilibrium may occur, setting the stage for the development of illness or disease. How individuals respond to *stress* is a major factor in the development of illness. Stress is discussed more fully in Chapter 18.

Environment

The second concept basic to professional nursing practice is **environment**. Environment includes all the circumstances, influences, and conditions that surround and affect individuals. The environment can be as small as a premature infant's incubator or as large as the universe. Included in environment are the social and cultural attitudes that profoundly shape human experience.

The environment can either promote or interfere with homeostasis and well-being of individuals. As seen in Maslow's hierarchy of needs, there is a dynamic interaction between a person's needs, which are internal, and the satisfaction of those needs, which is often environmentally determined. Environmental factors to be discussed are family, culture, social support, and community.

Family Influences

The most direct environmental influence on people is the family. The quality and amount of parenting provided to infants and growing children constitute a major determinant of health. Children who are nurtured when young and vulnerable, who are allowed to grow in independence and self-determination, and who are taught the skills they need for social living are likely to grow into strong, productive, autonomous adults.

For most of the history of humankind, immediate and **extended families** were relatively intact units that lived together or lived within close proximity to each other. Children were nurtured by a variety of relatives, as well as by their own parents. This closeness was profoundly affected by industrialization, which fostered urbanization. When families ceased farming, which was a family endeavor, and moved to cities where fathers worked in factories, the first dilution of family influence on children began. Former sources of nurturing such as grandparents, aunts and uncles, and other extended family members often stayed in rural areas, whereas the **nuclear family** (mother, father, and their children) moved away.

During World War II, more women began to work, taking them out of the home and away from young children for hours each day. The increased geographic mobility of families since World War II also had a destructive effect on the role of extended family in the lives of children since nuclear families often live half a continent or more away from grandparents and other family members. The intense attention children traditionally received from adult relatives diminished, sometimes to the detriment of the child's well-being.

Today there are more single-parent families in the United States than ever before, most of which are headed by women. The 1990 U.S. census revealed that there are over 10 million women with a total of 16 million children under age 21 and no father present (U.S. Bureau of the Census 1990, p. 20). This represents a 39 percent increase in such families in a decade. Only half of the single and divorced mothers are receiving child support due from absent fathers, according to the U.S. Census Bureau. Louis Sullivan, secretary of the Department of Health and Human Services, stated, "Many of this country's societal problems can be traced back to parents not supporting their children" ("Half of Single Moms" 1991). Lack of money often means adequate nutrition and health care are not attainable, adversely affecting the health status of all the family members.

In addition to single mothers, there are nearly 3 million single fathers in this country (U.S. Bureau of the Census 1990, p. 20). Life is challenging for single parents of both sexes who must perform traditional breadwinner roles as well as traditional nurturing roles in the family. The combination of bearing multiple roles over long periods of time can be extremely stressful, even exhausting, to single parents. Long-term stress affects the mental and physical health of these adults, which in turn affects their parenting abilities. Although many single parents manage stress well and are able to provide excellent parenting, some children's needs are neglected. The impact of this neglect can be seen in the behavior and school performance of children who have not learned the skills they need to be successful.

The examples given are only a few of the ways families influence the well-being of individuals. There are many others. Understanding a patient's family and home environment is part of a complete nursing assessment. Modification of the home environment may be needed, particularly when a person is returning home with a physical disability, in cases of child neglect, and in abuse cases. Nurses, social workers, and discharge planners often collaborate to ensure that needed changes occur before patients are discharged to homes and families.

Cultural Influences

Culture is another important environmental influence affecting individuals. Culture consists of the attitudes, beliefs, and behaviors of social and ethnic groups that have been perpetuated through generations. Patterns of dress, eating habits, activities of daily living, attitudes toward those outside the culture, health beliefs and values, spiritual beliefs or religious orientation, and attitudes toward children, women, men, work, and recreation all are influenced by culture.

Effective nurses learn to be aware of and to respect cultural influences on patients. Whenever possible, they pay attention to patients' cultural preferences. They recognize that some cultural groups attribute illness to bad fortune. Individuals from these cultures do not see themselves as active participants in their own health status. This attitude is a challenge for nurses who value the collaboration of patients in their own health care planning. This is merely one example of the influence of cultural beliefs on the nurse-patient interaction. Wise nurses realize that integration of a patient's cultural health beliefs into the individualized treatment plan can make a strong impact on that patient's desire and ability to get well.

Understanding the relationship between culture and health is the basis for "transcultural nursing," a term coined by nurse-sociologist Madeline Leininger, who has studied extensively in this field. A discussion of the influence of culture is included in Chapter 18.

Influence of the Social Environment

In addition to families and cultural groups, individuals are also influenced by the social environment in which they live. Social institutions such as families, neighborhoods, schools, churches, professional associations, civic groups, and recreational groups all may constitute a form of social support. Social support also includes such factors as presence in the home of a spouse; proximity to neighbors, children, and other supportive individuals; access to medical care; coping abilities; educational level; and so on.

Holmes and Rahe (1967) published a study of the relationship of social change to the subsequent development of illness. People with many social changes that disrupt social support, such as death of a loved one, divorce, job changes, moving, or unemployment, were much more likely to experience illness in the following 12 months than were people with few social changes. Both positive and negative changes created the need for social readjustment. Table 10–2 lists the 43 life events studied by Holmes and Rahe.

Broadhead et al., in a 1983 review of the literature, found additional evidence that social support has a direct relationship to health. They reviewed a number of studies that indicated that poor social support preceded declining health in the subjects studied. They concluded that further research is needed to determine more precisely the type(s) of social support people most need.

In assessing patients, nurses need to remember that the adequacy of social support is determined by the patient, not the nurse. Individuals vary in their need and desire for social support. When it is determined that strengthening social support is desirable, nurses can encourage patients to use interest groups, parenting classes, marriage enrichment groups, religious groups, formal and informal educational groups, and self-help groups to develop stronger support from the social environment.

Community, National, and World Influences

Community environment also influences the health status of people. The types and availability of jobs, housing, schools, and health care as well as the overall economic well-being of a community all profoundly affect its citizens. While it may not seem an obvious nursing role, nurses can be instrumental in improving community environment. Identifying health needs and bringing these to the attention of community planners, offering screening programs, serving on health-related committees and advisory boards, and lobbying political leaders all can bring about positive community change. Nurses also have become politically active by running for elected offices at local, state, and national levels. They can actively support political candidates who have sound environmental platforms. More about political activism in nursing is found in Chapter 22.

On a broader perspective, environment also includes the nation, the world, and the universe. An isolated incident such as a volcano eruption in the Philippines may have worldwide environmental repercussions. While nothing can be done to prevent natural disasters, nurses can contribute to a healthier world environment by promoting or participating in humanitarian responses to international disasters. And individual nurses, in the interest of world health, may choose to engage in a variety of environmentally sound practices and encourage others to do the same. These include recycling, using pump rather than aerosol sprayers, avoiding insecticides and unnecessary use of gardening chemicals, buying energy-efficient appliances and automobiles, walking when possible instead of driving, and boycotting companies that engage in environmentally unsound practices such as polluting air and water.

Table 10–2   Holmes and Rahe's Social
Readjustment Rating Scale
Each of the 43 life events is ranked in order of the
average length of time following the event it is
believed to take people to readjust. Notice that life
events include both positive and negative changes.

Rank	Life Event
1	Death of spouse
2	Divorce
3	Marital separation
4	Jail term
5	Death of close family member
6	Personal injury or illness
7	Marriage
8	Fired at work
9	Marital reconciliation
10	Retirement
11	Change in health of family member
12	Pregnancy
13	Sex difficulties
14	Gain of new family member
15	Business readjustment
16	Change in financial state
17	Death of close friend
18	Change to different line of work
19	Change in number of arguments with spouse
20	Mortgage over $10,000 [in 1967 dollars]
21	Foreclosure of mortgage or loan
22	Change in responsibilities at work
23	Son or daughter leaving home
24	Trouble with in-laws
25	Outstanding personal achievement
26	Wife begin or stop work
27	Begin or end school
28	Change in living conditions
29	Revision of personal habits
30	Trouble with boss
31	Change in work hours or conditions
32	Change in residence
33	Change in schools
34	Change in recreation
35	Change in church activities
36	Change in social activities
37	Mortgage or loan less than $10,000
38	Change in sleeping habits
39	Change in number of family get-togethers
40	Change in eating habits
41	Vacation
42	Christmas
43	Minor violations of the law

(From Holmes, T. H., and Rahe, R. H. (1967). The social readjustment rating scale. *Journal of Psychosomatic Research,* 11(2), 213–
218. Used by permission.)

Hospitals are among the highest producers of waste. In an effort to reduce environmental pollution, some hospitals have committees dedicated to identifying and recommending environmentally sound products. Nurses may wish to consider reducing the amount of solid waste generated by hospitals by recommending the purchase of fewer disposable products and avoiding products with wasteful packaging.

Health

Health is the third concept basic to the practice of professional nursing. Health can be viewed as a continuum, or series of events, rather than as an absolute state. Each individual's health status varies from day to day, depending on a variety of factors such as rest, nutrition, and stressors, as shown in Figure 10–4. Illness is also not an absolute state. People can have chronic illnesses such as diabetes or seizure disorders and still manage to work, take part in recreational activities, and maintain acceptably healthy lives.

Defining Health

There are numerous definitions of health. The World Health Organization (WHO) defined health as "a state of complete physical, mental and social well-being and not merely the absence of disease or infirmity" (1947, p. 29). This definition was the first modern recognition of health as multidimensional. The WHO definition presented a holistic view of health that reflected the interplay between the psychological, social, spiritual, and physical aspects of human life.

A holistic view of health focuses on the interrelationship of all the parts that make up a whole person. Jan Christian Smuts (1926) first introduced the concept of **holism** in modern Western thought by emphasizing the harmony between people and nature. When viewing health holistically, individual health

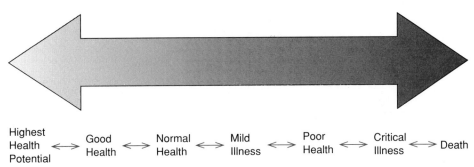

Highest Health Potential ⟷ Good Health ⟷ Normal Health ⟷ Mild Illness ⟷ Poor Health ⟷ Critical Illness ⟷ Death

Figure 10–4 The health-illness continuum—a holistic health model. (Adapted from Flynn, J., and Heffron, P. (1984). *Nursing: From concept to practice.* East Norwalk, CT: Appleton & Lange. Used by permission.)

practices must be taken into account. Health practices are culturally determined and include nutritional habits, type and amount of exercise and rest, how one copes with stress, quality of interpersonal relationships, and other life-style factors. As a profession, nurses value a holistic view of health.

Parsons (1959) defined health as "the state of optimum capacity of an individual for the effective performance of his roles and tasks." This definition focused on the roles individuals assume in life and the impact health or illness has on the fulfillment of those roles. A few examples of roles that are familiar may include the student role, the parent role, the breadwinner role, and the friend role. Given the activities inherent in each of these roles, it is easily seen that the state of health profoundly influences how people carry out their roles in life.

Yet another description of health is the opposite of illness (Dunn 1959). Dunn described health as a continuum with high-level wellness at one end and death at the other. He described **high-level wellness** as functioning at maximum potential in an integrated way within the environment. A prisoner of war kept in solitary confinement and given a diet of rice for many months certainly would have difficulty maintaining health. If he keeps active, both physically and mentally, and retains a positive outlook, however, he is likely to be healthier than the prisoner who does none of these things. Using Dunn's definition and taking his environment into consideration, the prisoner may even be said to have attained high-level wellness.

A National Health Initiative: Healthy People 2000

On September 6, 1990, the U.S. secretary of Health and Human Services, Louis W. Sullivan, released a report to the nation entitled *Healthy People 2000*. Heralded as an unprecedented cooperative effort, the preparation of the report involved government, private businesses, voluntary and professional associations, and concerned individual citizens. *Healthy People 2000* was designed to stimulate initiatives to improve significantly the health of all Americans in the last decade of the century. Three broad goals for health of the public in the 1990s were identified (U.S. Department of Health and Human Services 1990, p. 1):

1. "Increase the span of healthy life for Americans."
2. "Reduce health disparities among Americans."
3. "Achieve access to preventive services for all Americans."

In order to meet these goals, 300 objectives were identified in 22 different priority areas under the broad categories of health promotion, health protection, and preventive services. The report challenged American citizens, organizations, and communities to change behaviors and environments to support good health for all. U.S. public health agencies were charged with the responsibility for overseeing the initiatives in each of the 22 priority areas. Box 10–1 lists the *Healthy People 2000* priority areas.

It is the hope of those involved in preparing the report that it will stimulate sustained support from a diverse base of individuals, groups, communities, associations, and governmental agencies to improve health outcomes. Particular

+++++++++++++++++++++++ ■ +++++++++++++++++++++++

Box 10–1   *Healthy People 2000* Priority Areas

Physical Activity and Fitness
Nutrition
Tobacco
Alcohol and Other Drugs
Family Planning
Mental Health and Mental Disorders
Violent and Abusive Behavior
Educational and Community-Based
  Programs
Unintentional Injuries
Occupational Safety and Health
Environmental Health
Food and Drug Safety
Oral Health

Maternal and Infant Health
Heart Disease and Stroke
Cancer
Diabetes and Chronic Disabling Condi-
  tions
HIV [human immunodeficiency virus]
  Infection
Sexually Transmitted Diseases
Immunization and Infectious Diseases
Clinical Preventive Services
Surveillance and Data Systems

(From U.S. Department of Health and Human Services. (1990). *Healthy people 2000:
Fact sheet.* Washington, D.C.: Author.)

emphasis is placed on improving access to health care by the poor, minorities, and rural populations, all of whom have borne "a disproportionate burden of suffering compared to the total population" (p. 1).

Health Beliefs and Health Behaviors

Health is affected by **health beliefs** and **health behaviors**. Health behaviors include those choices and habitual actions that promote or diminish health, such as eating habits, frequency of exercise, use of tobacco products and alcohol, sexual practices, and adequacy of rest and sleep.

Rosenstock (1966) was interested in determining why some people change their health behaviors, whereas others do not. For example, when the surgeon general's report on smoking first came out in 1960, some people immediately quit smoking. Over the years, condemning evidence against smoking has accumulated and been widely communicated, yet many intelligent people still smoke. Rosenstock wondered why. He formulated a model of health beliefs that illustrates how people behave in relationship to health maintenance activities. His model included three components:

1. An evaluation of one's vulnerability to a condition and the seriousness of that condition.
2. An evaluation of how effective the health maintenance behavior might be.
3. The presence of a trigger event that precipitates the health maintenance behavior.

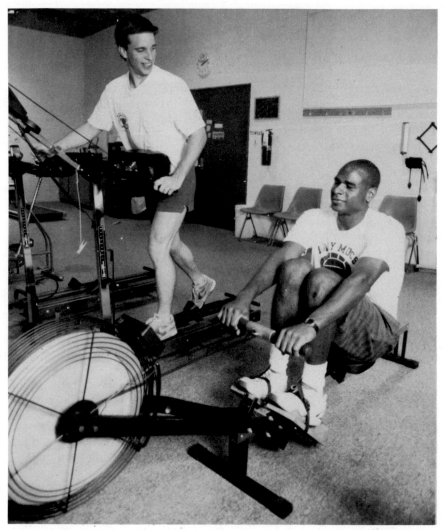

More Americans are engaging in health behaviors such as regular exercise.

Using Rosenstock's model, a man chooses to participate in a stop-smoking program depending on his perception of smoking-related heart disease and his personal susceptibility to it. If because of family history he believes he is very susceptible to heart disease and that it may cause his early death, and if he believes that not smoking will substantially reduce his risk, he is likely to participate in the program. If, however, the stop-smoking program is in an inconvenient location, scheduled at an inconvenient time, or not affordable, he is less likely to participate. If his older brother, who smokes, has a massive heart attack,

---

Box 10–2 Self-Assessment: Developing a Personal Plan for High-Level Wellness

Nurses' personal health behaviors send a powerful message to consumers of nursing care. Are you in a position to demonstrate that you practice what you preach? In answering the following questions, you can assess how well you are meeting your responsibilities in this area of nursing.

1. I weigh no more than five pounds over or under my ideal weight. T F

2. I eat a balanced diet including breakfast each day. T F

3. Of the total calories in my diet, less than 30 percent come from fat. T F

4. I exercise aerobically at least three times each week. T F

5. I get at least seven hours of sleep each night. T F

6. I do not smoke or use any other form of tobacco. T F

7. I use alcohol in moderation and take mood-altering medication only when prescribed by my physician. T F

8. I identify and control the sources of stress in my life. T F

9. I have a balanced life-style, with work and diversional activities both playing an important role. T F

10. I have friends, neighbors, and/or family members who are sources of social support for me. T F

11. I practice safe sex. T F

Directions for scoring: If you could not honestly answer "True" to all 11 questions, you need to set goals for yourself to enable you to do so.

1. On a piece of paper, begin your personal plan for high-level wellness. Write down at least two things you can do to address each "False" answer you gave to the self-assessment questions.

2. Share your health goals with one other person in your class. Make a contract with that person to serve as your "health coach."

3. Review your progress with your health coach at least once per week for the remainder of the term.

4. Begin your quest for high-level wellness today!

---

he may be motivated to attend the stop-smoking program in spite of the inconvenience and cost. The illness of his brother is what Rosenstock termed "a cue to action," or trigger event. A trigger event propels a previously unmotivated individual into changing health behaviors.

No one definition or theory of behavior can fully explain the complex state called health. It is important for nurses to recognize that health is relative, ever changing, affected by both genetics and environment, and affects the entire person physically, socially, psychologically, and spiritually.

Devising a Personal Plan for High-Level Wellness

Each individual nurse has a personal definition of health, certain health beliefs, and individual health behaviors. How nurses view health behaviors in their own lives has both direct and indirect impact on nursing practice. Sedentary nurses, for example, are less likely to encourage patients to become fit. This has a direct impact on their effectiveness as nurses. And since not exercising is a health behavior that most agree disqualifies people as healthy role models, being unfit also has an indirect effect by portraying a poor image of nursing.

Nurses have a professional responsibility to model positive health behaviors in their own lives, but nurses are people, too. Being or becoming a healthy role model may require some effort. Box 10-2 will help you get started.

Putting It All Together: Nursing

Nursing integrates concepts from person, environment, and health to form a meaningful whole. Nursing is an example of an open system that freely interacts with, influences, and is influenced by external and internal forces. Chapter 7 focused on a variety of definitions of nursing, and Chapter 9 discussed a number of beliefs about nursing. It will be helpful to review those chapters now.

Nursing is the provision of health care services that focus on maintaining, promoting, and restoring health. Nursing involves collaborating with patients and their families to help them cope and adapt to situations of disequilibrium in an effort to regain homeostasis. Nursing is also health and wellness promotion, including patient teaching to maximize rehabilitation and restoration of high-level wellness.

Nursing, a lifelong process, is integrally involved with people at points along the health-illness continuum. The purpose of nursing is to assist people in maintaining health, avoiding or minimizing disease and disability, restoring them to wellness, or assisting them to achieve a peaceful death. Nursing care is provided regardless of diagnosis, individual differences, age, beliefs, gender, sexual preference, or other factors. As a profession, nursing supports the value, dignity, and uniqueness of every person.

Nurses require advanced knowledge and skills; they also must care about their patients. Nursing requires concern, compassion, respect, and warmth as well as comprehensive, individualized planning of care in order to facilitate patients' growth toward wellness. Nursing links theory and research in an effort to answer difficult questions generated during nursing practice. Nursing's role is to assist patients to achieve health at the highest possible level.

CHAPTER SUMMARY

Nursing integrates three basic components—person, environment, and health—to form its focus. General systems theory and needs theory can be used to understand these components. Persons are viewed as unique open systems who are motivated by needs. Maslow organized human needs into a hierarchy consisting of five levels that range from basic physiological needs, which are common to all people, to self-actualization, which is attained by few. Environment consists of all the circumstances, influences, and conditions that affect an individual. The physical environment as well as family, cultural, social, and community environments have impact.

Health is dynamic and viewed as a continuum. There are numerous definitions of health. Nurses view health holistically, including its effect on an individual's physical, emotional, social, and spiritual functioning as well as the impact on the family. Health is affected by health beliefs and health behaviors.

Nursing integrates person, environment, and health into a meaningful whole. Nursing assists people to achieve health at the highest possible level, given their environmental and genetic constraints.

REVIEW/DISCUSSION QUESTIONS

1. Discuss general systems theory in relation to your family. What are the family equivalents of inputs, subsystems, suprasystems, outputs, evaluation, and feedback? Is your family an open or closed system?
2. Describe Maslow's hierarchy of needs and place yourself on the hierarchy today; one week ago; and when you were a senior in high school.
3. Write your own personal definition of health and share it with one other person. Evaluate your definition in terms of holism.
4. What are factors that influence an individual's personal health behaviors? Make a list of your health behaviors including those that promote health and those that diminish health. Analyze why you continue both the healthy and nonhealthy behaviors.
5. Conduct an assessment of your community in terms of one of the following: availability of jobs, quality of public education, availability of health services, environmental hazards, and quality of air and water. What is the impact of the factor you selected on the health of the community's citizens? What can you do to strengthen the environmental health of your community?
6. Look through the yellow pages of your local telephone book under "social services" and "organizations." What types of social support do you find that might be useful to patients?

REFERENCES

Broadhead, W. E., et al. (1983). The epidemiologic evidence for a relationship between social support and health. *American Journal of Epidemiology,* 117(5), 521–531.

Dunn, H. L. (1959). High-level wellness for man and society. *American Journal of Public Health,* 49(6), 786–792.

Flynn, J., and Heffron, P. (1984). *Nursing: From concept to practice.* East Norwalk, CT: Appleton & Lange.

Half of single moms get support. (1991). *Citizen-News* (Dalton, GA), October 14, 1991, p. 4A.

Holmes, T. H., and Rahe, R. H. (1967). The social readjustment rating scale. *Journal of Psychosomatic Research,* 11(2), 213–218.

Maslow, A. (1954). *Motivation and personality.* New York: Harper & Row.

Parsons, T. (1959). Definitions of health and illness in light of American values and social structure. In E. G. Jaco (Ed.), *Patients, physicians and illness* (pp. 165–187). New York: Free Press.

Rogers, C. (1961). *On becoming a person.* Boston: Houghton Mifflin.

Rosenstock, I. M. (1966). Why people use health services, part II. *Milbank Memorial Fund Quarterly,* 44(3), 94–124.

Smuts, J. C. (1926). *Holism and evolution.* New York: Macmillan.

U.S. Bureau of the Census. (1990). *Statistical abstract of the United States: 1990.* Washington, D.C.: Author.

U.S. Department of Health and Human Services. (1990). *Healthy people 2000: Fact sheet.* Washington, D.C.: Author.

von Bertalanffy, L. (1968). *General systems theory: Foundations, development, applications.* New York: George Braziller.

World Health Organization. (1947). *Constitution.* Geneva, Switzerland: Author.

SUGGESTED READINGS

Giger, J. N., et al. (1990). Contextual care: Religious considerations for culturally appropriate nursing care. *Advances in Clinical Care,* 5(4), 48–51.

Maslow, A. (1970). *Motivation and personality* (2nd. ed.). New York: Harper & Row.

McGuire, C. (1990). An overview of holistic nursing. *Imprint,* 37(3), 73–74.

Phillip, J. R. (1990). The different views of health. *Nursing Science Quarterly,* 3(3), 103–104.

Todd, T. (1990). Holistic nursing: A new paradigm for practice. *Imprint,* 37(3), 75, 78, 80.

Wolffe, H. G. (1950). *Life stress and body diseases.* Baltimore: Williams & Wilkins.

Chapter

11

*Theory as a Basis for Professional Nursing**

Pamela J. Holder

CHAPTER OBJECTIVES

What students should be able to do after studying this chapter:

1. Differentiate among conceptual frameworks, models, and theories.
2. Describe selected nonnursing theories including implications for nursing practice.
3. Compare and contrast selected models of nursing theory.
4. Explore the relationship of theory to nursing research and practice.
5. Describe how nurses can participate in theory development.
6. Explain the importance of theory-based nursing practice.

---

* The author would like to thank Ardyce Mercier, R.N., B.S.N., for her suggestions in writing this chapter.

VOCABULARY BUILDING

People and terms to know:

adaptation theory
concept
conceptual framework
coping mechanisms
developmental theory
growth
Virginia Henderson
model

Betty Neuman
Florence Nightingale
Dorothea Orem
peer review process
phenomena,
   phenomenon
proposition
Martha Rogers

Sister Callista Roy
stage theory
stressors
systems theory
theory

*A*s a science, nursing is in its infancy. Professional nurses are aware of this and conscious of the need for both nursing theory development and theory-based practice. As nursing comes of age, not only as a practice discipline but also as a scholarly discipline, there will be increasing interest in delineating the theory base for nursing. Some believe that theory development is "the most crucial task facing nursing" (Chinn and Jacobs 1978).

There are three reasons for this interest in theory. First, as seen in Chapter 6, one criterion for professions is a distinct body of knowledge upon which practice is based. There has long been interest in identifying a body of nursing knowledge that is essential to professional nursing practice. Theory development contributes to knowledge building and is seen as a means of establishing nursing as a profession.

Second, commitment to practice based on sound, reliable knowledge is intrinsically valuable to nursing. That is to say, knowledge is desirable by its very nature. The growth and enrichment of theory in and of itself is an important goal for nursing, as a scholarly discipline, to pursue.

And third, theory is useful. Nursing practice settings are complex, and the amount of data available to nurses is virtually endless. Nurses must analyze a tremendous amount of information about each patient and decide what to do. If a theory helps practicing nurses categorize and understand what is going on in nursing practice, if it helps them predict patients' responses to nursing care, and if it is helpful in clinical decision making, it is useful as a guide to practice.

This chapter defines and differentiates among various terms used in discussing theory, examines several theories that have implications for nursing practice, and briefly reviews several theoretical nursing models.

What Is Theory?

Theories are general explanations scholars use to explain, predict, control, and understand commonly occurring events. Theories provide a method of classifying and organizing data in a logical and meaningful manner.

Perhaps the best-known theory is Einstein's theory of relativity, which states that "matter and energy are equivalent and form the basis for nuclear energy and that space and time are relative rather than absolute concepts" (Flexner 1980, p. 743). While this theory may not be especially meaningful to non-physicists, it is clear that it is a logically connected group of general statements used as principles of explanation for a class of events. And that is a good working definition of theory.

It is important to remember that a theory is an explanation that has not yet been disproved. Until disproved, it may be useful. When more knowledge becomes available, theories that are no longer useful are discarded, and new ones are generated.

Theories are best understood as preliminary explanations that reflect the current understanding of events. For the purposes of this chapter, **theory** is defined as "a set of propositions used to describe, explain, predict, and control events."

Useful Definitions

Several other terms and descriptions are useful in discussing our definition of theory:

- *Set.* A group of circumstances, situations, and so on, joined and treated as a whole. In mathematics, for example, negative numbers are treated as a set.
- *Propositions.* Statements about how two or more concepts are related. For example, "Heart rate increases as anxiety increases" is a proposition.
- *Concepts.* Abstract classification of data. For example, "temperature" is a concept.
- *Describe.* To tell about in detail.
- *Explain.* To offer reasons for.
- *Predict.* To foretell.
- *Control.* To exercise a regulating influence over.
- *Phenomenon.* An occurrence or incident; event.

The Four Functions of Theory

Each of the four functions of theory—description, explanation, prediction, and control—represents a different phase of theory development. The perfect theory would do all four things well. However, no perfect theories exist in any discipline. Because science is evolving and because humans are fallible, that is, liable to make mistakes, theories are always changing. At any given point in time in a given area of study, theories in all stages of development can be found. This is certainly true in nursing, as will be seen later in this chapter.

Some theories are specifically designed as explanations, without having any intention of predicting. An example is the theory of evolution. Other theories are designed to predict but do not provide control. For example, plate tectonic theory may someday contribute to the ability of geologists to predict earthquakes, but it is doubtful that man can ever control them. The world of theory building is an imperfect but dynamic one, always in a state of evolution to higher levels of scientific thought.

Conceptual Frameworks and Models

People often use the terms **theory** and **conceptual framework** interchangeably. The term **model** may be used in the same discussion. This imprecise usage of terms results in a state of confusion in which terms have very little meaning. Nurses need a clear understanding of these terms to participate effectively in theory building.

CONCEPTUAL FRAMEWORKS

Conceptual frameworks and theories overlap somewhat since both utilize concepts as major developmental components (Polit and Hungler 1991). Fawcett (1984) defined a conceptual framework as "a set of concepts and those assumptions that integrate them into a meaningful configuration" (p. 2). A conceptual framework is not a theory. A conceptual framework is a less formal and somewhat more abstract explanatory framework than a theory. It is the degree of formality and abstractness that differentiates between theories and conceptual frameworks (Fawcett 1984).

MODELS

Model is a third term that frequently appears in nursing literature. A key idea in understanding models is that they are not the real thing but attempt to make concrete the concepts they represent. A model replicates reality with various degrees of precision. The symbolic form of a model may consist of words, mathematical notations, or physical material, as in a model airplane. Models use a minimal amount of language. They are useful in understanding concepts that cannot be directly observed or visualized. A visit to a planetarium, for example, allows one to gain an understanding of the universe, a phenomenon so vast that it could not otherwise be grasped. In theory building, theories are often graphically represented by means of models.

Nonnursing Theories Useful in Nursing Practice

The contributions of many theorists outside of nursing formed the knowledge base for nursing practice for many years. New disciplines are often slow to develop their own theories, and nursing was no exception. Even now, theories from the physical, biological, social, and behavioral sciences, in addition to more recent nursing models and theories, are used extensively in nursing practice.

Nurses use theories developed outside of nursing to understand, explain, and intervene in relationships among people. They also use these theories to understand, explain, and predict changes in health and the environment. Adaptation, systems, stress, developmental, role, and communication theories are all heavily used in nursing.

Several nonnursing theories used by nurses are covered elsewhere in this textbook: Systems theory is discussed in some detail in Chapter 10; Selye's (1976) stress theory is covered in Chapter 18; communication theory is discussed in Chapter 19; and theories of moral development are explored in Chapter 20. Even though they are not nursing theories, these theories are all relevant and useful in nursing practice.

Additional nonnursing theories that nurses use extensively are adaptation theories and developmental theories. These will be discussed to show how nonnursing theories enhance nursing practice.

Adaptation Theories

Adaptation theories are based on systems theory and view change in terms of cause and effect. People have to adjust to changes every day. Adaptation theories provide ways to understand how balance is maintained in the face of change and the possible effects of disturbed equilibrium. Adaptation theories have been widely used to explain, predict, and control biological responses of people.

In adaptation theory, the human body is seen as functioning as a whole. All body cells are affected by the activities of other cells. This communication is made possible because all cells are surrounded by the same fluids (e.g., blood, lymph, and interstitial fluid), which form an internal environment for the entire body. The internal environment provides a medium for the exchange of nutrients and wastes, and it provides a stable physiochemical environment for cell function.

Normal cells require that constancy of the body's internal environment be maintained within relatively narrow limits. These limits must be maintained even though the body is constantly responding to interactions between internal and external environments. Stability of the internal environment is maintained through feedback mechanisms. As changes occur in the internal environment, regulatory systems, such as the nervous system and the endocrine system, respond to keep the change within limits the body can tolerate. The word "homeostasis" was originally used by Cannon (1929) to describe a state of relative constancy of the body's internal environment due to the action of regulatory mechanisms. Constancy does not imply that the internal environment is static. It is constantly changing, but *relative* equilibrium is maintained. For example, when blood sugar drops, the endocrine system responds by secreting cortisone, which both decreases the rate at which cells use glucose and stimulates the conversion of amino acids into glucose. These compensatory actions cause blood sugar to rise. If blood sugar rises above acceptable limits, the endocrine system again responds by increasing insulin secretion, which increases the rate of glucose uptake by cells. These compensatory actions cause the blood glucose level to fall. In both situations, homeostasis is maintained.

STRESSORS

In adaptation theories, stimuli that tend to disturb equilibrium are called **stressors**. Stressors are anything that create change in the external or internal environments, thus placing demands on the body to compensate. Potential external stressors include such factors as environmental temperature and noise level. Internal stressors include such factors as hunger, joy, and infection. Stressors may be beneficial or harmful, but they all require the body to respond. The response of the body is called adaptation. As mentioned in Chapter 10, the ability to adapt effectively to changes in life events is believed to be a major factor in determining a person's potential for health or disease (Holmes and Rahe 1967).

COPING

One way that a person adapts is by means of coping mechanisms. **Coping mechanisms** are psychological devices a person uses when threat is perceived. A person's reaction to stress therefore occurs on two levels: (1) the cognitive level where appraisal of the stress occurs and resulting psychological coping methods are begun and (2) the physiological level where compensatory reactions occur.

USING ADAPTATION THEORIES IN NURSING PRACTICE

Adaptation theories are useful in nursing practice because they allow nurses to assess patients' stressors and abilities to cope. Illness is stressful, as is being hospitalized or otherwise unable to meet one's usual responsibilities. But not all people react the same to these stressors. Nurses familiar with adaptation theories can help patients realistically appraise their stressors, examine their usual coping responses, and if necessary, learn new ones. If a patient is newly diagnosed with a chronic health problem, such as diabetes, nurses using adaptation theories will help patients learn to anticipate and cope with the stress of life changes created by the disease.

Adaptation theories are also useful to nurses working in the area of health promotion. Predicting and eliminating stressors and strengthening coping abilities are valuable steps in promoting health.

Developmental Theories

Developmental theories, sometimes called theories of growth and development, assume that human growth is linear, has predictable irreversible direction, occurs in degrees (stages), and progresses toward maximum potential (Chin 1980). Nurses use developmental theories in planning future-oriented nursing interventions because knowing developmental theories makes it possible for nurses to describe and predict patient behavior.

GROWTH

In developmental theory, **growth** is defined as an increase in physical size and shape to a point of optimal maturity (Billingham 1982, p. 4). Because no change occurs in isolation, each modifies the individual as a whole. Thus, assessment of maturation requires data about all aspects of the individual—physical, intellectual, psychological, and social.

Growth is continuous and orderly, with regular trends in direction. For example, the direction of motor growth proceeds from the head to the extremities, and from the central part of the body toward the periphery. As a result, a child sits before standing and can control shoulder movements before those of the fingers. Although growth is patterned and continuous, it is not always smooth and gradual. Different aspects of a person develop at different rates. Adolescents, for example, sometimes experience pain in the long bones of their legs when growth spurts occur. This results when leg muscles do not develop as rapidly as the bones grow.

DEVELOPMENT

While growth is quantitative, development is related to functional changes that are usually qualitative. As with growth, multiple factors influence development, and authorities have differing opinions about the relative importance of maturational versus environmental influences on development. All aspects of human development are interrelated and integrated. Because development proceeds in a sequential pattern, realistic expectations for behavior can be predicted for various stages of development.

There are a number of theories about how development occurs. The classical approach is called "**stage theory**." This theory proposes that all people pass through a number of levels (stages). The stages differ in quality and duration, but the order is fixed, and a person cannot skip a stage or reorder the stages. Mastering the tasks of one stage forms the basis for mastering the tasks of the next. Individuals differ in the speed with which they move through these stages and in the level of development that they finally reach.

Various developmental or stage theorists such as Erikson, Kohlberg, and Piaget have described particular aspects of human development. Erikson described the stages of human development from birth to death, including the developmental "tasks" that must be accomplished at each stage. Kohlberg explored the stages of moral development. Piaget (1969) delineated the cognitive (intellectual) stages of development.

USING DEVELOPMENTAL THEORIES IN NURSING PRACTICE

The value of developmental theories in nursing practice is undeniable. They are particularly useful in assessing whether a child's growth pattern and developmental stage are keeping pace with his chronological age. There are broad

---

Research Note

Nursing students are introduced to a number of nursing and non-nursing theories during the educational process. Dr. Blenda Smith of the State University of New York at Binghamton, was interested in knowing more about how students link the theory they learn in class with the actual practice of nursing. She designed a study to test the usefulness of two learning strategies called Vee heuristics and concept mapping. These two learning strategies were designed to help students identify and make connections between the scientific theories they learn in class and basic nursing and assessment skills. Forty-two baccalaureate nursing students participated in the study. During the semester, some students were taught basic nursing skills using traditional methods and some were taught using the Vee heuristics and concept mapping. Then they were tested. Students who were taught using the experimental methods scored significantly higher than other students in identifying scientific principles underlying basic nursing skills.

(From Smith, B.E. (1992). Linking theory and practice in teaching basic nursing skills. *Journal of Nursing Education*, 31(1), 16–23.)

---

ranges of "normal" growth and development, but when children fall outside of these ranges, medical and nursing interventions are often required.

Growth and development theories are also quite useful to nurses teaching parents about what to expect from their children at certain ages and stages. Sometimes parents expect young children to have abilities beyond their level of maturation; for example, they may become frustrated when their nine-month-old is not toilet trained. Using developmental theories, nurses can explain that children do not have sufficient control of the muscles involved in toilet training until two years or even older. If the mother of a five-year-old child is concerned that the child tells "lies," it is helpful for the nurse to explain that a child of this age often has difficulty separating fact from fantasy and is not simply being "bad."

When studying developmental theories, nurses should remember that although knowing characteristic traits, developmental tasks, and stages is useful, each individual is unique in style and behavior.

Models of Nursing Theory

Until the 1950s, nursing knowledge was principally derived from social, biological, and medical theories. With the exception of the work of Florence Nightingale (1859), who—as you learned in Chapter 1—was ahead of her time, nursing theory began with the publication of Hildegarde Peplau's *Interpersonal Relations in Nursing* (1952). Peplau was the first to describe the phases of the nurse-patient relationship and the factors that influence that relationship.

With recognition of the importance that theory plays in developing a scientific discipline, and awareness that theories in other disciplines were insufficient to describe nursing, nurses began to develop their own theories. Descriptions of nursing and nursing models evolved from the personal, professional, and educational experiences of nurse theorists and reflect their perception of "ideal" nursing practice. Most theoretical models in nursing are based on the major concepts basic to nursing discussed in Chapter 10. They describe the nature of nursing, the individual recipient of care (patient), the context of nurse-patient interactions (environment), and health (Fawcett 1984). This section presents an overview of selected nursing models.

Nightingale's Environmental Model

Florence Nightingale conceptualized disease as a reparative process and described the nurse's role as manipulating the environment to facilitate this process. Her ideas regarding ventilation, warmth, light, diet, cleanliness, variety, and noise are presented in her classic nursing textbook *Notes on Nursing* (1859). Nightingale's intent was to describe nursing and provide guidelines for nursing practice and education. She defined nursing as a service to people and viewed a healthful environment as critically important.

MAJOR CONCEPTS AS DEFINED BY NIGHTINGALE

Patient	Individuals; responsible, creative, in control of their lives and health, and desiring good health.
Health	A state of being well; using one's powers to the fullest.
Illness	The reaction of nature against the conditions in which we have placed ourselves. Disease is a reparative mechanism, an effort of nature to remedy a process of decay.
Environment	External to the person, but affecting the health of both sick and well persons. The environment, one of the chief sources of infection, must include fresh air, fresh water, efficient drainage, cleanliness, and light.
Nursing	A service to people intended to relieve pain and suffering. The goal of nursing is to promote the reparative process by manipulating the environment.

Henderson's Model

Virginia Henderson viewed nursing as an art and a discipline separate from medicine. As discussed in Chapter 7, she believed that the "unique function of the nurse . . . is to assist the individual, sick or well in the performance of those activities contributing to health or its recovery (or a peaceful death) that he would perform unaided if he had the necessary strength, will or knowledge" (Henderson 1966, p. 15).

Box 11–1 **Fourteen Basic Needs of the Patient**

1. Breathe normally.
2. Eat and drink adequately.
3. Eliminate body wastes.
4. Move and maintain desirable position.
5. Sleep and rest.
6. Select suitable clothes—dress and undress.
7. Maintain body temperature within normal range by adjusting clothing and modifying the environment.
8. Keep the body clean and well groomed and protect the integument (skin).
9. Avoid dangers in the environment and avoid injuring others.
10. Communicate with others in expressing emotions, needs, fears, or opinions.
11. Worship according to one's faith.
12. Work in such a way that there is a sense of accomplishment.
13. Play or participate in various forms of recreation.
14. Learn, discover, or satisfy the curiosity that leads to normal development and health and use the available health facilities.

(From Henderson, V. (1966). *The nature of nursing: A definition and its implications for practice, research, and education.* New York: Macmillan.)

Henderson viewed the nurse's role as that of a substitute for the patient, a helper to the patient, and a partner with the patient. She listed 14 basic needs that nurses should assist patients with if patients are unable to perform them unaided. These basic needs compose Henderson's components of nursing care. Box 11–1 contains Henderson's 14 basic needs of patients.

MAJOR CONCEPTS AS DEFINED BY HENDERSON

Patient	Individual; requires assistance to achieve health and independence or a peaceful death. Individuals will achieve or maintain health if they have the necessary strength, will, or knowledge. The individual and family are viewed as a unit.
Health	A quality of life basic to human functioning. Equated with independence.
Illness	A lack of independence.
Environment	All external conditions and influences that affect life and development.
Nursing	A unique function of assisting sick or well individuals in a complementary role. The goal of nursing is to help the individual gain independence as rapidly as possible.

Orem's Self-Care Model

Dorothea Orem first published her concepts of nursing in 1959, refining them in 1980 and 1985 (Orem 1980, 1985). Originally, she designed her model for nursing school curricula to help students differentiate among nursing actions. This model focuses on identifying the patient's self-care needs and nursing actions designed to meet the patient's needs.

Today Orem's model is widely used in both nursing education and practice. It is useful for comprehensive assessment and analysis of individuals. The model is very useful for nurses working with chronically ill patients in the hospital or in other settings. It can also be used in health maintenance and illness prevention.

MAJOR CONCEPTS AS DEFINED BY OREM

Patient	Individual unable to continuously maintain self-care in sustaining life and health, in recovering from disease or injury, or in coping with their effects.
Health	Ability to meet self-care demands that contribute to the maintenance and promotion of structural integrity, functioning, and development.
Illness	Occurs when an individual is incapable of maintaining self-care as a result of health-related limitations.
Environment	Any setting in which a patient has unmet self-care needs.
Nursing	A service of deliberately selected and performed actions to assist individuals to maintain self-care, including structural integrity, functioning, and development.

Roy's Adaptation Model

Sister Callista Roy has continuously expanded her model from its inception in 1970 to the present (Roy 1970). Roy's model is based on general systems theory. She focused on the individual as a biopsychosocial adaptive system and described nursing as a humanistic discipline that "places emphasis on the person's own coping abilities" (Roy 1984, p. 32). According to Roy, the individual and the environment are sources of stimuli that require modification to promote adaptation. When the demands of environmental stimuli are too great or the person's adaptive mechanisms are too low, the person's behavioral responses are ineffective for coping. Effective adaptive responses promote the integrity of the individual by conserving energy and promoting the survival, growth, reproduction, and mastery of the human system.

MAJOR CONCEPTS AS DEFINED BY ROY

Patient	Person or family with unusual stressors or ineffective coping mechanisms.

Health ·	State and process of being and becoming integrated and whole.
Illness	A lack of integration.
Environment	All conditions, circumstances, and influences surrounding and affecting the development and behavior of persons or families.
Nursing	Promotion of the patient's effective coping and progress toward integration.

Roger's Model: Science of Unitary Human Beings

Martha Rogers first described her science of unitary human man in 1970 (Rogers 1970). She sought to develop a science unique to nursing and a basis for nursing practice, believing that without this body of knowledge, there was no need for higher education in nursing (Rogers 1991). Rogers defined *nursing* as a noun—a body of knowledge necessary for practice. She called this organized body of abstract knowledge "nursing science" and considered the imaginative and creative use of knowledge in practice as "art." As both science and art, nursing is described as a learned profession that focuses on the nature and direction of human development and human betterment. Rogers viewed the interaction between humans and their environments as the central focus of nursing.

MAJOR CONCEPTS AS DEFINED BY ROGERS

Patient	"Unitary human being"; human field; an irreducible, pan-dimensional energy field identified by pattern and manifesting characteristics that are specific to the whole and that cannot be predicted from knowledge of the parts.
Health*	Occurs when patterns of living are in harmony with environmental change.
Illness*	Occurs when patterns of living conflict with environmental change and are deemed unacceptable.
Environment	Environmental field; an irreducible, pan-dimensional energy field identified by pattern and integral with the human field.
Nursing	A learned profession; a science and an art. The science of nursing is an organized body of abstract knowledge; a synthesis of facts and ideas. The art of nursing refers to the use of this knowledge in the delivery of nursing care for human betterment.

---

* Rogers viewed the terms *health* and *illness* as value laden, arbitrarily defined, and culturally infused. She saw them not as dichotomous but as part of the same continuum.

Neuman's Health Care Systems Model

Betty Neuman developed a systems model in response to student requests. They expressed a need to focus on breadth rather than depth in understanding human variables in nursing problems. First published in 1972, this model was refined and published in its present form in *The Neuman Systems Model* in 1989 (Neuman 1989). This is a complex systems model, with a focus on stress reactions and stress reduction. This comprehensive model depicts the patient as the core of a circle with several protective layers. The patient is continuously exposed to internal and external stressors, which require lines of defense and reactions. Nursing interventions can occur before or after stressors and at three levels of prevention: primary, secondary, and tertiary.

Neuman's model is applicable to all phases of the nursing process. It can be applied across all clinical areas and is especially useful for individuals and families. It is a holistic approach because each system or subsystem cannot be isolated; rather, the influence of each system on the whole must be considered. The three levels of prevention are useful guides for planning nursing interventions.

MAJOR CONCEPTS AS DEFINED BY NEUMAN

Patient	Open system seeking balance and harmony. Composite of physiological, psychological, sociocultural, and developmental variables and viewed as a whole. Individuals, families, and communities.
Health	Dynamic equilibrium of the normal line of defense.
Illness	Due to reaction to stressors with lines of resistance.
Environment	Internal and external stressors and resistance factors.
Nursing	Reduction of stressors through prevention activities at three levels.

Ongoing Model Development

Each of these nurse theorists has made significant contributions to the development of nursing's unique body of knowledge. Offering an assortment of perspectives, these models of nursing theory vary in their level of abstraction and their conceptualization of the patient, health, illness, environment, and nursing. To describe any of the existing nursing models as a "theory" may be going too far. As in other disciplines, models of nursing theory are found at various stages of development, but no comprehensive theory is yet in existence. Some nurse theorists continue to develop and refine their models, whereas others no longer actively work on theory development. Each theoretical model has followers who continue to expand, clarify, and refine the original work.

In the future, nursing models must clearly differentiate activities that are unique to nursing and different from other disciplines. Nursing must distinguish a separate body of knowledge or a distinct manner of applying shared knowl-

---

Box 11–2   Using Nursing Science in Practice: Observations

In this abstract system [the Rogerian model], the key is always listening to clients and allowing exploration of whatever they bring. Modalities I use to assist people in the discovery process and in creating change include therapeutic touch (TT), imagery, hypnosis, poetry, music, humor, bibliotherapy, and journaling.

Therapeutic touch is based on the therapeutic use of hands, a human function that goes back to depictions in cave paintings calculated to be more than 15,000 years old. The basic skill in therapeutic touch is centering, a process of finely focusing one's consciousness. The centered nurse is attuned to the cli-ent's patterning process and with the client can assist in identifying direction for creative change. The goal is to regain balance, or repatterning.

My practice includes working with undergraduate nursing students in the home health setting, directing the Therapeutic Touch and Centering Clinic at the Arizona State University College of Nursing, and private practice. Using Rogers's science of unitary human beings in practice is health promoting, fulfilling, and exciting—for the nurse as well as the client!

(Courtesy of Katherine E. Rapacz, Ph.D., R.N., Arizona State University, 1992.)

---

edge. Future nursing theorists will strive to describe, explain, predict, and control patient outcomes. Theories will facilitate the prevention of illness, and the maintenance, promotion, and restoration of the patient's optimum health potential.

Relationship of Theory to Nursing Practice and Research

Nurses have traditionally based their practices on intuition, experience, or "the way I was taught." These methods lead to unimaginative, rote, and stereotypical practice. To move nursing practice forward and to improve the quality of nursing care, theory development and research were undertaken.

Theory-Based Practice

How is theory translated into practice? The answer to that question lies with theory-based practice. Theory-based practice enables nurses to challenge conventional views of patients, the health-illness continuum, and traditional nursing interventions. Theory-based practice encourages hypothesis formation, testing of hypotheses, drawing conclusions about nursing actions, and evaluating nursing actions.

Nurses who engage in theory-based practice must feed their findings back to nurse theorists and nurse researchers for theory, research, and practice to continue to energize each other and advance the science of nursing. Box 11–2 contains the observations of a nurse who uses Rogers's science of unitary human beings as a basis for her teaching and practice.

Research

Nursing research is conducted to test and refine nursing's developing scientific base. Research is the best means to test and validate the usefulness of knowledge necessary for nursing practice. Ultimately, research will enable nurses to reliably predict how nursing actions influence patient outcomes. Research is the future of nursing and is so important that an entire chapter in this textbook is devoted to understanding the research process.

It is important for nurses to understand that theory, nursing practice, and research are interrelated. Each stimulates, improves, and advances the others. Figure 11–1 illustrates the circularity of theory, research, and practice in nursing.

How Nurses Can Participate in Theory Development

Theory development is not a mysterious activity, nor is it restricted to a few nursing scholars. To the extent that nurses continue to think, read, study, and develop nursing practice, they are *all* scholars of nursing.

Many nurses have developed their ideas about nursing and continue to develop nursing assumptions based on experience, observation, and reading. Most nurses do not talk explicitly about their personal theories, although these theories probably influence the way these individuals practice nursing. Personal theories, however, tend to be incomplete or inconsistent. Therefore, using personal theory as a basis for practice is probably ineffective.

Public, systematic development of nursing theory is necessary to advance nursing. Nurses who devise theories of nursing must present them for public review by nursing colleagues, thus engaging in the **peer review process** essential to advancing theory development.

Theory building involves discovery and creativity. The aspiring theorist who approaches theory construction in a mechanical way through structured procedures will have limited success. While it is possible to teach specific theory-building techniques, how to facilitate creativity and originality is unknown. It has been said, "You can teach someone how to look, but not how to see; how to search, but not how to find" (Rosenberg 1978, p. 2). A sense of imagination, playfulness, and participation is essential not only for theorists but also for readers who seek to understand theories.

In addition to imagination, developing and presenting theories require personal discipline. Novel ideas tend to occur in a vague, disconnected, and tenuous form (Mills 1959). Self-discipline is required to work with the idea, develop it, and express it in written form for others to review.

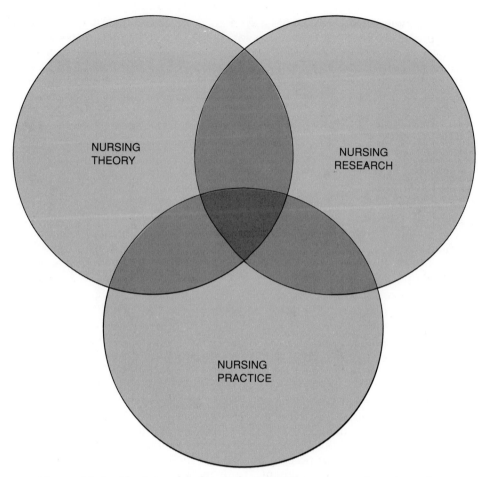

Figure 11–1 The interrelatedness of nursing theory, research, and practice.

Astute observations and clinical interventions of nurses in practice settings can advance progress toward a distinct knowledge base for nursing. Nursing theorists rely on practicing nurses to test the usefulness of theories. Such clinical investigations cannot take place without the widespread support of practicing nurses who recognize the importance of theory-based practice. Professional nurses must participate in research investigations whenever possible. Their insights and observations about patients and nursing care provide invaluable contributions to nursing theory.

CHAPTER SUMMARY

Theory improves nursing practice by describing, explaining, predicting, and controlling phenomena of interest to nurses. Nurses who have and use theoretical knowledge are more likely to be reliably effective than those using trial and error, intuition, or ritual. Nurses who base their practices on theory can justify their decisions and explain them to others. This facilitates the transmission of nursing knowledge to students and neophytes in the profession as well as to those outside the profession.

Theory allows professional autonomy by guiding the practice, education, and research functions of the profession. The study of theory helps develop analytical skills, challenges thinking, and clarifies values and assumptions.

Building a sound nursing knowledge base requires that nurses test theory in practice. Contributions of practicing nurses through their active participation in research are of significant value to the development of nursing theory.

When nursing develops its own theory, validates research knowledge in the practice setting, and relies on this knowledge to direct nursing practice, it will be recognized as an independent, autonomous profession. At that point, nursing will no longer rely on knowledge from other disciplines but will use its own knowledge base, called nursing science, to guide nursing practice.

REVIEW/DISCUSSION QUESTIONS

1. Why is theory development important to the profession of nursing?
2. From the brief summaries given, do any of the nursing theoretical models described in this chapter appeal to you? Do any evoke a negative response from you? Identify the attractive and unattractive features of each.
3. Recognizing that your understanding of nursing theories is preliminary, make some predictions about how nurses using each model might behave.
4. Interview nurses to determine what nonnursing and nursing theories and theoretical models they use. Ask how theory is useful in their practices.

REFERENCES

Billingham, K. (1982). *Developmental psychology for the health care professions.* Boulder: Westview Press.

Cannon, W. (1929). The sympathetic division of the autonomic system in relation to homeostasis. *Archives of Neurological Psychology, 22,* 282–294.

Chin, R. (1980). The utility of systems models and developmental models for practitioners. In J. Riehl and C. Roy (Eds.), *Conceptual models for nursing practice* (2nd ed.) (pp. 21–37). New York: Appleton-Century-Crofts.

Chinn, P., and Jacobs, M. (1978). A model for theory development in nursing. *Advances in Nursing Science,* 1(1), 1–11.

Fawcett, J. (1984). *Analysis and evaluation of conceptual models of nursing.* Philadelphia: F.A. Davis.

Flexner, S. B. (Ed.). (1980). *The Random House dictionary.* New York: Random House.

Henderson, V. (1966). *The nature of nursing: A definition and its implications for practice, research, and education.* New York: Macmillan.

Holmes, T., and Rahe, R. (1967). The social readjustment rating scale. *Journal of Psychosomatic Research,* 11(2), 213–218.

Mills, C. (1959). On intellectual craftsmanship. In L. Gross (Ed.). *Symposium on sociological theory*. Evanston, IL: Row, Peterson.

Neuman, B. (1989). *The Neuman systems model: Application to nursing theory and practice*. Norwalk: Appleton-Century-Crofts.

Nightingale, F. (1969 facsimile of 1859 edition). *Notes on nursing: What it is and what it is not*. New York: Dover Publications.

Orem, D. (1980). *Nursing: Concepts of practice* (2nd ed.). New York: McGraw-Hill.

Orem, D. (1985). *Nursing: Concepts of practice* (3rd ed.). New York: McGraw-Hill.

Peplau, H. (1952). *Interpersonal relations in nursing*. New York: G.P. Putnam's Sons.

Piaget, J. (1969). *The psychology of the child*. New York: Basic Books.

Polit, D., and Hungler, B. (1991). *Nursing research: Principles and methods* (4th ed.). Philadelphia: J.B. Lippincott.

Rapacz, K. (1992). Personal communication.

Rogers, M. (1970). *An introduction to the theoretical basis of nursing*. Philadelphia: F.A. Davis.

Rogers, M. (1991). Personal communication.

Rosenberg, J. (1978). *The practice of philosophy*. Englewood Cliffs, NJ: Prentice-Hall.

Roy, Sr. C. (1970). Adaptation: A conceptual framework for nursing. *Nursing Outlook*, 18, 254–257.

Roy, Sr. C. (1984). *Introduction to nursing: An adaptation model* (2nd ed.). Englewood Cliffs, NJ: Prentice-Hall.

Selye, H. (1976). *The stress of life*. New York: McGraw-Hill.

SUGGESTED READINGS

Andreoli, K., and Thompson, C. (1977). The nature of science in nursing. *Image*, 9, 32–37.

Auger, J. (1976). *Behavioral systems and nursing*. Englewood Cliffs, NJ: Prentice-Hall.

Baltes, P., Reese, H., and Nesselroade, J. (1977). *Life-span developmental psychology: Introduction to research methods*. Monterey, CA: Brookes/Cole.

Brodbeck, M. (1968). Models, meaning and theories. In M. Brodbeck (Ed.), *Readings in the philosophy of the social sciences* (pp. 579–600). New York: Macmillan.

Chinn, P., and Jacobs, M. (1987). *Theory and nursing—a systematic approach* (2nd ed.). St. Louis: C.V. Mosby.

Chinn, P., and Kramer, M. (1991). *Theory and nursing: A systematic approach* (3rd ed.). St. Louis: C.V. Mosby.

Erikson, E. (1968). *Identity, youth and crisis*. New York: W.W. Norton.

Freud, S. (1949). *An outline of psychoanalysis*. New York: W.W. Norton.

Kohlberg, L. (1978). The cognitive developmental approach to moral education. In P. Scharf (Ed.), *Readings in moral education* (pp. 36–51). Minneapolis, MN: Winston Press.

Maslow, A. (1968). *Toward a psychology of being* (2nd ed.). New York: Van Nostrand Reinhold.

Newman, M. (1979). *Theory development in nursing.* Philadelphia: F.A. Davis.

Sills, G., and Hall, J. (1977). A general systems perspective for nursing. In J. Hall and B. Weaver (Eds.), *Distributive nursing practice: A systems approach to community health.* Philadelphia: J.B. Lippincott.

Sullivan, H. S. (1953). *The collected works.* New York: W.W. Norton.

von Bertalanffy, L. (1968). *General systems theory: Foundations, development, applications.* New York: George Braziller.

Walker, L., and Avant, K. (1983). *Strategies for theory construction in nursing.* Norwalk: Appleton-Century-Crofts.

Chapter

Understanding Nursing Research

Carol T. Bush

CHAPTER OBJECTIVES

What students should be able to do after studying this chapter:

1. Differentiate between problem solving and research.
2. List the steps in the research process.
3. Discuss contributions nursing research has made to nursing practice and to health care.
4. Describe the relationship of nursing research to nursing theory and practice.
5. Describe the four phases in the development of nursing research.
6. Identify sources of support for nursing research.
7. Discuss the roles of nurses in research.

VOCABULARY BUILDING

Terms to know:

conceptual framework
confidentiality
experimental design
generalizable
hypothesis
informed consent

infrastructure
institutional review
  board
nonexperimental
  design
nursing research

peer review
phenomena
population
problem solving
protocol
qualitative research

quantitative research   research process   subjects
reliable   sample   valid
replication

Most college students' only exposure to research is in introductory psychology or sociology courses where they are subjects in a professor's research project. All they see of research are the boring forms they fill out or the nonsense syllables they memorize. This kind of orientation leads them to wonder what research could have to do with their ability to care for patients.

Before students of nursing write research off altogether, they should consider an example or two. Consider premature infants—those wriggling little creatures that look so frail and sometimes weigh fewer than three pounds. Nurses are the key to life or death for some of those fragile beings.

What do nurses need to know to tip the balance in favor of life for those babies? A nurse at the University of Florida, Gene Cranston Anderson (Anderson, Gill, and Bodo 1988), has considered this question. She wondered what impact sucking had on survival of premature babies. Anderson wondered if, in addition to obtaining nutrition, sucking was helpful in other ways. Most babies like pacifiers even though they provide no nourishment. Are pacifiers good for premature babies? Do premature infants rest more if they are given pacifiers, or does sucking on pacifiers take too much of their limited stores of energy?

Anderson undertook a research project to answer these questions. She and her research partner had called sucking a pacifier "non-nutritive sucking" in an earlier study (Measel and Anderson 1979). Anderson (Anderson, Gill, and Bodo 1988) found that premature babies who engaged in nonnutritive sucking behavior decreased their crying activity. Aside from the pleasant atmosphere in the newborn nursery that peaceful infants created, the babies that cried less gained weight faster and went home earlier than babies who were not given pacifiers. Going home quicker saves money for parents, insurance companies, and hospitals. Other possible advantages of earlier discharge from the hospital include quicker and more effective bonding (emotional attachment) of the infant with the mother and father. When the savings in hospital costs of one premature infant going home earlier is multiplied by the thousands of premature infants born each year, an annual savings of hundreds of thousands of dollars could be realized. This is one example of nursing research that is practical and scientific, and has the potential to save discomfort, inconvenience, and money.

Here is another example, this time at the other end of the age continuum. Some older persons use walkers or canes due to hip fractures and other injuries suffered during falls. Fractures can be set and hips surgically replaced, but wouldn't it be wonderful if older people didn't fall, and fractured bones occurred less frequently? Some researchers wondered, "How can falls in older people best be prevented?"

Elizabeth McNeely (1991), an Emory University nurse researcher, is involved in a study in which elderly individuals learn "tai chi," a martial art form, to see if those who practice tai chi fall less often than others. The moves performed in tai chi exercises promote balance and strengthen muscles. When elderly people have better balance and are stronger, they are not as likely to fall, and they may avoid breaking bones. This study, still in progress, may have an impact on the health of the elderly in the future.

Another example is provided by Marilyn Hochenberry-Eaton (1991), also at Emory University, who uses imagery to decrease the nausea and vomiting of children who are receiving cancer treatment. Imagery involves creating positive mental images that counteract unpleasant reality. It is sometimes used in stress reduction exercises. Hochenberry-Eaton designs individual imagery programs for the children with whom she works. For children who like *Star Wars*, she makes a tape with *Star Wars* music in the background and talks the patient into relaxing while listening to the music. For children who have a favorite recording artist, Hockenberry-Eaton plays that artist's recordings and talks the children through a sequence of pleasant mental images. Children who have cancer respond in a positive way to music and images to which they can relate and tolerate their treatments better.

This chapter describes some very basic concepts of nursing research. The purpose is to introduce nursing research, demonstrate that nursing research has merit, and provide a beginning vocabulary for nursing research. The ultimate goal is for nurses to participate in the research process and apply research findings to clinical practice.

What Is Nursing Research?

Nursing research is the systematic investigation of **phenomena** (events or circumstances) related to improving nursing care. When nurses have a question that they believe is necessary to answer in order to provide better care for patients, and they have the time, money, skill, and energy to study that question, they do nursing research. Although it does not have to be a topic that others are interested in for it to be an appropriate research question, there is much to be gained from choosing research problems that are connected to work already done. This builds nursing knowledge.

Research problems should be pursued only if they meet all three of the following tests:

1. Is there a **conceptual framework;** that is, do the researchers' ideas about the problem fit logically and dovetail with what is already known about the topic?
2. Is the proposed research project based on related research findings written up in professional journals?
3. Is the proposed research carefully designed so that the results will be applicable in similar situations?

If the answer to all three of these questions is not yes, the research will not be soundly based and should be reconsidered.

In addition to building nursing knowledge, studies that build on previous work are more likely to receive financial support. Research is expensive and often requires funding beyond what one nurse, hospital, or college can supply. Nurses who want to do research usually find it necessary to obtain outside funding or compete with other aspiring researchers for limited internal (from within the agency) funding. Therefore, to receive funding, nurses must do research that interests others and that a funding agency is willing to support.

The agencies that fund nursing research look for ideas that will build on and advance nursing knowledge. So while nursing research may be broadly defined as anything that interests nurses and helps them provide better care, controversy exists as to what can legitimately be included. When choosing a topic, the wise nurse researcher considers the important issues of background and support.

Research is different from **problem solving**. Problem solving is specific to a given situation and is designed for immediate action, whereas research is **generalizable** (transferable) to other situations and deals with long-term solutions rather than immediate ones. For example, Mrs. Abney is an elderly patient who frequently was found wandering in the halls of the nursing home, unable to find her way back to her room. This was quite distressing to her and time-consuming for the nursing staff who helped her find her way "home." A nurse noticed that Mrs. Abney had no difficulty recognizing her daughter, so she taped a photograph of the daughter to Mrs. Abney's door. Now Mrs. Abney can find her room easily. She is less agitated, and the nursing staff time can be spent on other priorities.

This is an example of problem solving. It is effective in one set of circumstances and has immediate application. But the solution that worked for Mrs. Abney may not work for all confused patients. Table 12–1 compares problem solving and research.

The Research Process

The nursing research process is the same as any other research process; it simply addresses a nursing-related problem. Research starts with a problem or stimulus. The stimulus for a research project may be the feeling that something needs to be addressed, that something is not right. It may be that there are insufficient data

Table 12–1 Comparison of Problem Solving and Research

Characteristic	Research	Problem Solving
Type of problems addressed:	Widely experienced	Situation specific
Conceptual basis:	Theoretical framework	Whatever works
Knowledge base needed:	Review of literature	Practical knowledge, common sense, and experience
Scope of application:	Generalizable to similar situations	Useful mainly in the immediate situation

for resolving a problem, or that the literature is unclear, or the data presented in the literature are conflicting. When there is a need for more information and no adequate information exists, research is in order.

There are two major categories of research: quantitative and qualitative. **Quantitative research** is generally considered objective and uses data-gathering techniques that can be repeated by others and verified. Data collected are quantifiable; that is, they can be counted, measured with standardized instruments, or observed with a high degree of agreement among observers.

Qualitative research is more subjective. Questions that cannot be answered by quantitative designs must be addressed by qualitative methods. Answering "why" questions requires the use of qualitative approaches. Why do persons with diabetes choose not to follow the diet prescribed for them? Why do chronically mentally ill individuals choose not to take the medications that would reduce psychotic symptoms? Qualitative research is useful in understanding perceptions and feelings.

Whether quantitative or qualitative, all research must be rigorously planned, carefully implemented, and scrupulously analyzed. Therefore, most research follows a formal process known as the **research process.** Students in baccalaureate nursing programs usually take a course in nursing research in which both qualitative and quantitative methods are described. For the purposes of this chapter, we will look at the steps in the quantitative research process.

There are several steps in the process:

1. Identification of a research problem.
2. Review of literature.
3. Formulation of the research question or hypothesis.
4. Design of the study.
5. Implementation.
6. Drawing conclusions based on findings.
7. Discussion of implications.
8. Dissemination of findings.

Each step will be briefly described.

IDENTIFICATION OF A RESEARCH PROBLEM

Problems generally come from three sources: clinical situations, the literature, or theories. Clinical situations are rich sources for research problems. Nurses want to prevent elderly clients from wandering off the unit and getting lost. How can they do it? Asking this question can lead to a research problem.

Sometimes researchers become interested in a problem because it is written about in the literature. They may find a study or two to replicate (repeat) or may design a new one.

The third source of research problems, theory, relates to testing theoretical models. Chapter 11 discussed several models of nursing theory that have been developed. If a theoretical model is designed to predict patients' responses to nursing actions, whether or not it *does* predict patients' responses can be tested through research. The researcher can create certain conditions and see if, in fact, the events happen as the theoretical model predicted.

Most ideas for nursing research projects come from one of these three sources.

REVIEW OF LITERATURE

Once a problem is identified, the professional literature must be reviewed. A review of the literature is comprehensive and covers all relevant research and supporting documents in print. Doing a thorough review of the literature requires a lot of library time and detective work. Computer-generated searches of the literature can assist tremendously with this step but cannot totally replace the efforts of a dedicated researcher.

The literature review is essential to locate similar or related studies that have already been completed and upon which a new study can build. The review is helpful in creating a **conceptual framework,** or organization of supporting ideas, upon which to base the study. At this point, you may want to review the brief discussion of conceptual frameworks in Chapter 11.

FORMULATION OF THE RESEARCH QUESTION OR HYPOTHESIS

Once researchers have identified a research problem, are intimately acquainted with the relevant literature, and have chosen a conceptual framework that helps to focus the topic, they need to formulate the research question. The question may be stated in one of three forms: a statement, a question, or a hypothesis. If researchers are going to describe something, they may make a statement, such as: "The purpose of this study is to identify the five most frequently expressed needs of family members in intensive care unit waiting rooms." They could also ask a question, such as: "What are the characteristics of mothers who have difficulty bonding to their newborn babies?" If comparing the relationship of two variables, a question might be asked, such as: "What is the relationship of time spent studying and grade point averages?" If conducting an experiment, researchers must have a **hypothesis** (educated guess) as to what the outcome will be so that hypothesis-testing statistics may later be applied. For example, "First-time mothers who attend childbirth classes will demonstrate earlier bonding with their newborn babies than mothers who do not attend the classes" is a testable hypothesis. Whatever the form used, the research question must be expressed succinctly and clearly.

DESIGN OF THE STUDY

Once the research question is identified, the study must be designed. There are two broad categories of research designs: **experimental** and **nonexperimental**. If the researcher influences the **subjects** (participants) in any way, the research is experimental. If not, the research is nonexperimental. There are numerous types of research under each of these two categories, but the main difference between experimental and nonexperimental research is whether the researcher manipulates, or influences, the subjects.

True experimental designs provide evidence of a cause-and-effect relationship between actions. For example, testing the hypothesis "Patients who receive preoperative teaching need less pain medication in the first 72 hours postoperatively" would provide evidence of a cause-and-effect relationship between teaching and pain. Sometimes it is impossible to conduct a true experimental study with human beings because to do so might endanger them in some way. In those instances, modified experimental studies are used.

Nonexperimental designs are frequently referred to as *descriptive designs* because the researcher describes what the situation is or was at some point in the past. There are many types of nonexperimental designs: surveys, descriptive comparisons, evaluation studies, exploratory studies, and historical-documentary research.

Whether the researcher chooses an experimental or nonexperimental design will influence the data collection process. The data collection process includes: selection of data collection instruments; design of the data collection protocol; the data analysis plan; subject selection; and informed consent and institutional review plans.

Data Collection Instruments. When designing a study, researchers must answer the question, "How will we collect the data?" Data collection instruments, sometimes called data collection tools, range from simple survey forms to complex radiographic scanning devices. The instrument used must be **reliable,** or accurate. A reliable instrument is one that will yield the same values dependably each time the instrument is used to measure the same thing. The tool must also be **valid,** which means it must measure what it is supposed to be measuring. If body temperature is being measured, a thermometer would be an obvious data collection tool. But when measuring an abstract factor, such as anxiety or depression, the best data collection tool will not be as clear. To minimize measurement errors, beginning researchers usually choose instruments with published reliability and validity, rather than designing their own.

Data Collection Protocol. Another aspect of designing the study is deciding on the data collection **protocol** (procedure). The quality of the data depends on strict adherence to the plan. If, for example, the plan calls for administering a questionnaire to renal dialysis clients after their dialysis treatments, the data collectors must be very sure that they give the questionnaires to all subjects only *after* their treatments. The data collection protocol answers the question, "How will we go about gathering our data?"

Data Analysis Plan. It may seem premature to decide how the data will be analyzed before it is even collected, but careful planning is very important. The research design is developed with data analysis in mind. The analysis must be part of the planning process because what data are collected and the protocols for collecting the data depend on how the data will be analyzed. The data analysis plan answers the question, "What will we do with the data once we gather it?"

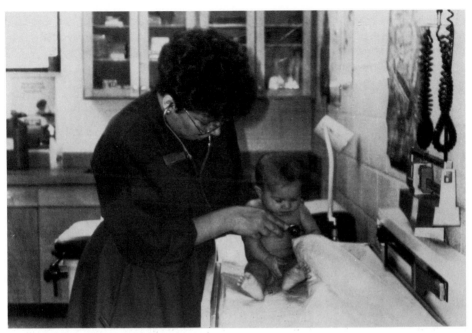

Research subjects are selected based on factors such as age, sex, condition, and location. (Courtesy of *Tennessee Nurse.*)

Subject Selection.   Once the researcher knows what is to be done, the specifics of who is to be included are decided. The individual people or laboratory animals being studied are known as research subjects. If the researchers plan to study pain control in postoperative patients, for example, they will have to decide the specific type of surgery, the age, sex, and geographic location of the patients, as well as a variety of other factors in planning the subject selection. Subject selection answers the question, "Who qualifies to be a participant in this study?"

Rarely, all subjects in a particular group are studied, but this is usually impossible. The term **population** refers to all subjects who meet the selection criteria. Usually, researchers have to use a sample of the entire population, however, and valid results can be obtained if the **sample** is properly selected.

Informed Consent and Institutional Review.   Next, researchers who use human subjects must plan to protect the rights of those subjects. Research subjects must be asked to sign a subject consent form that describes the details of the study and what participation means for the subjects. Any risks involved in participating must be explained. No one should be pressured in any way to participate, and the **confidentiality** (privacy) of participants must be assured.

A related step when using human subjects is submitting the proposal to the institution, such as a hospital or clinic, where the research will take place. It must be approved by the **institutional review board** (IRB). This board exists to ensure that research is well designed and ethical and does not violate the policies and procedures of the institution. Only after the IRB approves the proposal can the study begin.

IMPLEMENTATION

Up until this point, only planning has taken place. In the implementation phase the actual study is conducted. The two main tasks during this phase are data collection and data analysis.

Data Collection. Data should only be collected by those who understand the study. All research assistants should understand the purpose of the data and the importance of accuracy and careful record keeping. No matter who is collecting the data, however, the integrity of the project is ultimately the responsibility of the primary researcher.

Data Analysis. If all goes well, the data will be analyzed exactly as proposed. In analyzing the data, most researchers use the same statistics consultants who assisted in planning the study. The researcher is well advised to work closely with the statistician in interpreting as well as analyzing the data. The nurse researcher is in charge, however, and he or she has the final word on what interpretations are made.

DRAWING CONCLUSIONS BASED ON FINDINGS

In writing the research report, the findings directly related to the research question are presented first. Findings are presented factually—without value judgments. The facts must speak for themselves. Simple presentation of the facts is all that is required. After findings related to the research question are reported, unexpected findings can be reported. Conclusions are then drawn. Conclusions answer the question, "What do these findings mean?" Here researchers can be more subjective and inject some of their own thinking but should stay within the boundaries of the study.

DISCUSSION OF IMPLICATIONS

Researchers are always on the lookout for the implications of their studies. Implications are suggestions of things that should be done in the future. Every good study raises more questions than it answers. In nursing studies, there may be indications for modifications in nursing education or nursing practice. Nearly every study has implications for further research, and if the findings are as expected, almost all studies should be carefully replicated. **Replication** can answer these and other questions: What needs to be known to develop more confidence in the findings? Will the research instrument produce similar results in a similar population in a different part of the country? Will the procedure be effective with patients having a slightly different type of surgery? Will age make a difference? What else do we need to know to improve the care of patients?

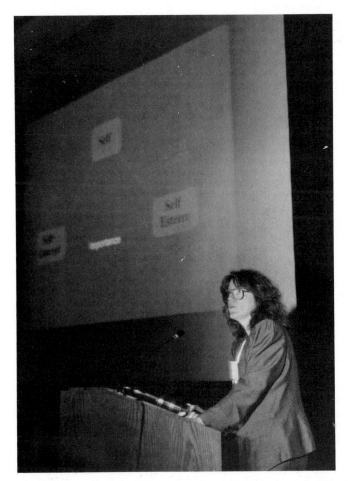

Researcher Maureen Killeen presents her research at the Third State of the Art and Science of Psychiatric Nursing Conference, February 20, 1992. (Courtesy of Maureen Killeen.)

DISSEMINATION OF FINDINGS

A study is not completed until the results are communicated to others who may find it useful. Most funding agencies want to know in advance how the researcher plans to disseminate the findings. The two major vehicles for knowledge dissemination are articles in professional journals and presentations at conferences. Examples of nursing research journals include *Clinical Nursing Research, Image, Nursing Research, Research in Nursing and Health Care,* and the *Western Journal of Nursing Research.* Since there are relatively few research journals in nursing, the competition for publishing might seem fierce, but editors say they have great difficulty getting well-written manuscripts on topics of interest to readers. Most research that is carefully conceived, conducted, and presented can get published, although the researcher must be persistent and resilient in taking criticism and reworking manuscripts.

A somewhat easier, yet still discriminating, route to dissemination is presentation at one or more of the numerous nursing research conferences. In general, the proportion of abstracts (summaries of research) chosen for presentation at conferences is higher than the proportion of manuscripts chosen for publication.

Whether research is published or presented, it is important to disseminate research results to other nurses who may choose to use it to improve patient care practices.

Interviews with Nurse Researchers

The field of nursing research is growing, and many nurses are actively involved in research. Listen to what two nurse researchers say about their work.

Research on Self-Esteem in Children

The first interview is with Maureen Killeen (1991), an associate professor of nursing at the Medical College of Georgia.

INTERVIEWER: Maureen, your research is with children and self-esteem; exactly what do you do?

RESEARCHER: I go into people's homes and ask children about themselves, and I ask the parents about the children. I ask, "What kinds of things are you good at?" And I ask them how important certain words are to them.

INTERVIEWER: What are some examples of the important words?

RESEARCHER: *Pretty, smart, honest, messy, lazy, active, careful, happy*—things like that. In another study, I am interested in the relationship between obesity and self-esteem. I go into a fifth-grade classroom and give everyone a self-concept scale and measure height and weight. I ask if they are heavier or thinner than others their age.

INTERVIEWER: How do you happen to be doing what you are doing?

RESEARCHER: I read about research on self-esteem in a "Social Psychology and the Self" course I took in graduate school. I read a lot of studies, and every study indicated that if you think of yourself in a certain way, this leads to certain behaviors. But there was nothing about how people come to think of themselves in certain ways. What are the characteristics or traits that get people thinking that way? I wanted to know the answer to that question.

INTERVIEWER: What impact do you hope your research will have on the care of children?

RESEARCHER: If we can figure out how other people affect children's ideas about themselves, how talk *about* children and talk *to* children affects them, then we can teach parents how to talk more effectively with their children. We can increase the relevance of treatment and therapy. We will know how to change how people feel about themselves. That is the treatment implication of this research.

INTERVIEWER: What has been most helpful to you in the process of becoming a nurse researcher?

RESEARCHER: Mentoring by more experienced researchers. I have benefited from the kindness of senior researchers who shared ideas. Experience is the best teacher, and I have been fortunate to have had good mentoring. Also—getting a funded grant to pay the bills while I do research has helped a lot!

INTERVIEWER: With regard to your professional life, what is the most fun for you?

RESEARCHER: Some aspects of research are the most fun, but teaching is close behind. If I can use my research in teaching—that's a *lot* of fun!

INTERVIEWER: What do you like the least of the things you have to do?

RESEARCHER: Writing. Writing is hard. There are constant revisions. I'm not sure it ever gets done.

INTERVIEWER: What would you like to say about research to nursing students?

RESEARCHER: Research can be a lot of fun. Hook up with someone who believes it's fun and asks interesting questions. It's very exciting!

Research on Decreasing Falls in the Elderly

The second nurse researcher interviewed was Elizabeth McNeely (1991), who does the tai chi research with older people mentioned earlier in this chapter. Dr. McNeely is an assistant professor in Emory University's Nell Hodgson Woodruff School of Nursing. Her research collaborators are in the Emory School of Medicine and the Atlanta Veterans Administration Medical Center.

INTERVIEWER: How did you happen to become a nurse researcher?

RESEARCHER: Accidentally. It was the last thing I envisioned. I happened to have a specialization in a field [gerontology] where research was growing. I became recognized as an expert in the field. My supervisor told me one day to go to a meeting where my expertise was needed. The meeting turned out to be a planning meeting for the multidisciplinary [involving professionals from several fields] research I do now.

INTERVIEWER: How do you believe your research has contributed to better patient care?

RESEARCHER: There are so many things people do because they "know" they work. But this knowledge doesn't get communicated beyond the walls of the institution. With hard data that comes from research, the information can be published so others can know how to do it. This improves patient care.

INTERVIEWER: What are some examples?

RESEARCHER: This tai chi grant. They have been doing tai chi in China for hundreds of years. But thousands of testimonials to the benefits won't lead to its being recommended by medical professionals in this country. We have to study the effects systematically before it will be supported by the medical profession.

INTERVIEWER: How do you like your work as a nurse researcher?

RESEARCHER: It's intriguing. Everyone needs to realize the importance of getting hard data to support practice.

INTERVIEWER: What do you like best about your work?

RESEARCHER: The air of excitement and discovery that comes when we see that some of our ideas are working. Also, my association with other researchers and the opportunities for thinking.

INTERVIEWER: What do you like the least?

RESEARCHER: There is a lot of tedium. It's hard to realize how long it takes to get from idea to publication. You have to be "long-term" oriented.

INTERVIEWER: What would you like to say to nursing students?
RESEARCHER: I would tell them that nurses have a unique contribution to make to the multidisciplinary research team. The problems are complex and require complex approaches, including the nursing perspective.

These interviews demonstrate how two nurse researchers feel about the work they do. Nationwide there are hundreds of nurses who, like Dr. Killeen and Dr. McNeely, are excited about nursing research and the contributions it makes to improving nursing practice.

Relationship of Nursing Research to Nursing Theory and Practice

Relationships among nursing research, practice, and theory are circular. As mentioned earlier in this chapter, research ideas are generated from three sources: (1) clinical practice, (2) literature, and (3) theory.

Questions about how best to deal with patient problems regularly arise in clinical situations. As shown in the example of Mrs. Abney, the elderly lady who couldn't find her room, problems often can be "solved" for the present. But when the same questions repeatedly recur, long-term answers may be needed. Research develops solutions that can be used with confidence in different situations.

Published articles about nursing research often generate interest in further studies. If there is published research literature on a particular nursing care problem, other researchers may be stimulated to investigate further and refine the solutions. This is how nursing knowledge builds.

Nursing theorists also generate research ideas. They piece together postulates or premises that "explain" what has been discovered. The explanation will be "tested" to see if it is robust or strong enough to be useful. If so, there may be more implications for applications in clinical practice.

Nursing research journals are full of clinical studies that have made a difference in patient care. A few examples of changes in nursing practice stimulated by research include:

1. Improved care of patients with skin breakdown from pressure ulcers.
2. Decreasing light and noise in critical care units to prevent sleep deprivation.
3. Using caps on newborns to decrease heat loss and stabilize body temperature.
4. Positioning patients following chest surgery to facilitate respiration.
5. Scheduling pain medication more frequently following surgery.
6. Preoperative teaching to facilitate postsurgery recovery.

Nursing research findings not only improve patient care but also impact the health care system itself. For example, research studies have demonstrated the cost-effectiveness of nurses as health care providers. You will learn more about this in Chapter 14.

Another contribution of nursing research to practice is in the area of power. A person who possesses knowledge that is useful to others has power. Nurses

---

Box 12-1   Relating Nursing Research, Practice, and Theory

Behavior theory suggests that behavior can be modified with reinforcement (reward or punishment). Incontinence is behavior characterized by involuntary urination before the patient can get to the bathroom or get positioned on a bedpan or with a urinal. Some researchers wondered, "Can incontinence be modified with positive reinforcements such as a special treat or additional time in the television room?" Specifically, they believed that patients could be "taught" to control urination if effective reinforcers were applied. Several studies suggest that patients *can* learn to control incontinence in specific situations. In this case, a theory—behavior theory—was useful in planning research, the results of which were directly applicable to clinical nursing care.

---

gain much knowledge through clinical practice. But practical knowledge, as important as it is, lacks the power of research-validated knowledge. Research can be used to demonstrate, for example, that one nursing action is more effective than another. When knowledge from practice is validated through research, that knowledge is more powerful. Thus, it could be said that research *empowers* practice.

A final point about the influence of research on practice has to do with professionalism. In Chapter 6, the characteristics of professions were given. One of the criteria commonly mentioned is a scientific body of knowledge that is expanded through research. Nursing research enhances the status of nursing as a profession by expanding nursing's scientific knowledge base.

A brief example that may clarify the interplay between nursing research, practice, and theory is found in Box 12-1.

Four Phases in the Development of Nursing Research

Lisa Marchette (1987) clarified the four phases that nursing research has taken in the course of its 30-year history. The phases Marchette identified are:

1. The stimulated phase.
2. The individualistic phase.
3. The unified phase.
4. The balanced phase.

She described the goal of the stimulated phase as sensitizing and exciting nurses about the importance of nursing research. This phase was predominant in the 1960s and 1970s in university schools of nursing. Hospitals caught the excitement during the late 1970s and early 1980s. In the stimulated phase a number of books and articles were written about nursing research, but little research was actually done.

During the individualistic phase of the mid-1970s, some schools of nursing hired statisticians and directors of nursing research to provide support and technical help to encourage researchers. In this phase, hospital based nurses struggled in isolation to conduct studies on topics of individual interest. In large medical centers, research facilitators were sometimes employed to design a program of nursing research. Even though nurses conducted clinical research during this phase, the studies tended to be fragmented and contributed little to nursing science.

The unified phase, spanning the late 1970s and 1980s in universities and extending into the l990s in hospitals, was characterized by organized basic internal support networks. These networks are the **infrastructure** for nursing research. Infrastructure refers to financial support, having resource people available "in-house" for consultation, the expectation of teamwork, and established peer review processes. **Peer review** refers to the process of having colleagues look at a research design and provide constructive criticism or suggestions for improvement. A type of research characteristic of the unified phase is the cluster study. Cluster studies consist of research projects that use the same theme but are carried out by different researchers working in a network.

The l990s may be the era when nursing research moves into what Marchette called the balanced phase. This phase is characterized by the expectations of focused, scholarly nursing research conducted with adequate support. Collaboration between nursing and other disciplines is the hallmark of the balanced phase. This goal is a worthy one toward which nursing must strive. Table 12–2 provides an overview of the four phases in the development of nursing research.

Table 12–2 Characteristics of Marchette's Phases of Nursing Research Development

Phase	Characteristics

Stimulated (1960s and early 1970s)	Excitement; articles and books *about* research; few actual studies.
	   Leininger (1968)*
	   Wandelt (1970)*

Individualistic (mid-1970s)	Early clinical studies begun; isolated efforts; increasing interest in nursing research
	   Lindeman (1976)*
	   Martinson et al. (1978)*

Unified (1980s)	Organized research support networks (infrastructures) developed; cluster studies
	   Horsley, Crane, and Haller (1981)*
	   Kramer, Albrecht, and Miller (1985)*

Balanced (1990s)	Focused, scholarly research; collaboration; adequate support
	   Bock (1990)*
	   Fitzpatrick, Wykle, and Morris (1990)*

* Characteristic studies of this phase of development. See References for full citations on these studies.
(Data from Marchette, L. (1987). Research: The big picture. *Perioperative Nursing Quarterly*, 3(3), 67–72.)

News Note "Beyond Tender Loving Care, Nurses Are a Force in Research"

The Florence Nightingales of the nation are busily adding a Louis Pasteur research component to their profession. And nursing's distinctly human, low-tech studies are bringing better and less costly medical care to millions of patients as well as helping relatives who care for them at home.

In the five years since Congress established the National Center for Nursing Research over President Reagan's veto, federally financed studies by nurses have made important strides toward closing gaps in patient care that often lead to physical and emotional complications, prolonged hospital stays or failure to adapt to disease or its treatment.

. . . Nurse researchers at the University of Rochester found that when nurses or family members provided moral support for heart patients during their transfer out of the coronary care unit, fewer cardiovascular complications occurred and the patients stayed in the hospital an average of four days fewer than similar patients who weathered the transfer without added support.

A study by nurses at Ohio State University showed that several weeks of aerobic exercise before surgery and chemotherapy for breast cancer speeded the patient's ability to return to normal activities.

. . . A recent analysis of 84 studies conducted by nurse researchers among a total of 4,146 patients prompted Dr. Barbara S. Heater, associate professor of nursing at the University of Missouri in St. Louis, to conclude that "research-based nursing interventions can produce 28 percent better outcomes for 72 percent of patients" and save money by shortening hospital stays. . . .

. . . nurse researchers are carving out new territories in health promotion and disease prevention that have been all but ignored by physicians. Studies by nurses look, for example, at factors that help patients follow doctor's orders to change their living habits after a heart attack, reasons many elderly patients fail to take influenza seriously, ways to help families cope with high cholesterol levels in children and circumstances that keep women from following an exercise routine.

—Jane E. Brody From *The New York Times*, Tuesday, August 13, 1991. Copyright © 1991 by the New York Times Company. Reprinted by permission.

Sources of Support for Nursing Research

Nursing research is expensive, and support takes many forms. It can include encouragement, consultation, computer and library resources, money, and release time from researchers' regular work responsibilities. Each of these forms of support is important, but none alone is adequate. Early in the development of nursing research, encouragement was often the only support available, and not all nurse researchers had that. Gradually over the years funding sources have developed, but financial support is still difficult to obtain, particularly for new researchers.

The National Center for Nursing Research (NCNR) was founded in 1986 as part of the National Institutes of Health. The purpose of the NCNR is to support nursing research. In the years of NCNR's existence, its budget has quadrupled, but it still is able to fund only a small portion of the proposals it receives. Several other federal agencies, while not specifically for nurses, also accept proposals that meet their funding guidelines when submitted by qualified nurse researchers. These include the National Institute on Aging, the National Cancer Institute, and the National Institute of Mental Health.

Nursing associations also fund nursing research. The American Nurses Foundation, Sigma Theta Tau, and many of the clinical specialty organizations provide research awards. State and local nursing associations sometimes have seed money for pilot projects. Universities, schools of nursing, and large hospitals also may provide small amounts of research funds. Generally, however, adequate funding for large-scale studies continues to be a problem faced by nurse researchers.

Roles of Nurses in Research

The *Code for Nurses* states, "The nurse participates in activities that contribute to the ongoing development of the profession's body of knowledge" (American Nurses Association 1985). In an ideal world, every nurse would be involved in research. In the real world, all nurses should, as a minimum, use research results to improve their practices. Professional nurses should not practice nursing without staying abreast of the current literature, especially studies done in their areas of clinical practice.

In addition to using research to improve practice, all professional nurses can contribute to one or more aspects of the research process (Table 12–3). Baccalaureate nurses can read, interpret, and evaluate research for applicability to

Table 12–3 Levels of Educational Preparation and Levels of Participation in Nursing Research

Level of Preparation	Level of Research Participation
Student nurse	Consumer
B.S.N. nurse	Data collector Problem identifier
M.S.N. nurse	Replicator Concept tester
Doctoral nurse	Theory generator
Postdoctoral nurse	Funded program director

B.S.N. = Bachelor of science in nursing.
M.S.N. = Master of science in nursing.

nursing practice. Through clinical practice, they can identify nursing problems that need to be investigated. They can participate in the implementation of scientific studies by helping principal researchers collect data in clinical settings or elsewhere. This beginning level of researcher must know enough about the purpose of the research to follow the research protocols (procedures) explicitly or know when it is necessary to deviate from the protocol for a patient's well-being. Baccalaureate nurses also can help disseminate research-based knowledge by sharing useful research findings with colleagues.

The master's prepared nurse may be ready to replicate (repeat) studies that have been previously conducted. Replication is very important. Researchers cannot be sure that their findings are what they seem to be until studies are repeated with similar results. It is not necessary (or even desirable) to generate a totally new and disconnected idea to do research. As mentioned earlier in the chapter, in order to be most useful, research must be based on a conceptual framework (organized ideas) and related to previous research.

Depending on education, clinical and research experiences, and interests, some nurses at the master's level are better prepared to conduct research than are others. In addition to education and experience, a crucial factor is the support system the nurse has available. To do research, nurses need time, money, consultation, and subjects. With rich resources in a research environment, master's prepared nurses can and do make vital research contributions.

Usually, to be a nationally recognized researcher and obtain federal funding for a research program, nurses need doctoral and even postdoctoral preparation. Researchers nationwide in all professions compete for a limited pool of research dollars available each year. Only those nurses with strong academic and experiential backgrounds and the best proposals succeed in obtaining federal funding.

Nurses who aspire to careers as competitive nurse researchers would do well to plan a specific program of research. May Wykle (Wykle 1986; Dunkle and Wykle 1988; Fitzpatrick, Wykle, and Morris 1990), who is at Case Western Reserve, has a research program producing stimulating studies about persons who care for their elderly dependent relatives. Sandra Dunbar (1991), who is at Emory University, is focusing her research program on circadian rhythms (physiological patterns occurring approximately every 24 hours) in various populations. These researchers realize that only by becoming specialists in a particular area of research will they receive the kind of funding they need to support their research and the national recognition it takes to get the results of their studies published so they can have the desired impact—improvement in nursing care.

CHAPTER SUMMARY

This chapter provided an overview of nursing research for the professional nursing student. Nursing research was defined as the systematic investigation of phenomena related to improving nursing care. The major steps in the research process were reviewed. They are identification of a research problem, review of the literature, formulation of the research question, design of the study, implementation, drawing conclusions based on findings, discussion of implications, and dissemination of findings. Examples of significant contributions of selected nurse researchers were highlighted. The circular relationship of nursing research to nursing theory and practice was described. Four phases of nursing research development were examined. The phases are stimulated, individualistic, unified, and balanced. Sources of funding for nursing research were identified. The research roles of nurses with differing educational backgrounds were described.

REVIEW/DISCUSSION QUESTIONS

1. Go to the college library and see which nursing research journals are in the collection. Thumb through some recent issues and notice the types of studies reported.
2. Read a research article that interests you. See if you can identify each of the steps in the research process. If not, what is missing? Discuss with your teacher and class what the significance of the missing steps might be.
3. Find out what research is being done in your school or hospital. If possible, talk with those involved including data collectors, data analysts, research directors, subjects, families of subjects, and/or nurses who work on units where research is being conducted. What do they know about the research? What are their concerns? What do they hope will be learned from the research?
4. Obtain job descriptions for nurses at varying experience levels at different agencies. Are research functions included in the job descriptions? If not, what research functions do you think might appropriately be included?
5. Of the studies below, identify which are nursing research and which are not, giving your rationale for each:
   a. The investigation of optimum staffing patterns in a long-term care facility.
   b. A study of effective methods of clinical supervision of nursing students.
   c. A comparison of two behavioral techniques for managing incontinence in spinal cord–injured patients.

REFERENCES

American Nurses Association. (1985). *Code for nurses with interpretive statements.* St. Louis, MO: Author.

Anderson, G. C., Gill, N. E., and Bodo, T. L. (1988). Self-regulatory feeding and nonnutritive sucking: Effect of regular sleep after beginning bottlefeeding in preterm infants. Paper presented at the biennial research conference of the Nurses Association of the American College of Obstetricians and Gynecologists, Toronto, Ontario, Canada, June 1988.

Bock, L. R. (1990). From research to utilization: Bridging the gap. *Nursing Management,* 21(3), 50–51.

Dunbar, S. (1991). Personal communication.

Dunkle, R. E., and Wykle, M. L. (1988). *Decision making in long-term care: Factors in planning.* New York: Springer.

Fitzpatrick, J. J., Wykle, M. L., and Morris, D. L. (1990). Collaboration in care and research. *Archives of Psychiatric Nursing,* 4(1), 53–61.

Hochenberry-Eaton, M. (1991). Personal communication.

Horsley, J. A., Crane, J., and Haller, K. B. (1981). *Conduct and utilization of research in nursing projects.* New York: Grune & Stratton.

Killeen, M. (1991). Personal communication.

Kramer, M. A., Albrecht, S., and Miller, R. A. (1985). A team approach to nursing practice. *Nursing Forum,* 22(1), 19–21.

Leininger, M. M. (1968). The research critique: Nature, function, and art. *Nursing Research,* 17(5), 444–449.

Lindeman, C. (1976). Implementing nursing research in a critical care setting. *Journal of Nursing Administration,* 6, 14–17.

Marchette, L. (1987). Research: The big picture. *Perioperative Nursing Quarterly,* 3(3), 67–72.

Martinson, I. M., et al. (1978). Facilitating home care for children dying of cancer. *Cancer Nursing,* 1, 41–45.

McNeely, E. (1991). Personal communication.

Measel, C. P., and Anderson, G. C. (1979). Nonnutritive sucking during tube feedings: Effect upon clinical course in premature infants. *Journal of Obstetric Gynecologic and Neonatal Nursing,* 8, 265–272.

Wandelt, M. A. (1970). *A guide for the beginning researcher.* New York: Appleton-Century-Crofts.

Wykle, M. L. (1986). Mental health nursing: Research in nursing homes. In M. S. Harper and B. Lebowitz (Eds.), *Mental illness in nursing homes: A research agenda* (pp. 221–234). (Publication No. [Adm] 86–1459). Rockville, MD: U.S. Department of Health and Human Services.

SUGGESTED READINGS

Abdellah, F. G., and Levine, E. (1979). *Better patient care through nursing research* (2nd ed.). New York: Macmillan.

Clinton, J., and McCormick, K. (1987). *Research in nursing: Toward a science of nursing.* Kansas City, MO: American Nurses Association.

Moody, L. E. (1990). *Advancing nursing science through research* (vols. 1 and 2). Newbury Park, CA: Sage Publications.

Notter, L. E., and Hott, J. R. (1988). *Essentials of nursing research* (4th ed.). New York: Springer.

Chapter

13 The Health Care Delivery System

Jennifer E. Jenkins

CHAPTER OBJECTIVES

What students should be able to do after studying this chapter:

1. Describe the four types of services provided by the health care delivery system.
2. Differentiate between the activities of health promotion and illness prevention.
3. Explain the organizational structure of a typical hospital.
4. Describe how major health care agencies are classified.
5. Identify the roles of key members of the health care team.
6. Cite examples of the roles of the nurse on the health care team.

VOCABULARY BUILDING

Terms to know:

case manager	counselor	governmental (public)
change agent	delegate	agency
clinical director	diagnosis	health care team
collaborator	entrepreneur	health promotion
continuous quality	for-profit agency	home health agency
improvement (CQI)	governance	illness prevention

institutional structure
managed care
manager
not-for-profit agency
nurse executive
nurse manager
patient advocate

primary care
professional
  governance
provider
rehabilitation services
secondary care
teacher

tertiary care
total quality
  management
  (TQM)
voluntary (private)
  agency

*T*he health care delivery system in the United States has traditionally been a system of illness care delivery. It is complex, which makes it difficult for patients to negotiate. It is extremely expensive, with multiple types of financing. The technology and sophisticated procedures available are the best in the world, but many people don't have access to even the most basic care. It is a system in crisis.

There are encouraging signs that it may be different in the future. Health care reform is clearly necessary. Experts predict that reform will take place before the year 2000 and certainly early in the professional careers of today's students. Therefore, this chapter will describe the health care delivery system of the present and make some predictions about the future.

The very words *health care delivery system* speak to the nature of change in how the health and illness needs of patients will be met in the twenty-first century. Most planners believe that one of the essential parts of an improved health care system will be an emphasis on prevention and the active participation of patients in their own health choices. While scientists will continue to search for and find cures to many illnesses, health care services will increasingly emphasize the importance of holism (treating the whole person, not just the diseased part). Another prediction is that health care professionals and governmental officials will work together to return the environment to a healthier balance, thus reducing pollution-related disease.

The delivery system of the future needs to be more efficient than the current one is. Life-threatening illnesses and injuries will continue to be treated in centers where the technology and intensive care are available. People with noncritical injuries and illnesses will be cared for in homes or at work, in the schools, and in community-based facilities such as neighborhood clinics. Health care workers will be educated to provide, holistic, efficient, and cost-effective care.

A system that answers the following questions will ensure that these objectives for the future are met:

1. What services does the patient need and want?
2. Who can best provide these services (patient, health care worker, family, others)?
3. Where is the most effective and efficient place to provide these services?
4. How will these services affect the quality of care, the cost, and both patient and health care worker satisfaction?

Box 13–1   Healthy People 2000 Goals

1. Increase the span of healthy life for Americans.
2. Reduce health disparities among Americans.
3. Achieve access to preventive services for all Americans.

(From U.S. Department of Health and Human Services. (1990). *Healthy people 2000: National health promotion and disease prevention objectives.* Washington, D.C.: Author.)

The American government has not yet devised a definitive health policy. However, an important first step has been taken. You will remember from Chapter 10 that in 1990 a consortium of nearly 300 national health organizations, the U.S. Public Health Service, and state health departments joined to draft goals and objectives for improving the health of the nation's citizens by the year 2000. The resulting report, *Healthy People 2000: National Health Promotion and Disease Prevention Objectives,* sets out three main goals, as outlined in Box 13–1 (U.S. Department of Health and Human Services 1990). How well these goals are met will be determined by the commitment of health care providers and citizens and the degree to which government officials (elected and appointed) can continue to focus on desired health outcomes rather than becoming side-tracked with political maneuvering.

With this brief look at the future, let us now take a look at the health care delivery system you will encounter and build a framework for understanding tomorrow's system.

Types of Health Care Services

There are four major types of health services: health promotion, illness prevention, diagnosis and treatment, and rehabilitation and long-term care. Each will be briefly explained.

Health Promotion

Health promotion services assist patients to remain healthy, prevent diseases and injuries, and promote healthier life-styles. These services require patients' active participation and cannot be performed solely by a health care provider. Health promotion services are based on the assumption that patients who participate in certain life-style changes are likely to avoid heart attacks, lung cancers, and other life-style–related diseases.

Box 13–2   Illness Prevention and Health Promotion Activities

ILLNESS PREVENTION

Periodical histories/physicals
Identification of familial/environmental
  risk factors
Community health programs
Promotion of healthy life-styles to
  counteract risk factors
Occupational safety programs (use of
  eye guards for work that endangers
  the eyes)
Environmental safety programs (proper
  disposal of hazardous waste)
Legislation that prevents injury/disease
  (seat restraint laws)

HEALTH PROMOTION/MAINTENANCE

Health education programs (prenatal
  classes)
Exercise programs
Health fairs
Wellness programs (worksite/school)
Proper nutrition
Learning how to balance one's life

An example of health promotion services are prenatal classes. By learning good nutritional habits, an expectant mother can take care of both herself and her baby during pregnancy and after delivery. This increases the chances of a normal pregnancy and the birth of a healthy baby. Other examples include aerobic exercise classes and "stop-smoking" classes aimed at increasing the health of an individual's cardiovascular and respiratory systems.

Illness Prevention

When risk factors, such as a family history of heart disease, are identified, **illness prevention** services assist patients in reducing the impact of those risk factors on their health and well-being. These services also involve the patients' active participation.

Prevention services differ from health promotion services in that they address health problems *after* risk factors are identified, whereas health promotion services seek to *prevent* development of risk factors. For example, a health promotion program might teach the detrimental effects of alcohol and drugs on the person's health in order to prevent the person from using alcohol and drugs. Illness prevention services would be used when the patient has been using alcohol or drugs and is at risk for developing health problems as a result. In reality, the boundary between health promotion and illness prevention is often blurred. Box 13–2 gives examples of activities in these two areas.

Diagnosis and Treatment

Traditionally in our health care system, there was heavy emphasis on diagnosis and treatment. Early **diagnosis**, that is, detecting disease as soon as the first signs occur, has been the focus of most physicians' efforts. Modern technology has enabled the medical profession to refine the acts of diagnosing illnesses and disorders and to treat them more effectively.

Health care technology has allowed physicians to cure illnesses and disorders that have plagued humans for thousands of years. As a result, much human suffering has been avoided. Newer scientific advances permit many tests and treatments to be performed noninvasively, that is, without cutting into the body. Examples include the use of ultrasound to examine unborn fetuses to determine if they are developing normally and lithotripsy, which disintegrates kidney stones so they can be expelled in the urine. The future promises more "high tech" noninvasive technologies.

On the negative side, high-tech services can lead patients to feel dehumanized. This occurs when the care givers focus on machines rather than on patients. Nurses must remember that patients benefit most when they understand their diagnoses and treatments and when they can be active participants in the development and implementation of their own treatment plans.

Rehabilitation and Long-Term Care

Rehabilitation services are those that help restore the patient to the fullest possible level of function and independence following injury or illness. Rehabilitation programs deal with conditions that leave patients with less than full functioning, such as strokes, broken bones, or severe burns. Both patients and their families must be active participants in this care if it is to be successful. Rehabilitation services should begin immediately after the patient's condition has stabilized following an injury or stroke. These services may be provided in institutional settings such as hospitals, in special rehabilitation facilities, in long-term care facilities such as nursing homes, and in the home and the community. The objectives are to assist patients to achieve their potential and to return them to a level of functioning that permits them to be contributing members of society again.

Organization and Structure of Hospitals

The health care delivery system consists of entities such as hospitals, clinics, associations, and **home health agencies** that provide any of the four major types of health services: health promotion, illness prevention, diagnosis and treatment, and rehabilitation and long-term care. The most complex of these are hospitals. In this section, we will examine how most hospitals are organized and look at the place of nursing in the hospital structure.

Institutional Structure

Institutional structure means how an agency is organized to do what it is intended to do. The institutional structure of most hospitals includes a governing body, a board of trustees, also called a board of directors.

THE BOARD OF TRUSTEES

In the past, board members were often chosen from two groups: community philanthropists, who were expected to donate generously to the facility, and physicians who practiced there. Boards were large, met infrequently, and had mainly ceremonial functions.

As the health care environment became more complex, board members were chosen to represent various business and political interests of the community. They were expected to bring knowledge and expertise from the larger business world as well as have an appreciation and understanding of hospitals and how they operate. Boards now tend to be smaller and carry significant responsibility for the mission of the organization, the quality of services provided, and the financial status of the organization. Boards are not involved in the day-to-day running of the hospital, but they are responsible for establishing policies governing operations and for ensuring that the policies are executed. They **delegate** responsibility for running the hospital to the chief executive officer.

THE CHIEF EXECUTIVE OFFICER

The hospital chief executive officer (CEO) is the individual responsible for the overall operation on a daily basis. He or she usually has a master's degree in business or hospital administration. The CEO's responsibilities include making sure that the hospital runs efficiently, is cost-effective, and carries out the policies established by the board. The CEO usually sits on the board of trustees.

THE MEDICAL STAFF

A hospital's medical staff (physicians) may be either employees or independent practitioners. In either case, they must be granted privileges by the board of trustees to see patients at that particular institution. They may not simply decide to admit patients to a hospital. They must submit evidence that they are qualified and competent and must give evidence periodically that they have kept their skills and knowledge updated.

Medical staffs are usually organized by service (e.g., Department of Surgery, Department of Medicine, Department of Pulmonary Medicine). A chief of staff is usually elected by the entire medical staff. Together with the chiefs of the various services the chief of staff makes important decisions regarding medical policy for the institution. Bylaws govern these activities. The actions of the medical staff must be approved by the board of trustees, to whom the physicians are responsible.

THE NURSING STAFF

The top nurse in a hospital is known as the **nurse executive**, vice president for nursing, or director of nursing. Once excluded from decision making, nurse executives of today are often members of the board of trustees. Many hospitals now consider the nurse executive and the chief of the medical staff of equal stature.

The educational preparation for nurse executives includes a master's degree in nursing administration or business administration. Nurse executives are responsible for overseeing all the nursing care provided in the hospital and serve as clinical leaders as well as administrators. Nurse executives supervise the largest group of hospital employees, the nursing staff.

The nursing staff consists of all the registered nurses (R.N.s), licensed practical nurses (L.P.N.s)/licensed vocational nurses (L.V.N.s), and nursing assistants employed by the department of nursing. They are usually organized according to the units on which they work. The typical nursing unit consists of a **nurse manager**, or head nurse, several assistant managers, and a number of staff nurses, L.P.N.s/L.V.N.s, and nursing assistants.

Staff nurses are the direct, bedside care givers. They are responsible for planning, delivering, and evaluating care of a group of patients. They are also responsible for delegating to and supervising L.P.N.s/L.V.N.s and unlicensed personnel. Staff nurses are the backbone of hospital nursing.

Each nursing unit has its own budget and staff for which the nurse manager is responsible. The nurse manager is also a communication link between the nursing staff and the next level, middle management.

Between the nurse executive and the nurse manager of a unit are middle-management nurses, known as **clinical directors** or supervisors. They have responsibility for multiple units or for specific projects or programs. Their role is changing to one of coach and facilitator. These nurses ensure that nursing is integrated with other hospital services. As middle managers, they often have roles that resemble project managers. That is, they ensure that plans are in place, assignments are made and carried out, timetables are kept, and progress is evaluated on a regular basis. They serve as the communication link between the nurse managers and the nurse executive.

Some nurses employed in hospitals have limited direct patient care responsibilities and management responsibilities. They include nurse educators, nurse researchers, clinical nurse specialists, infection control nurses, and others. Nurses in these roles support direct care nurses and serve as resources to them.

OTHER HOSPITAL PERSONNEL

Hospitals employ far more than doctors and nurses. Doctors, nurses, and all the other individuals who work with patients are called the **health care team**, or interdisciplinary team. They are supported in their work by a number of other departments such as dietetics, housekeeping, laundry, and many others. Some key health providers will be discussed later in this chapter.

Hospitals are very complex facilities. The way they are organized varies somewhat from hospital to hospital. Every hospital has an organizational chart that shows its unique structure and explains lines of authority.

Hospital Accreditation

As you learned in Chapter 2, schools of nursing may choose to participate in a process called accreditation. Hospitals, too, are accredited. Their accrediting body is the Joint Commission on the Accreditation of Healthcare Organizations (JCAHO). JCAHO accreditation is very important for hospitals and requires that they meet a number of standards in every hospital department. The goal of accreditation is to improve patient outcomes (results). The way most hospitals have chosen to work toward improvement in patient outcomes is through **continuous quality improvement** (CQI).

CONTINUOUS QUALITY IMPROVEMENT/TOTAL QUALITY MANAGEMENT

In the 1940s, W. Edwards Deming (1982, 1986) proposed that groups of employees, rather than managers, be allowed to make decisions regarding how work was to be done. He called the employee groups "quality circles." Deming's ideas were discussed in the United States but did not receive widespread acceptance here. There *was* interest in Deming's ideas elsewhere, however. The Japanese government asked him to help them rebuild their workplaces, which were devastated by World War II, and Deming went to Japan.

By the 1970s, consumers worldwide recognized that certain Japanese-made products were superior to their American-made counterparts. American businesses began to discuss and imitate Japanese management techniques. These were really Deming's ideas brought back to us through Japan.

Today's health care systems have borrowed management concepts from industry and are very interested in CQI, also called **total quality management** (TQM). Rather than trying to identify mistakes after they have occurred, these systems focus on establishing procedures for assuring high-quality patient care.

Using quality improvement concepts, groups of employees from different hospital departments decide how care will be provided. They decide what outcomes are desired and design systems and assign roles and activities to best create those outcomes. Every effort is made to anticipate potential problems and prevent their occurrence. Hospital management delegates (gives) authority to the providers of services to plan and carry out quality improvement programs. CQI/TQM programs reinforce the belief that quality is everyone's responsibility.

Nurses are actively involved both in quality improvement and in accreditation processes, but these activities are not the responsibility of nursing managers alone. They are hospitalwide initiatives, and everyone at all levels gets involved. Working together to improve patient care in the institution builds cooperation among departments and boosts morale.

Nursing's New Organization and Structure

Nursing in hospitals is being transformed by the CQI/TQM movement. Putting quality improvement programs into place has required a reorganization of nursing administration.

DECENTRALIZATION

The key to nursing's new organization and structure is decentralization. Rather than decision-making authority being closely held by a few top nurses, decisions are made by those nurses most affected by the decision. This does not simply mean fewer layers in an organizational chart but also refers to the philosophy that all professionals should be encouraged to use their talents fully.

Decentralization empowers nurses, allowing them to exercise their own good judgment rather than being told what to do. For empowerment to be effective, the hospital board and top executives must clearly articulate their vision, goals, and expectations so that each member of the organization knows where the organization is going and what his or her part in it is. In the most decentralized model, employees at all levels are involved in the process of developing the hospital's vision and goals.

Decentralization and empowerment involve the development and use of three skills: (1) consensus decision making, (2) positive discipline, and (3) independence and interdependence. Once decisions are made, responsibility is given and accepted, commensurate authority is granted, and a system of accountability (evaluation of outcomes) ensures the responsibility was met. Figure 13–1 shows a model of decentralization and empowerment.

Perhaps one of the areas that is least clear in decentralized decision making is authority. Who has the final authority for decisions? The knowledge, experience, and maturity of individuals determine how much authority can be delegated to them. Four levels of authority are outlined in Box 13–3.

PROFESSIONAL GOVERNANCE

When hospitals accept the concept of decentralized decision making, the bureaucratic structures of the past no longer work. A system of **professional governance** is needed. Professional governance is founded on the philosophy that employees have both a right and a responsibility to govern their own work and time within a financially secure, patient-centered system. A common structure used for professional governance in nursing is the council model.

In the council model, there is a coordinating council made up of the chief nurse executive and the chairpersons of four subcouncils (clinical practice council, education council, administrative affairs council, and quality of care/research council). The coordinating council coordinates nursing activities, sets broad goals and objectives, and facilitates communication about nursing's vision. This group also ensures that successes are shared and that learning rather than punishment is the result of risk taking.

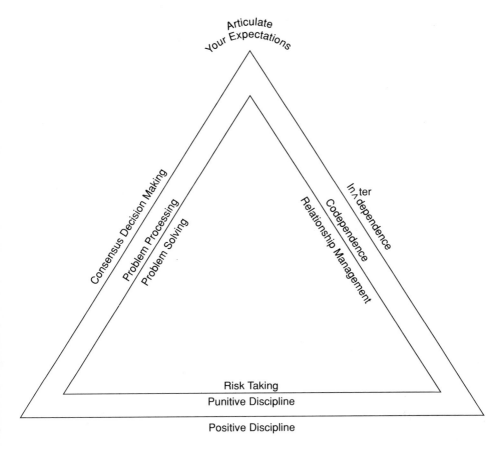

Figure 13–1 Empowerment triangle. (From Manthey, M. (1991). *Leaders empower staff.* Minneapolis, MN: Creative Nursing Management. Used by permission.)

The other councils have the responsibility, authority, and accountability within their designated areas—clinical, administrative, education, and quality of practice—for setting the standards, policies, procedures, and behaviors necessary for nursing to carry on its work. Each council works closely with the others to ensure that decisions are well thought out. At the patient care unit level, a unit committee (or council) is elected by the staff to represent all jobs and shifts on that unit. This group is authorized to translate the organizational council decisions at the unit level.

To show how the council model of professional governance works, the clinical practice council might set a standard that all patients will know their

Box 13-3 Levels of Authority

LEVEL I: GATHERING DATA/COMPLETING TASKS

In this level, people have limited knowledge or skill and will not be making the decisions.

LEVEL II: GATHER DATA/COMPLETE TASKS + MAKE RECOMMENDATIONS TO THE DECISION MAKER(S)

As people gain experience and knowledge, they begin to learn how things fit together, and they will be asked for recommendations. This does not mean that they will make the decisions but will contribute to the idea generation and options the decision maker has to choose from.

LEVEL III: GATHER DATA/COMPLETE TASKS + MAKE RECOMMENDATIONS* DECIDE AND ACT

The delegator is interested in building the delegatee's confidence in decision making. The delegatee is authorized to make the decision and take action. However, the asterisk (*) indicates that the delegatee must consult or negotiate with someone or communicate information to someone or a group before the decision is made. It does not mean that the delegatee can take the decision-making authority back just because he or she would make a different decision. The asterisk (*) simply means that the delegatee must know the parameters and limitations placed on the decision.

LEVEL IV: ACT ON YOUR OWN OR ON MY BEHALF

At this level of authority the delegator is very comfortable with the skill level of the delegatee. The delegatee is given full authority and responsibility for the decision-making process. This includes evaluating the effectiveness and appropriateness of the decision (accountability).

nurse's name and what they can expect from the nurse. The unit committees would then decide how that will be done and report back to the practice council on how they plan to implement the new standard on their particular unit. Figure 13-2 shows the council model for professional governance.

The council model is only one of several possible ways nursing departments in hospitals are structured to perform professional-governance functions. An issue with professional governance is that nurses tend to be action-oriented people who may not value committee work. They need to realize that professional governance is important to nursing as a profession and that they must participate if nursing is to have a voice in the way hospitals are run.

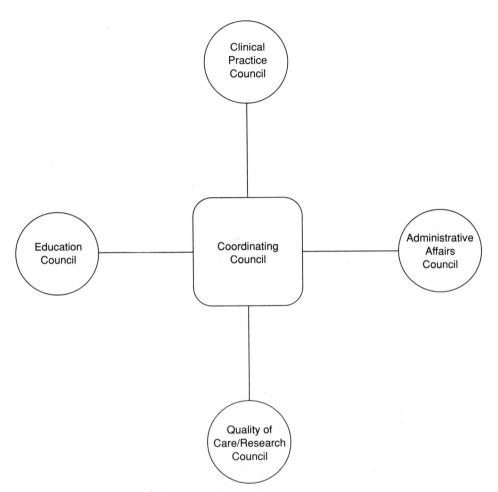

Figure 13–2 Council model for professional governance. (From Jenkins, J. E. (1991). Professional governance: The missing link. *Nursing Management,* 22(8), 30. Used by permission.)

Classifications of Health Care Agencies

Although much health care is delivered in hospital settings, there are many other agencies involved in the total health care delivery system. Organizations that deliver care can be classified in several ways: as governmental or voluntary agencies, as not-for-profit or for-profit agencies, and by the level of health care services they provide.

Governmental or Public Agencies

There are many **governmental**, or public, **agencies** that contribute to the health and well-being of our citizens. All are primarily supported by taxes, administered by elected or appointed officials, and tailored to the needs of the communities served.

LOCAL AGENCIES

Local agencies serve one community, county, or a few nearby counties. They provide services to both paying and nonpaying citizens. Public health departments are examples of local governmental agencies found in almost every county in the nation. All citizens, whether or not they can pay, are eligible for health care through local public health departments. These services usually include immunizations, prenatal care and counseling, well-baby and -child clinics, sexually transmitted disease clinics, tuberculosis clinics, and others. Public health nurses sometimes make home visits as well.

STATE AGENCIES

State health agencies oversee programs that affect the health of citizens across the state. Examples of state governmental health agencies include state departments of health and environment, departments that regulate and license health professionals such as state boards of nursing, and those that administer Medicaid insurance programs for the poor. These agencies are not typically involved in providing direct patient care but support local agencies that do provide direct care.

FEDERAL AGENCIES

Federal agencies focus on the health of all the nation's citizens. They promote and conduct health and illness research, provide funding to train health care workers, and assist communities in health care services planning. They also develop health programs and services and provide financial and personnel support to staff them. They establish standards of practice and safety for health care workers and conduct national health education programs on subjects such as the benefits of nonsmoking, prevention of acquired immunodeficiency syndrome (AIDS), need for prenatal care, and many others. Examples of federal agencies are the U.S. Public Health Service (PHS), the National Institutes of Health (NIH), the U.S. Department of Health and Human Services (DHHS), the Occupational Safety and Health Administration (OSHA), and the Centers for Disease Control (CDC).

In addition, the federal government operates hospitals providing direct care to active duty military personnel and veterans. A little known but important branch of the PHS is the Indian Health Service, which provides health care to native Americans who live on federal reservations.

Voluntary or Private Agencies

Citizens often voluntarily support the work of agencies working to promote or restore health. When an agency providing health care is supported by private volunteers, it is called a **voluntary** or **private agency**. Support is generally through private donations, although many of these agencies apply for governmental grants to support some of their activities.

Voluntary agencies often begin when a group of individuals band together to address a health problem. All their services may initially be performed by volunteers. Later, they may obtain enough donations to hire personnel, staff an office, and expand services. They may be able to secure ongoing funding through grants or organizations like the United Way. Examples of voluntary health agencies are the Visiting Nurses Association, the American Heart Association, Hospice, the American Cancer Society, and the Mental Health Association.

Not-for-Profit and For-Profit Agencies

Another way to classify health service delivery agencies is by what is done with the income earned by the agency. A **not-for-profit agency** is one that uses profits to pay personnel, improve services, advertise services, provide educational programs, or otherwise contribute to the mission of the agency. A common misconception is that not-for-profit agencies do not ever make a profit. The reality is that they may make profits, but the profits must be used for the improvement of the agency. Most voluntary agencies, such as the ones listed above, are not-for-profit, as are many private hospitals.

For-profit, or proprietary, **agencies**, on the other hand, may distribute profits to partners or shareholders. The growth in for-profit health care agencies has mushroomed over the past decade. Health care is big business and has the potential to be very profitable.

For-profit agencies include numerous home health care companies that send nurses and other health personnel to care for patients at home. There are also several large national chains of for-profit hospitals such as Humana and Hospital Corporation of America that have demonstrated that it is possible to provide quality patient care and make a profit while doing so. An issue hotly debated is that for-profit hospitals do not typically treat nonpaying patients. These people must go to public hospitals that are rapidly becoming overburdened with patients who are unable to pay their bills.

Level of Health Care Services Provided

A third way health care services are classified is by the level of health care services provided.

PRIMARY CARE SERVICES

The point at which a patient first enters the health care system is considered **primary care**. This may be a student health clinic, health centers in the com-

Box 13–4   Examples of Primary Care Agencies

Ambulatory care centers.   These centers provide a variety of services ranging from diagnostic to therapeutic; nurse practitioners and clinical nurse specialists may have pivotal roles in providing services in these centers.

Crisis centers and hotlines.   Hospitals and communities typically offer services to assist citizens experiencing things like suicide, AIDS (acquired immunodeficiency syndrome), herpes, abuse, psychiatric crisis, and so on; hotlines generally provide information and support; crisis centers may provide telephone hotlines, direct counseling, limited first aid, ongoing support, and guidance.

Day care centers.   Formerly thought of for children only, these now also serve the elderly and medically/emotionally impaired; usually open during daytime hours, some may offer extended hours when there is a need; they also provide respite care for families who need a break from caring for family members in the home or who need help while they work.

Employment settings.   As managers and employees recognize the benefits of healthy employees, nurses are very much in demand to run employee health clinics at the worksite; services may include histories/physicals, health teaching/promotion, health screens, and occupational safety programs.

Home health care agencies.   A fast-growing service, nurses and other health care team members (social workers, physical therapists, respiratory therapists, pharmacists, and others) provide services traditionally provided in both the home and hospital; even acute care services (home ventilators, intravenous therapy, chemotherapy) are provided.

Managed care organizations.   To hold down health care costs, many businesses use managed care organizations to provide health care to employees at a prearranged fee; examples of these are:

* Health maintenance organizations (HMOs)—group health agencies providing basic and supplemental services to enrollees at a fixed rate; clients generally may not have much choice as to which physician will care for them; preventive care is stressed.
* Preferred provider organizations (PPOs)—groups of physicians/hospital that provide services at a discounted rate; the client chooses which physician in the group he or she wishes to see.
* Individual practice associations (IPAs)—"middlemen" in the system; clients pay the IPA for services at a fixed rate, and the IPA pays the providers; profits are shared with the providers, and losses are absorbed by the IPA.

Neighborhood health centers.   These centers are usually found in areas where citizens are underserved, financially stressed, and at risk; a variety of health care workers provide basic health care and social services support; a recent addition to this category is a health care center run primarily by volunteers to provide health services to the "working poor" (those who have jobs but cannot afford health care insurance).

Physicians' offices. In general, people seek the services of the physician when they are ill; nurses working in these settings register clients, give medications, take vital signs, assist with examinations, and provide information and education.

Support Groups. These groups assist individuals with ongoing coping and life-style changes; Reach for Recovery assists women who have had mastectomies; Alcoholics Anonymous helps alcoholics stop drinking through a 12-step program; the Dream Machine helps children who are terminally ill have one of their wishes come true; some of these are well funded by agencies, and others are purely voluntary.

munity, an emergency room, physicians' offices, nurse practitioners' clinics, health clinics at work, and many more. Aydelotte (1983, p. 812) defined the major goals of the primary health care system as providing:

1. Entry into the system.
2. Emergency care.
3. Health maintenance.
4. Long-term and chronic care.
5. Treatment of temporary malfunctioning that does not require hospitalization.

In addition to treating common health problems, primary care centers are, for many citizens, where much of the prevention and health promotion work takes place. These centers are plagued by many problems, such as lack of adequate financing, staffing, space, and community support. The unfortunate truth is that preventive services are not well reimbursed by insurance, which prevents people from seeking them and contributes to growing health costs. See Box 13–4 for examples of primary care agencies.

SECONDARY CARE SERVICES

Secondary care agencies assist in the prevention of complications from disease, treat temporary dysfunction requiring hospitalization, evaluate long-term care or chronic patients who may need treatment changes, and provide counseling and therapy that are not available in primary settings (Aydelotte 1983, p. 813). Hospitals have traditionally been associated with this level of care.

In addition to hospitals, agencies that provide secondary health services are the home health agencies, ambulatory care agencies, and surgical centers. These agencies offer skilled personnel, easy access, convenient parking, compact equipment and monitoring systems, medications and anesthesia services, and a financial reimbursement program that rewards shorter lengths of stay and home/community care. It is expected that the trend toward providing community-based secondary care will continue well into the next century.

TERTIARY CARE SERVICES

Tertiary care services are those provided to acutely ill patients, to those requiring long-term care, and to those needing rehabilitation services. Tertiary care also includes provision of care to the terminally ill. It usually involves many health professionals working together on multidisciplinary teams to design treatment plans.

Examples of tertiary agencies are specialized hospitals such as trauma centers and specialized pediatric centers; long-term care facilities (skilled nursing, intermediate care, and supportive care); rehabilitation centers; and hospices (care is provided to the terminally ill and their families either in the hospital, in the home, or in special centers).

The Health Care Team

At one time doctors and nurses were the only members of the health care team. As health care became more complex and technology expanded, a number of other health disciplines developed. Today there are many different health care team members who come from a variety of backgrounds. Deciding which of these various personnel need to be involved in the care of a patient depends on the patient outcomes that must be achieved.

Once physicians were the only coordinators of patient care. In contemporary practice, the coordination of services is likely to be governed by an individual known as a **case manager**. Case managers, who are often nurses, recognize the contribution of each discipline in achieving the desired outcomes and bring a team together to plan, deliver, and evaluate the desired outcomes in the most cost-effective manner.

Key Members of the Health Care Team

In addition to nurses, who will be discussed in detail later in the chapter, there are dozens of health care workers who serve from time to time on interdisciplinary health care teams. Several of the key members who are most likely to be involved in the care of patients in hospitals will be mentioned.

PHYSICIANS

Physicians have completed college and three to four years of medical school and are licensed by a state board of medical examiners. Although it is not required to practice medicine in all states, most physicians have also completed a residency in a hospital setting, and many do postgraduate work in a specialty area.

Physicians are responsible for the medical diagnosis and medical therapies designed to restore health. Increasingly, physicians are specializing in an area of medicine and see only patients with that particular problem. This means one patient may have five or more doctors, each treating a different body system.

While physicians have traditionally been involved mainly in restorative care, many are coming to recognize the value of illness/injury prevention and health promotion. These activities have not been reimbursed by most insurance companies and there has been little financial incentive to do so. However, recent changes in some physician reimbursement plans have dramatically increased reimbursement for preventive care.

DIETICIANS

Many patients, particularly in hospitals, require management of their nutritional intake as part of the healing process. Others need to know how to prepare and eat a healthy diet. Dieticians have baccalaureate degrees and may have completed internships. They understand how the diet (oral or intravenous) may affect a patient's recovery and promote and maintain health. They focus on the therapeutic value of foods and on teaching people about therapeutic diets.

PHARMACISTS

Pharmacists prepare and dispense medications, instruct patients and other health workers about the medications, monitor the use of controlled substances such as narcotics, and work to reduce medication errors. The number and complexity of drugs available today require special education and training in their preparation, dispensing, monitoring, and evaluation of actions and effects on patients.

Pharmacists may pursue either a bachelor's degree in pharmacy, which takes five years, or a doctor of pharmacy, which takes six years. Depending on state licensing requirements, they may also be required to do an internship.

Pharmacists are an integral part of the interdisciplinary team. They serve as resources to physicians, nurses, and patients; administer intravenous medications and nutrition (antibiotics, cancer drugs, and liquid nutrients) in hospitals and homes; and monitor patients for actual and potential drug interactions.

PARAMEDICAL PERSONNEL

A number of personnel are educated to assist the physician in the diagnosis of patient problems. This connection with medicine identifies them as "paramedical" staff.

Laboratory technologists handle patient specimens such as blood, sputum, feces, urine, and body tissues to be examined for cancer or other abnormalities. Laboratory technologists carefully subject these body substances to various tests to determine whether or not the patient needs treatment. Technologists have at least a bachelor's degree and are often assisted by laboratory technicians, who have two-year degrees. They must pass a licensing examination in order to practice.

Radiologic technologists perform X-ray procedures. While patients still need routine X rays, technology in this field has become very sophisticated. Subspecialties such as computerized axial tomography (CAT), magnetic resonance imaging (MRI), and positron emission tomography (PET) have evolved. These are all ways of "seeing" what is going on inside the body without surgery. All require specially educated technicians who operate multimillion-dollar equipment. Although some radiology technicians are still trained "on the job," most are educated in formal programs lasting from one to four years. Radiologic technologists have a bachelor's degree. They must be registered with the state in which they practice.

RESPIRATORY TECHNOLOGISTS

Acutely ill or injured patients often require assistance in breathing. Respiratory technologists operate equipment such as ventilators, oxygen therapy devices, and intermittent positive pressure breathing machines. They also perform some diagnostic procedures such as pulmonary function tests and, in some facilities, blood gases. With the increase in respiratory care in the home and community, these health care team members are working very closely with home health agencies and community health centers. They must complete either a two-year (technician) or four-year (technologist) educational program and in some states must complete an internship.

SOCIAL WORKERS

The impact of illness and injury on patients and their families can often be profound. Financial problems may arise if the breadwinner cannot work or if insurance benefits are inadequate. Interruption of the normal family relationships may produce family crises. Lack of knowledge about community support systems may hinder discharge of a patient from the hospital.

The social services worker is specifically educated and trained to assist patients and their families with these and many other life and social challenges. They hold either a bachelor's or master's degree. Social workers serve as liaisons between hospitalized patients and the resources and services available in the community. In addition, social workers frequently are called upon to assist other health care personnel to cope more effectively with the stresses associated with caring for patients in crisis.

THERAPISTS

Several types of therapists help patients with special challenges. Physical therapists, or physiotherapists, assist patients to regain maximum possible physical activity and strength. They focus on assessing pre-illness or -injury function, current damage, and potential for recovery. They then develop a long-term plan for gradual return to function through exercise, rest, heat, and hydrotherapy. Physical therapists, who have a minimum of a bachelor's degree, also supervise physical therapy assistants, who hold associate degrees.

Occupational therapists work with physical therapists to develop plans to assist patients in resuming the activities of daily living following illness or injury. They may help patients learn how to cook, take care of their own hygiene, or

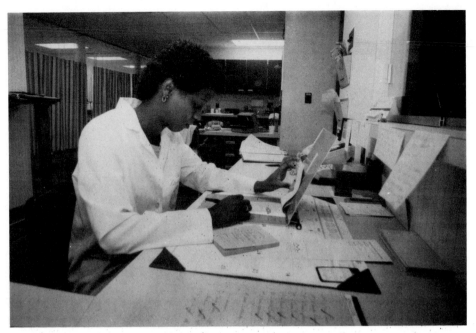

Administrative support personnel, such as this unit clerk, perform nonnursing functions. (Courtesy of Memorial Hospital, Chattanooga, TN.)

drive a specially equipped car with the physical capacity left to them. In addition, they assist patients to learn skills to return to previous employment or retrain patients for new employment options. Occupational therapists have bachelor's degrees.

ADMINISTRATIVE SUPPORT PERSONNEL

In all organizations, there are administrative functions that must be performed: payroll, billing, filing insurance claims, filing forms, paying bills, system support, and others. These activities require considerable time. By hiring administrative staff, the clinical staff is freed to concentrate on direct patient care services.

The administrative staff ensures that the operations of the facility run smoothly and that clinicians have the resources necessary to meet patient needs. They also educate the clinical staff on the financial realities of the environment and work with the staff to find ways to provide quality care at least cost.

Nurse's Role on the Health Care Team and in the Health Care Delivery System

Nurses fulfill a number of roles on the health care team. They are perhaps the most flexible of health professionals and do a number of things well. This section will provide an overview of several aspects of the nursing role.

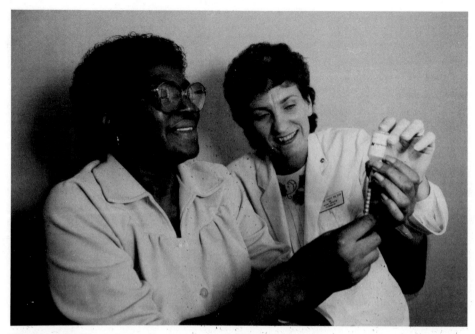

The nurse fulfills a vital role as patient teacher. (Courtesy of Memorial Hospital, Chattanooga, TN.)

PROVIDER OF CARE

Nurses provide direct, hands-on care to patients in all health care agencies and settings. They take an active role in illness prevention and health promotion and maintenance. They offer health screenings, home health services, and an array of health care services in schools, workplaces, clinics, doctors' offices, and other settings. They are instrumental in the high survival rates in trauma centers and newborn intensive care units.

TEACHER

Nurse educators teach patients and families, the community, other health care team members, students, businesses, and government. In hospital settings as patient/family educators, nurses provide information about illnesses and teach about medications, treatments, and rehabilitation needs. They help patients understand how to deal with the life changes necessitated by chronic illnesses. Nurses also teach how to adapt care to the home setting when that is required.

In community settings, nurses offer classes in injury/illness prevention and health promotion. Often these classes are jointly taught with other health care team members. For example, a nutritionist and a nurse may teach a group of expectant parents on how to prepare and feed their infants. Nurses have a responsibility to understand and teach how the health or dysfunction of the environment may affect both the short- and long-term health of the community.

Nurses are often the key educators on the health care team. They teach other team members about the patient and family and why different interventions may have varying degrees of success. Nurses help other team members find cost-effective, quality interventions that are desired and needed by the patient rather than wasting resources on ineffective, inefficient, undesired, or unneeded services.

Nurses also serve as teachers of the next generation of nurses. Nursing students need educators who set high standards and ideals but also who help students understand the ethical choices that all health care providers must make.

COUNSELOR

People who experience illness or injury often have strong emotional responses. It is clear that the relationship between emotions, the mind, and the body is critical to promotion of and restoration to health. As counselors, nurses provide basic counseling and support to patients and their families.

Using therapeutic communication techniques, nurses encourage people to discuss their feelings, to explore possible options and solutions to their unique problems, and to choose for themselves the best alternatives for action. They also serve as bereavement counselors to terminally ill patients and their families. Nurses may, with advanced education and certification, provide psychotherapy services, which extend beyond the basic counseling role.

The nurse's role as counselor often overlaps with the roles of social workers, psychiatrists, spiritual advisers, and mental health specialists. But because nurses are with patients more, they have opportunities to respond to the emotional needs of patients as they occur.

MANAGER

The effective management of nursing resources is essential. With budgets ranging from hundreds of thousands to many million dollars, nurse managers (head nurses) of patient care units in hospitals manage "businesses" larger than many small companies. Nurse managers must have strong leadership, financial, marketing, systems, and organizational behavior skills.

Chief nurse executives may manage over a thousand employees and multi-million-dollar budgets. They interact with other top executives and community leaders, often sitting on the hospital's board of directors. Nurse executives must ensure the quality of nursing care within financial, regulatory, and legislative constraints.

All nurses are managers, however. The bedside staff nurse must manage the care of a group of patients and decide what priorities are, which staff members to assign to patients, and how to accomplish all the activities during an 8- or 12-hour period. Nurses are also involved in case management or **managed care**. In this role, nurses review patient cases and coordinate services so that quality care can be achieved at the lowest cost. With health care costs escalating, managed care is one way to distribute scarce resources to the greatest number of patients.

Self-Assessment: How Intrapreneurial Are You?

If you answer "yes" to more of these questions than you answer "no," then you have the personality characteristics to become an intrapreneur.

Do you like to spend time thinking of ways to make things work better?

Are you willing to take risks that you view as reasonable?

Do you enjoy ambiguity because it stimulates your creativity?

Do you think of new ideas while driving to work, taking a shower, or exercising?

When you have a new idea, can you visualize the steps to take to get it done?

Do you have more energy than most people you know?

Do you like the challenge of new tasks and projects?

Are you willing to work extremely hard at problems or tasks when you be-lieve you can make a difference in how they turn out?

Are you good at influencing others to accept new ways of doing things?

Do you have a good sense of humor? Can you laugh at yourself?

Do you like to consider the possibilities rather than the limitations in a situation?

Can you mobilize the necessary resources (time, energy, people, materials) when a job needs to be done?

Can you work collaboratively with others on your ideas?

Do you learn from your failures?

Have you found ways to give yourself positive feedback so you are less reliant on the feedback of others?

Adapted, with permission, from: Manion, J. (1991). Nurse intrapreneurs: The heroes of health care's future. *Nursing Outlook,* 39(1), 18–21.

RESEARCHER

As you learned in Chapter 12, whether research is a nurse's primary responsibility or not, all nurses should be involved in nursing research. Nurse researchers investigate whether current or potential nursing actions achieve their expected outcomes, what options for care may be available, and how best to provide care. Nursing research looks at patient outcomes, the nursing process, and the systems that support nursing services. Participation by all nurses in research is essential to the growth and development of the nursing profession.

COLLABORATOR

With so many health care workers involved in providing patient care, collaboration among the professions is very important. The **collaborator** role is an important one for nurses who work with others to ensure that everyone has the same patient outcomes in mind. Collaboration requires that nurses understand and appreciate what other health professionals have to offer. They must also be able to interpret to others the nursing needs of patients.

Box 13–5 Interview with Nurse Entrepreneur

The following interview was held with Margaret Fizer, B.S.N., R.N. (president of Fizer & Associates), a wellness consultant who promotes healthy employees as an integral way to promote the health and viability of a business. This means she contracts with businesses to provide workshops and classes to employees on how to attain and maintain high-level wellness. With over 15 years in the health care field, her thoughts are typical of the growing group of nurse entrepreneurs who are finding new ways for nursing to promote health for all citizens.

Q: Why did you choose to become a nurse entrepreneur?
A: For three reasons: First, I recognized that my life's purpose had changed, and I could not fulfill this purpose in the hospital setting. Second, it fit my changing life-style as my family grew. Third, I had a growing need to fulfill some creative energies that were not being met in the hospital setting. I often use the phrase "feeling haunted" to describe the force within me which required expression in new settings and formats. I believe we all have this "voice" within us which tells us what we need to do. Many people don't listen and so continue to do things they no longer find satisfying.
Q: In what ways are you better able to affect positive patient outcomes in your current position?
A: I am able to affect the lives of my patients in many ways. Sometimes it is immediately, sometimes far in the future. While I teach groups of people and can reach many more individuals this way, my impact is clearly on the individual. As a result of my work, individ-

uals may immediately apply new habits which improve their life-styles. For those who are already applying health principles in their lives, my presentations may spark them to take the next step in their quest for health. For others this may be their first exposure to alternative approaches which they can implement themselves. Many patients have told me they are very affected by my philosophy that "if you don't move today, you'll be in the same place tomorrow."
Q: What are two of the biggest challenges for nursing in the next decade?
A: First is how to look at the same things you have always seen and see them and think about them differently. Second is to change our paradigms. I believe the first leads to the second, but not everyone is willing to see things differently or change their beliefs (paradigms).
Q: What do nurses need to do to meet these challenges?
A: Nurses must be honest with themselves and not afraid of the answers to their questions. The answers may challenge how they view themselves and others, but only if they are willing to use these insights to update their beliefs and behaviors will nurses be able to truly be full partners in the future of health care. They must also start seeing things differently in their own lives, their communities, states, country, and the world.
Q: What advice do you have for nurses who would like to be nurse entrepreneurs?
A: Don't be afraid and have a vision. You need to "follow your bliss and doors will open where there were no

doors before." This is a quote from Joseph Campbell, who believed that individuals who were committed to a purpose, visualized it daily, and kept working to achieve it experienced a "power of the mind." That is, as they focused their thoughts on their goals and visualized them, they were more likely to achieve them. This has proven to be true for me over and over again. It is really trusting yourself.

Q: How will nursing's role on the health care team and within the health care delivery system change in the next decade?

A: Nurses will be more knowledge based, especially in assessments, decisions, and their suggestions for change. They will be trusted as peers with other disciplines, stretched, and challenged. They will work in many more places than now; this will only be limited by the scope of society's and nursing's vision. The things which nurses possess which will make this happen are (1) the ability to care, (2) ethical standards, and (3) intuition.

Q: What skills will nurses need to have to best demonstrate this role?

A: Intelligence. The ability to think as others think and to see their point of view while remaining able to then move into the nurse's shoes and use nursing knowledge, intelligence, critical thinking, caring, and skills to help others find solutions to their health needs.

Q: Why have you remained a part of the health care team/system instead of going into business outside of health care?

A: This is how I can best be a nurse, affecting people's lives, caring for them, and remaining intact as a person. I am able to see a need, design approaches to meet that need, and yet maintain a healthy distance and perspective. I have a wonderful ability to remember what it was like before I became a nurse and yet use what I know as a nurse to help others find solutions to their needs. I work hard to maintain this perspective and to be able to move easily between knowing and not knowing the answers. It helps me find creative solutions which may not be obvious to others. I find my ability and opportunity to find this in health care to be very satisfying.

(From Fizer, M. (1991). Personal communication. Used by permission.)

An often overlooked collaborative function of nurses is collaboration with patients and families. In planning nursing care, patients should always be involved to the full extent of their interests and abilities. Involving patients and their families in the plan of care from the very beginning is the best way to ensure their cooperation, enthusiasm, and willingness to work toward the best patient outcomes.

CHANGE AGENT (INTRAPRENEUR)

When changes are needed in the nursing system, nurses themselves can serve as agents of change. Most professional nursing education programs include change theory as part of their management courses, and graduates are prepared to become **change agents** in their work settings. The role of change agent is one that requires a combination of tact, energy, creativity, and interpersonal skills. Change is often resisted, particularly if people are comfortable with the "old

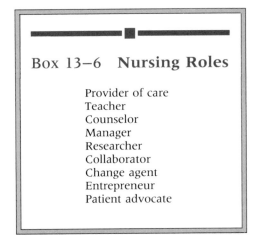

Box 13–6   Nursing Roles

Provider of care
Teacher
Counselor
Manager
Researcher
Collaborator
Change agent
Entrepreneur
Patient advocate

way" and believe it works. The role of change agent within a health care organization has been dubbed "intrapreneurship" (Manion 1990) in the belief that it requires the same kind of initiative and risk taking that entrepreneurship requires. (See "How Intrapreneurial Are You?" p. 252.)

ENTREPRENEUR

Nurse entrepreneurs are becoming more and more common. As you learned in Chapter 5, nurses now have businesses of their own that provide direct patient services in hospitals, community settings, businesses, schools, homes, and many other settings. Nurse entrepreneurs provide consultation and education services to nurses and other health team members. They provide services to businesses by conducting worksite wellness programs and by advising human resource staff on how to provide high quality health benefits to employees while reducing their costs.

To better understand this exciting new role for nurses, a nurse entrepreneur who provides workplace wellness programs to businesses was interviewed. The interview is included in Box 13–5.

PATIENT ADVOCATE

Since hospitals and the entire health care system are so complex, patients sometimes "fall through the cracks." Others need someone to help them negotiate the way through the system. They need to know how to cut through the levels of bureaucracy and red tape to get what they need when they need it.

Health care institutions often have special positions for **patient advocates**. Nurses who occupy these positions must value patient self-determination, that is, patient independence and decision making. In this role, nurses sometimes help patients bend the rules when it is in the patient's best interests and no one else will be harmed by doing so. Patient advocates are nurses who realize that policies are important and govern most situations well but that policies occasionally can, and should, be broken. For example, special care units often have strict visiting hours. Family members may only be allowed in to see the patient for ten minutes each hour. If a patient's recovery will be faster if the family is present, the nurse, serving as a patient advocate, will allow the family members more generous visitation than the policy provides.

Box 13–6 lists the roles nurses fulfill.

CHAPTER SUMMARY

The health care delivery system is a complex system that provides illness prevention, health promotion and maintenance, diagnosis and treatment, and rehabilitative and long-term care. Health care agencies are classified as governmental or voluntary, for-profit or not-for-profit, or according to level of care provided. The interdisciplinary health care team consists of an array of professionals. Each member has an important part to play in ensuring the best patient outcomes.

Nurses often serve as liaisons between the health care system and patients and their families. In doing so, they use a variety of roles such as provider, teacher, counselor, manager, researcher, collaborator, change agent, and patient advocate in meeting patients' needs.

REVIEW/DISCUSSION QUESTIONS

1. Using the yellow pages of your telephone directory or a directory of social services, identify local health services falling in the categories of health promotion, illness prevention, diagnosis and treatment, and rehabilitation and long-term care. Judging from the numbers of each, where does the health care emphasis in your community seem to be?
2. Obtain the organizational chart of a local hospital. Examine it to see how nursing fits into the overall structure. Who reports to the nurse executive, and to whom does the nurse executive report? What other administrative staff members are on the same level with the nurse executive?
3. Identify at least one local health care agency in your community that falls into each of the following classifications: governmental, voluntary, for-profit, not-for-profit, primary care, secondary care, and tertiary care. Check with classmates or your teacher to make sure you understand these classifications.
4. Interview a nurse and one nonnurse health professional. Ask them to share some of their experiences as members of interdisciplinary health care teams. What do they see as the advantages and disadvantages of the team concept?
5. From your own experiences as a consumer of nursing care, identify all the nursing roles you have encountered. Share these with at least one classmate.

REFERENCES

Aydelotte, M. K. (1983). The future health care delivery system in the United States. In N. L. Chaska (Ed.), *The nursing profession: A time to speak.* New York: McGraw-Hill.

Deming, W. E. (1982). *Quality, productivity, and competitive position.* Cambridge, MA: Massachusetts Institute of Technology, Center for Advanced Engineering Study.

Deming, W. E. (1986). *Out of the crisis.* Cambridge, MA: Massachusetts Institute of Technology, Center for Advanced Engineering Study.

Fizer, M. (1991). Personal communication.

Jenkins, J. E. (1991). Professional governance: The missing link. *Nursing Management.* 22(8), 26–28, 30.

Manion, J. (1990). *Change from within: Nurse intrapreneurs as health care innovators.* Kansas City, MO: American Nurses Association.

Manthey, M. (1991). *Leaders empower staff.* Minneapolis, MN: Creative Nursing Management.

U.S. Department of Health and Human Services. (1990). *Healthy people 2000: National health promotion and disease prevention objectives.* Washington, D.C.: Author.

SUGGESTED READINGS

Anderson, C. A., and Daigh, R. D. (1991). Quality mind-set overcomes barriers to success. *Healthcare Financial Management, 91*(2), 21–32.

Capuzzi, C., and Garland, M. (1990). The Oregon plan: Increasing access to health care. *Nursing Outlook, 38*(6), 258–263.

Caruso, L. A., and Payne, D. F. (1990). Collaborative management: A nursing practice model. *Journal of Nursing Administration, 20*(12), 28–32.

Cohen, E. L. (1991). Nursing case management: Does it pay? *Journal of Nursing Administration, 21*(4), 20–25.

Drew, J. C. (1990). Health maintenance organizations: History, evolution and survival. *Nursing & Health Care, 11*(3), 145–149.

Hawkins, J. W., et al. (1988). An interdisciplinary team in a nurse managed center. *Nursing Management, 19*(4), 58–64.

Jenkins, J. (1988). A nursing governance and practice model: What are the costs? *Nursing Economic$, 6*(6), 302–311.

Porter-O'Grady, T. (1991). A nurse on the board. *Journal of Nursing Administration, 21*(1), 40–46.

Ryan, S. A. (1990). A new decade of leadership. *Nursing Clinics of North America, 25*(3), 597–605.

Chapter

Financing Health Care

Kay K. Chitty

CHAPTER OBJECTIVES

What students should be able to do after studying this chapter:

1. Explain the economic principle of supply and demand and its relevance to health care costs.

2. Cite examples of causes of health care cost escalation.

3. Describe the major methods of payment for health care.

4. Explain cost containment efforts since 1975 and their impact on nursing practice.

5. Describe the relationship between cost containment and quality management initiatives.

6. Identify general guidelines for evaluating national health insurance proposals.

VOCABULARY BUILDING

Terms to know:

acuity
certificate of need
  (CON)
cost containment
deductible

diagnosis-related
  groups (DRGs)
Health Care Financing
  Administration
  (HCFA)

health maintenance
  organization
  (HMO)
Hill-Burton Act
Medicaid

Medicare
out-of-pocket
  payment
patient classification
  system (PCS)
personal payment
preferred provider
  organization
  (PPO)

premium
private insurance
professional review
  organization (PRO)
prospective payment
  system (PPS)
quality management
retrospective
  reimbursement

skill mix
third-party payment
worker's
  compensation

*T*he public debate over financing health care in the United States has waxed and waned since the mid-1970s. The dilemma faced by the nation is how to provide high-quality health care services while keeping costs down.

Evidence of public concern about rising health care costs was seen in a cover story in the November 25, 1991, issue of *Time* magazine. That story began with the statement: "There are two kinds of prices in America today: regular prices and health care prices" (Castro 1991, p. 34). It seems that at a time when health care miracles are at an all-time high, public support for the system that created those miracles is eroding. Finding an answer to the health care finance dilemma is a challenge that will not be easily resolved.

The following letter, published in *Rate Controls*, a health care finance newsletter, summarizes some of the reasons behind upwardly spiraling health care costs.

An Open Letter to the American Public*

[Dear Fellow Citizens:]

I can't stand it any longer—it's me—I am guilty—I did it. I listened to your demands for more of everything, and I supplied them. You wanted more and better educated people to take care of you, and I supplied them. You wanted new and higher levels of care, and I brought them to you. The pressure to create bright, beautiful facilities became a goal for you, and I have responded. You wanted more time in life and I gave it to you. You wanted me close by—and you wanted me to be ready for anything at any time—and I am. You wanted to sell me new technologies, and I bought them. You wanted me to pull you into this life and you want me to gently caress your hand as you leave it, and I do. And yes, it costs. It costs a lot more than you like and much more than I would like—and I will continue to create the best possible system for you to use. And I will

---

*(From Silver, A. (1987). We'd like to be more optimistic about 1987—but. *Rate Controls*, 2 (2a), 1. Used by permission.)

always be aware of the resources I consume and the financial burden I contribute to—but I will be here—it's me—I did it—I'm guilty.

[Yours truly,]

"Your American Health Care System"

Most Americans believe that health care is a right, not a privilege. President George Bush, in his 1992 "State of the Union" address, affirmed that belief with his statement, "Good health is every American's right." In spite of this affirmation by the highest elected official in the nation, the statistics are disturbing.

In 1991, an estimated 37 million Americans had no health insurance, and millions more were underinsured (Castro 1991). Health care consumed 17 percent of the gross national product (GNP), more than any other single entity. Over $2 billion per day is spent on medical care in the United States, a staggering amount.

During 1990, employee health care benefits consumed 26 cents of every dollar of business profits (Cuniff 1991). General Motors alone spent $3.2 billion, more than it spent on steel, to provide health coverage for employees, their dependents, and retirees (Castro 1991). All these figures are expected to increase, with no end in sight. If this trend is allowed to continue until the year 2010, one third of all national resources will be spent on health care. As a result of upwardly spiraling costs, almost everyone agrees that there is a crisis in health care and that reform is needed.

Nurses and nursing practice are profoundly affected by financial issues. Therefore, students of professional nursing need to understand the overall economic context in which nursing care is provided. This chapter will explore several major concepts necessary to understanding health care finance: basic economic theory, a brief historical review of the causes of health care cost escalation, current methods of payment, cost containment efforts, the economics of nursing care, and the impact of cost containment on nursing care. Criteria by which to evaluate proposals for national health reform will be summarized.

Basic Economic Theory

Nursing school curricula do not typically require undergraduates to take courses in economics, yet there is an urgent need for nurses to understand the economic context in which they practice.

Supply and Demand

A basic economic theory is the "law of supply and demand." According to this theory, a normal economic system consists of two parts: suppliers, who provide goods and services, and consumers, who demand and use goods and services. In a monetary environment, that is, one in which money is used as a unit of exchange, consumers exchange money for desired goods and services.

Figure 14–1   Price sensitivity in a normal economic environment.

In an efficient marketplace, the market price of goods and services serves to create an equilibrium in which supply roughly equals demand, and demand roughly equals supply. When demand exceeds supply, prices rise. When supply exceeds demand, prices fall. The relationship between price and equilibrium can be seen at the clothing store. During an unusually mild winter, for example, the demand for heavy coats is likely to be low. Since demand is low, manufacturers cut back on production, and retailers stop ordering coats and place their current stock of coats on sale. If the sale price is low enough, however, people will continue to buy coats. Through fluctuations in supply and demand, created by price, equilibrium is approached. This example illustrates the principle of price sensitivity, that is, that "the change in demand for goods or services is a function of the change in the price of those goods or services" (Ward 1988, p. 7). Figure 14–1 illustrates the relationship between price and demand.

Price Sensitivity in Health Care

In pre–health insurance days when people paid their own medical bills, doctors and hospitals set their fees with some sensitivity to what patients could pay. When costs were high, patients complained. But health insurance created a system that removed price sensitivity from the concern of most health care consumers because they pay only a small portion of the real costs; a third party (the employer or insurance company) pays the rest.

Following the principle of price sensitivity to its extreme, which would occur if price were to diminish to zero, demand for goods and services theoretically would increase to the point of being insatiable (Ward 1988, p. 6). But even when price remains constant or even increases, if someone other than the consumer pays, demand can still become insatiable because the consumer is insensitive to cost. This is an important point to keep in mind when reviewing the history of health care finance. History has demonstrated that when there is little or no out-of-pocket expense to the consumer, economic equilibrium is upset.

History of Health Care Finance

Prior to 1940, more than 90 percent of Americans either paid directly from their own pockets for health care or depended on charity care. Fewer than 10 percent had private health insurance. Public insurance programs, such as Medicare and Medicaid, had not yet come into existence (Eason, Lee, and Spickerman 1988). Following World War II, most industrialized countries began publicly financed health care systems that provided care for all citizens to the extent each country could afford to do so. The United States, however, did not adopt a public, universal access system, choosing instead to continue the private, fee-for-service system.

Growth of Private Insurance

In 1943, the Internal Revenue Service (IRS) ruled that people did not have to pay income tax on health benefits paid by their employers. Since wage controls were imposed during the war to keep the wartime economy stable, providing employer-paid health benefits was a new way employers could reward employees without violating wage controls. And when states chose to grant tax-exempt status for hospital- and physician-owned private insurance companies, such as Blue Cross and Blue Shield, these private insurers grew dramatically. By 1960, two thirds of nonelderly Americans had private health insurance, mostly paid for by employers.

The Hill-Burton Act

In 1946, the U.S. Congress passed the Hospital Survey and Construction Act. Called the **Hill-Burton Act** after the congressmen who sponsored it, this law called for and funded surveys of states' needs for hospitals, paid for planning hospitals and public health centers, and provided partial funding for constructing and equipping them. Small towns, which could not have afforded community hospitals on their own, were encouraged by this legislation to build them, and many did. The scope of the Hill-Burton Act expanded until the late 1960s. With accessible, new, well-equipped hospitals in many towns and employer-paid health insurance a standard job benefit, the stage was set for dramatic increases in the utilization of hospitals and health care services.

The Rise of Public Insurance Programs

The problem of paying for health care for the unemployed and the elderly was not solved by private insurance, and many continued to receive inadequate care. But in 1965, Congress approved two public insurance programs to cover these groups: **Medicare**, which is for the elderly and certain disabled people, and **Medicaid**, which is for the poor. They were designed to ensure that citizens who were uninsured by employers and unable to afford their own private health insurance would be protected. At that point in time, a unique public-private partnership system of insurance that would care for all seemed to be in place. Unfortunately, that partnership has not lived up to anyone's expectations.

Retrospective Reimbursement

Originally, both public and private insurance plans were based on **retrospective** (after-the-fact) **reimbursement**. This meant that when Mrs. Johnson went to the hospital with pneumonia, a request for reimbursement for whatever services were rendered (chest X rays, blood work, physical examinations, antibiotic therapy) was sent to the insurer. Depending on the terms of her insurance policy and the level of Mrs. Johnson's **deductible** (the portion she has to pay personally), the hospital was reimbursed for much, or even most, of the charges. Using retrospective reimbursement, the cost of services to insured consumers of health care was extremely low or zero. Since neither the orderers of health care (physicians) nor the consumers (patients) were concerned about cost, the demand for health care services became virtually insatiable, driving costs up dramatically (Ward 1988).

Dramatic Rise in Health Care Costs Lead to Cost Containment Initiatives

From 1960 to 1983, state and federal government spending for health care nearly doubled, rising from 5.3 percent of the GNP to 10.8 percent (Lampe 1987). In the late 1960s, the Hill-Burton legislation was replaced with legislation calling for comprehensive health planning agencies. At least one agency per state was established and empowered to review the health care needs of communities. In order to build or expand existing facilities, a **certificate of need (CON)** had to be approved by the health planning agency. Utilization of existing facilities and needs of the public were examined closely before CONs were issued. The result of this attempt to cut costs was a dramatic slowing in the construction and expansion of hospitals and public health facilities nationwide (Lampe 1987).

By 1975, additional serious cost containment efforts were under way, stimulated by concerns about costs on the part of politicians, consumer groups, and employers. After-the-fact payment for services was gradually changed to prospective payment systems in which providers, such as physicians and hospitals, received payment on a per-case basis, regardless of the cost to the provider to deliver the services (Lampe 1987). There is more about this and other cost containment initiatives later in this chapter.

Continued Escalation of Health Care Costs

In spite of comprehensive health planning efforts, health care costs continued to rise. One of the reasons for the rise in costs is related to the development of technologies. New technologies are extremely costly: A single X-ray machine can cost $250,000, and more advanced types of diagnostic imaging machines can cost up to $2 million each. In 1991, a single dose of a drug used to treat heart attacks cost $2500 per dose (Castro 1991). Box 14–1 itemizes a sampling of medical charges in 1991.

The United States has experienced increases in both the aging and non-elderly-but-uninsured populations. The members of both groups desire and re-

---

Box 14–1   Some Examples of Medical Charges, 1991

- "Annual dose of human growth hormones for a child with a severe deficiency—$20,000."
- "Coronary bypass surgery for a 50-year-old man—$49,000."
- "Cost of a Bufferin tablet for a patient in a psychiatric hospital—$3.75."
- "Price of a modified radical mastectomy—$7900."
- "One day's intensive care for a crack baby—$2000."
- "A 50-minute session with an elite psychotherapist—$160."
- "Delivery of a baby by Caesarean section—$7500."

(Data from Castro, J. (1991). Condition: Critical. *Time*, November 25, 1991, 34.)

---

quire increasing amounts of health care, creating additional cost escalation. Another reason for increasing costs is that expanding employment opportunities for health care personnel outside of hospitals has caused shortages of such personnel in hospitals and nursing homes. These shortages in turn have resulted in increased salary and benefit costs.

Fraud and abuse of the payment system account for part of the problem as well. An estimated $75 billion of the United States's annual health expenditures may be due to fraud, including as much as 20 percent of all worker's compensation claims (Kerr 1991). Health care providers such as doctors, clinics, and hospitals are on the honor system, but some find ways to cheat the system. In June 1991, for example, a $1 billion scheme was uncovered in California. After offering free tests in order to learn patients' insurance information, sham "clinics" sent insurers phony bills without the awareness of the insured patients.

The result of upwardly spiraling costs, fueled by technology, demographic changes, and fraud, is that health care costs accounted for 17 percent of the GNP in 1991. Unable to pay for employees' health care, some employers have either left the system and insured their own employees (called self-insurance), scaled back or eliminated health benefits, or passed more and more of the costs of insurance on to employees. In 1989, 78 percent of all labor union strike activity was stimulated by employers eliminating previously provided health care benefits (Horine 1990).

In 1990, an estimated 37 million Americans, two thirds of whom were employed, had no health insurance (Horine 1990). This figure represented 15.5 percent of the noninstitutionalized nonmilitary population (Ward 1990). At the same time, more than 100 million people were either underinsured or unable to pay their portion of the coverage available to them.

Current Methods of Payment for Health Care

Putting aside for a moment the problems associated with increasing health care costs, the major current methods of payment for health services in use today will be examined next. There are five major methods: personal payment, worker's compensation, Medicare, Medicaid, and private insurance.

Personal Payment

Personal payment for services is the least common method. Few people can afford **out-of-pocket** payment for more than the most basic health services. At today's prices, an illness or injury severe enough to require hospitalization can quickly exhaust a family's financial reserves, forcing them into bankruptcy. Generally, only those people without access to some form of private group insurance or public insurance rely on personal payment. The number of uninsured Americans is growing rapidly and is a grave national concern.

Worker's Compensation

Worker's compensation varies from state to state but generally covers only workers who are injured on the job. It usually covers both treatment for injuries and weekly payments during the time the worker is absent from work for injury-related causes. In the case of accidental death, the worker's family receives compensation. Companies are required by law to contribute to a compensation fund from which money is withdrawn when accidental injuries or deaths occur (Black 1988).

Medicare

Medicare, or Title XVIII of the Social Security Act, is a nationwide federal health insurance program established in 1965. Medicare is available to people aged 65 and over, regardless of the recipient's income. It also covers certain disabled individuals and people requiring dialysis or kidney transplants. Medicare has two separate but coordinated programs. The first, known as Part A, is a hospitalization insurance program. Part B is a supplementary medical insurance program that covers visits to physicians' offices and other outpatient services. Originally intended to be a no-cost or low-cost program for the elderly, the cost of participating in Medicare has risen steadily. In 1992, Part A required participants to pay a $652 deductible for hospitalization, and Part B required a $100 fee per year plus a monthly premium of $31.80 (Ables 1992). Ironically, many elderly people find they cannot afford to participate in Medicare.

Medicaid

Medicaid, or Title XIX of the Social Security Act, is a group of jointly-funded federal-state programs for low-income, elderly, blind, and disabled individuals. It, too, was established in 1965. There are broad federal guidelines, but states have some flexibility in how they administer the program. People must meet

Box 14–2   Facts About Medicare and Medicaid

	MEDICARE	MEDICAID
Funded by:	Federal government	Federal and state governments
Administered by:	Federal government	State governments
Who is eligible?	People over 65	Poor and disabled
Level of benefits:	Same nationwide	Varies from state to state
Payment by recipients?	Required	Not required
Coverage:	Hospitalization; outpatient care; no prescriptions or optical care	Comprehensive, including prescriptions and optical care

eligibility requirements determined by each state. Eligibility depends on income and varies from state to state. Rates of payment also vary, with some states providing far higher payments than others. The amount the federal government contributes to Medicaid varies from a minimum of 50 percent of total costs to a maximum of 75 percent. The differences in eligibility and payment rates lead to wide variations in the level of care provided to the poor in different states. Unlike those on Medicare, people who receive Medicaid are not required to pay any fees to participate. Box 14–2 highlights the similarities and differences in the Medicare and Medicaid programs.

Private Insurance

Private insurance, also called voluntary insurance, is a system wherein insurance premiums are either paid by insured individuals or their employers or shared between individuals and employers. Periodic payments (**premiums**) are paid into the insurance plan, and certain health care benefits are covered as long as the premiums are paid. Early in the development of private insurance, many treatments were covered only if they were performed in an inpatient (hospital) setting. This was one of the features that tended to drive up the cost of services. Today most insurers stipulate that costs of hospitalization are reimbursable only if treatment *cannot* be performed on an outpatient basis.

Cost Containment Measures Revisited

Spiraling health care costs have caused both public and private insurers to examine their practices and to institute a variety of measures designed to reduce costs. This initiative is referred to as **cost containment**.

Box 14–3   Medicare and Medicaid Costs, 1967 and 1991

Facts about Medicare

Costs in first full year (1967) = $ 5 billion
Costs in 1991   = $110 billion
Those helped   = All elderly, regardless of family resources

Facts about Medicaid

Costs in first full year (1967) = $ 2.3 billion
Costs in 1991   = $158.7 billion
Those helped in 1980   = 65 percent of the poor
           in 1991   = 40 percent of the poor
Medicaid is the fastest-growing spending program in the United States

(Data from Health care expenditures and other data: An international compendium from the Organization for Economic Cooperation and Development. (1989). *Health Care Financing Review*, annual supplement, 111–195.)

As discussed earlier, the 1970s saw attempts to control health care costs through legislation designed to regulate costs and monitor the quality of care. Comprehensive health planning agencies and CONs were two mechanisms used. Some states also practiced rate setting, in which the state set limits on reimbursements. Yet costs continued to rise. The retrospective payment method for Medicare and Medicaid had become uncontrollable. It was apparent that basic changes in payment mechanisms were required. Box 14–3 contains information about the dramatic increases in costs to taxpayers of Medicare and Medicaid since they were implemented in 1967.

The passage of the Tax Equity and Fiscal Responsibility Act (TEFRA) in 1982 stimulated a dramatic restructuring of health care delivery in this country. Through this act, the federal government changed the payment method for Medicare from the retrospective system, which was uncontrollable, to a **prospective payment system (PPS)** based on **diagnosis-related groups (DRGs)**. DRGs will be described later in this chapter. Prospective payment was designed to create a more competitive environment and resulted in an emphasis on efficiency, cost effectiveness, and financial accountability. It also stimulated competition among health care providers. For the first time, providers had incentives to operate in a cost-effective manner.

Entire governmental agencies have been created to monitor and administer cost containment programs. Private insurers have also gotten on the cost containment bandwagon. There are several cost containment entities students should be aware of.

Federal Cost Containment Programs

There are three main federal cost containment programs that are noteworthy: the Health Care Financing Administration, professional review organizations, and diagnostic related groups. Each will be reviewed briefly.

THE HEALTH CARE FINANCING ADMINISTRATION

The **Health Care Financing Administration (HCFA,** pronounced hic'-fa) is a federal cost containment agency created to administer the Medicare and Medicaid programs. Briefly stated, HCFA's goals are:

1. To develop and establish standards to ensure that quality care is rendered to recipients of Medicare and Medicaid.
2. To improve the efficiency and responsiveness of Medicare and Medicaid and to promote beneficiary awareness.
3. To enforce standards for hospitals, nursing homes and other long-term care facilities, laboratories, clinics, and other health care facilities.

PROFESSIONAL REVIEW ORGANIZATIONS

Professional review organizations (PROs) review every Medicare hospital admission to make sure that patients meet criteria for hospitalization and that their health care needs cannot be met on an outpatient basis or in a community-based setting. PROs also monitor all Medicare patients' lengths of stay. If a patient is hospitalized longer than the PRO determines is appropriate, or if procedures are performed that the PRO determines are unnecessary, the hospital is denied reimbursement for the extra days and the unnecessary procedures (Dougherty 1989). This causes hospitals to be very careful about who they admit, how long they allow patients to stay, and what procedures are performed while they are hospitalized.

DIAGNOSIS-RELATED GROUPS

DRGs represent all possible known disease entities classified according to medical diagnosis. Each disease is combined with similar diseases into nearly 500 DRGs for Medicare reimbursement purposes. For each DRG, the Medicare system has predetermined a fair price for hospital services. This represents the amount the hospital is paid by Medicare to treat patients in that particular DRG. If the hospital's costs exceed the preestablished reimbursement rate, it loses money. If the hospital is able to successfully treat the patient for less than the established reimbursement rate, it can keep the excess. This type of reimbursement system is an example of a PPS.

Private Cost Containment Programs

Private insurers have benefited from federal cost containment initiatives because they tend to establish private reimbursement rates at the same level the federal

News Note "Think Your Hospital Care Has Changed? It Has!"

Q: What exactly is a DRG?

A: The government (via Medicare and Medicaid) grouped all illnesses and symptoms into approximately 460 groups. The assumption is that every hospital stay will fall into a category (diagnostic related group). The hospital, then, is paid a flat fee for that group, rather than being paid for the actual services any individual patient receives. If a patient is admitted for a urinary infection, for instance, the hospital knows in advance how many days they will be reimbursed for treating that illness. The hospital stops getting paid at the expiration of that time, no matter how long the patient actually stays. Conversely, if the patient can be treated in less time, the hospital still gets the same amount. This has the effect of creating a powerful profit-loss situation for hospitals that is dependent on how quickly they can get the patient discharged. . . .

Q: Am I understanding that how long I may stay in the hospital is now a predetermined, known factor?

A: To a large extent, yes. One example is DRG-179 which is a category for people with digestive disorders. Regulations for DRG-179 allow 9.6 days of hospitalization. Hospitals are paid for 9.6 days when any patient is admitted with that diagnosis. If the patient has complications that cause more involved treatment or a prolonged stay, the hospital is losing money after 9.6 days. If the patient can be discharged in less time than 9.6 days, the hospital is nevertheless paid for the full 9.6 days. Clearly there is an incentive for hospitals to discharge early.

Q: What is the result of this payment method on me?

A: You will probably feel great pressure to be discharged from a hospital more quickly than you once did. Your physician is also under intense pressure to discharge patients at or before the time limit. Critics of the system charge that patients are being discharged sooner and sicker because of these financial considerations. . . .

Q: How are hospitals responding to the new standards?

A: Hospitals have reduced the amount of time nurses spend with each patient, have reduced services that are expensive . . . use less expensive medications, limit allowable tests, discourage inpatient acute care hospitalizations in favor of day surgery and outpatient care, and refer patients to home nursing agencies for needed care. . . .

The DRG system is here to stay. Implementation of the system in 1985 was to reduce waste in the medical system and bring skyrocketing costs to a halt.

Proponents claim we are receiving lower cost, more efficient medical care. Opponents feel the system has caused a significant downfall in quality of patient care and inappropriate profit motive. In any regard, it changes the way your health care is being delivered and deserves patient knowledge and attention.

(Excerpted from Black, C. (1989). Think your hospital care has changed? It has! *Accent on Living*, 33(2), 46–48. Used by permission.)

government uses for reimbursing hospitals for Medicare DRGs. Two additional types of programs designed to lower health care costs have been established by private insurers.

Preferred provider organizations (PPOs) are groups of physicians or institutions to which insurance companies direct their policyholders for care. These providers have agreed to provide services at somewhat lower-than-usual cost. Policyholders are provided a list of "preferred providers" from whom to choose. If they choose to use providers not on the list, they usually must pay a larger share of the costs of care.

Health maintenance organizations (HMOs) are networks or groups of providers who agree to provide certain basic health care services for a single predetermined yearly fee. The voluntarily enrolled participants in HMOs pay the same amount regardless of the amount and kind of services they actually receive. HMOs benefit financially when their patients stay well. Therefore, they have an incentive to promote health maintenance and prevention of illness in their enrolled participants.

The Economics of Nursing Care

Traditionally nurses were unconcerned with the cost of care, believing all patients were entitled to high-quality nursing care regardless of ability to pay. Until fairly recently, few efforts were made to determine the actual cost of nursing care. The average hospital bill included the cost of nursing services in the general category of "room rate," just as housekeeping services are included in the room rate. In the past, the hospital census (number of patients) was used to determine the number of nurses needed. This worked fairly well when payment was retrospective. With the advent of prospective payment, however, it was imperative for hospitals to determine their staffing needs more efficiently.

It has long been recognized that different patients require different amounts of nursing time, depending in large part on how sick they are. Conner, working at Johns Hopkins Hospital in 1960, developed a **patient classification system (PCS)** that identified patients' needs for nursing care in quantitative terms. It was a new idea that patient needs were quantifiable, were predictable, and could help hospitals determine the need for nursing resources. For the first time, patient needs, as opposed to hospital census, could be used as criteria for determining the number of nurses needed (DiVestea 1985). Since that time, different PCSs have been developed, most of which depend on patient *acuity*, or degree of illness, and the resulting amount and complexity of nursing care required.

Initiatives called "costing nursing services" are under way to determine the cost of nursing care precisely. It is believed that this will solve one dilemma of

Box 14–4   Quality Management and Cost Containment: An Interview

Gail Ward, M.S., R.N., is Vice President, Quality Management and Charlene Robertson, M.S.N., R.N., is Assistant Vice President, Nursing, at a private not-for-profit hospital in a midsized city in the southeastern United States.

Q: Tell me a little about the hospital, its size, services, and the number of nurses employed here.

A: Robertson: This is a 365-bed hospital. We have all services except obstetrics and pediatrics. There are 610 members of the nursing staff, which includes 405 R.N.s [registered nurses], 70 L.P.N.s [licensed practical nurses], and 135 nursing assistants.

Q: What specific cost containment programs have been started here in the past few years that have influenced nursing care?

A: Robertson: We instituted a program called "Winners" that invites all employees to submit suggestions for reducing costs, improving quality, or increasing patient or staff satisfaction. The ideas are examined by our management engineer, and if an idea is selected, the employee who suggested it receives a monetary award. Some people have received $1000 or more. This kind of program makes everybody aware of costs and keeps them alert to possibilities for reducing costs without sacrificing quality.

Q: What has been done to relieve nurses of nonnursing tasks?

A: Robertson: Two things come immediately to mind. Our pharmacy now premixes intravenous [IV] medications to save nurses time. Now the IV fluids for a particular patient come to the unit ready to administer. This has also reduced errors. Another example is that the housekeeping department has taken over some responsibilities that nurses used to assume.

Q: What is the goal of quality management?

A: Ward: The focus of quality management, or continuous quality improvement, is to take a positive rather than a negative approach. We look for ways to improve rather than trying to figure out who or what went wrong. When people find out that they are being helped to improve rather than punished for errors, they willingly participate and aren't fearful of reporting problems or errors.

Q: Who participates in quality management?

A: Ward: Everyone. We have a medical staff program and a hospitalwide program. We take a multidisciplinary approach. The goal is for everyone, even the lowest person in the hospital, to have input into quality management. This is a slow process and does not occur overnight, but it is the goal.

Q: How are nurses involved in quality management?

A: Robertson: About two years ago we reorganized nursing and decentralized certain functions. We now have a council of quality management, a clinical council, and a professional council. Each unit has a representative on these councils, and they meet monthly. When our hospitalwide and unit-specific quality monitoring programs reveal a problem, we develop an action plan that is implemented on each unit. For example, we decided we needed to reduce our patient falls. Now, each of our patients is assessed upon admission for their potential to fall. Medium- to high-risk patients wear green arm bands, their doors have green magnets on them, and their charts are marked with green stickers. Every member of the nursing staff is then alerted that this person might fall, and they pay attention to certain safety precautions. Through this program, we have cut our patient falls by two thirds.

Q: How does quality management impact the way nursing care is provided?

A: Ward: When nurses have been closely involved in quality monitoring, they are acutely aware of all the potential areas for problems. They are much more conscious of safety, prevention of irregular events, and so on. They are very interested in collaborating with other disciplines to improve patient care.

Q: What would you like to say about cost containment and quality management to students of professional nursing around the nation?

A: Ward: They should realize that dollars are tight but that health care consumers still expect improvement in quality of care. You might say customer expectations are high and increasing. Nurses have to be prepared to meet these demands and understand nursing's role in cost containment. Cost containment and quality management are inseparable. Nurses can achieve a higher level of satisfaction knowing that they are providing high-quality care while conserving our precious health care resources.

(From interviews: Robertson, C. (1992). Personal communication; and Ward, G. (1992). Personal communication.)

contemporary nurses who find themselves torn between two conflicting goals: first, their own desire to provide comprehensive patient care in the tradition of the past, when cost was no object; and second, pressure from financial managers to provide only services that are reimbursible under insurance regulations.

Not knowing the exact costs of nursing services limits nurses' ability to determine what high-quality nursing care costs and to calculate the number of hours of nursing care it takes to maintain it for each DRG. Determining the best **skill mix**, that is, the ratio of registered nurses to licensed practical nurses and nursing assistants on each hospital unit, is also impaired when the cost of nursing care is unknown.

In the past it was assumed that the cost of nurses was a major part of hospital costs. When tough economic times came, the first cost reduction efforts were therefore aimed at nursing. Studies by the American Nurses Association Center for Nursing Research (McKibben 1985) found that nursing accounts for only 20 to 28 percent of the costs of hospitalization for two thirds of DRGs examined. Costing nursing services and developing standardized reimbursements based on cost will enhance the ability of nurse managers to control nursing resources and negotiate for a fair share of hospital financial resources.

Since 1983 many studies have been undertaken to determine the actual costs of nursing care. Listed in the Suggested Readings at the end of this chapter are articles that explain more about this fascinating research that will profoundly affect nursing practice in the future.

The Impact of Cost Containment on Nursing Care

When the drive to provide high-quality nursing care meets the constraints of cost containment head-on, something has to give. What nurses hope, as both providers and consumers of health care, is that quality has not and will not suffer due to the emphasis on "the bottom line." The financial realities that affect the institutions in which 68 percent of nurses practice—hospitals—cannot be ignored (Bocchino 1990). In order to stay in business, hospitals must make at least enough money to pay personnel costs, maintain buildings and equipment, and pay suppliers of goods and services.

The financial vitality of a hospital depends in large measure on attracting physicians who will use that hospital's inpatient and outpatient services in providing medical care to their patients. A 1991 study done for the American College of Healthcare Executives by Arthur Andersen & Company examined the factors that influence physicians to seek affiliation with hospitals. When asked to rank factors, a panel of physicians ranked "quality of nursing staff" as the number-one factor affecting this choice (Arthur Andersen & Company and American College of Healthcare Executives 1991). If attracting physicians is essential to the financial stability of hospitals, and attracting physicians depends in large measure on the quality of the nursing staff, attaining or maintaining quality nursing care is of critical importance to the survival of hospitals.

COST CONTAINMENT AND QUALITY MANAGEMENT

Many agree that there is potential for disaster if low cost is the only outcome that matters in the health care system. The challenge is to balance the cost-effectiveness and quality patient care. Concern for maintaining high-quality services in the face of cost constraints has led to the development of a new health care initiative called "**quality management**." This field is growing and changing rapidly and creating change within hospitals. The interview in Box 14–4 with two nurses (Robertson 1992; Ward 1992) involved in quality management gives insights into the complexities and satisfactions of participation in quality management.

Health Care Reform and National Health Insurance

In 1992, the United States and South Africa were the only two industrialized nations not providing universal access to health care to all citizens (Johnson 1990). Despite the fact that 1990 health care expenditures averaged $2354 per person, infant mortality ranked twenty-second—lower than many countries with far fewer national resources. Two thirds of inner-city children under four years of age did not have the full series of immunizations that could protect them from preventable childhood diseases (Johnson 1990). There is no established minimum set of health services available to the entire population, but neither is there a maximum (Ward 1990). Some people cannot pay for even the most basic services, whereas others can afford any procedure, no matter how expensive.

News Note   "Pay More Now to Save More Later?"

The thorny pay-now-save-later dilemma facing health care reformers begs for an analogy from real life:

Say you've got an old clunker of a car that not only breaks down at the worst possible moment (the health care access problem) but costs astonishingly more every month to keep going (the health care cost inflation problem).

You contemplate buying a new car, figuring the breakdown problem would be solved and, in the long run, it would cost less to operate. But to buy the new car, you've got to pony up money now for a down payment—money you haven't got; also, the new car's monthly note is at the moment more than you're spending to fix your clunker.

Getting thorny? Now imagine that you also can't know for sure the new car payments won't also soar. And you don't know the odds the new car will be a lemon.

That's the kind of complex dilemma health care reform presents, says health policy expert Dallas Salisbury. That "lemon" factor, he adds, is driving mainstream reformers to middle-ground strategies—pay-or-play, tax incentives, insurance reforms—to fix the system rather than trash it, as national health or extreme free-market plans would.

"There may well be severe problems with the existing system" that will make fundamental change inevitable, he says. "But at least people have a sense of how the system we have works. With the middle-ground plans, there's a sense that you're not taking a chance on buying that lemon."

—Kevin Anderson

(From Anderson, K. (1992). Pay more now to save more later? *USA TODAY*, January 23, 1992, page 11-A. Copyright 1992, USA Today. Reprinted with permission.)

Soaring costs
Projected U.S. health care expenditures:

$2 trillion — $2.0

$1.5

$666 billion — $1.0

$0.5

0

'90¹   '95   2000
1-actual
Source: Commerce Dept.

By Rod Little, USA TODAY

A 1991 *Time*/Cable News Network poll of 1000 adults found that 91 percent believed that "fundamental change" in the health care system was needed, 75 percent felt costs were higher than necessary, and 83 percent advocated limiting physicians' fees. Two thirds said health care is a right, and 70 percent would be willing to pay more taxes to make sure all Americans have access to care (Castro

News Note   "Nurses Get Public's Vote as Best Bet to Cut Costs"

HEALTH COSTS
By Ron Winslow

FRIDAY, SEPTEMBER 21, 1990

The nation's nurses may hold one of the keys to lowering health-care costs.

Most people think nurses are far more likely to play a "constructive" role in reducing medical costs than doctors, hospital administrators or insurers, according to a poll conducted by Peter D. Hart Research Associates Inc. for the National League of Nursing.

Other health research indicates nurses can provide such routine services as screenings and physicals more cost-effectively than doctors, says Claire Fagin, dean at the University of Pennsylvania School of Nursing. And the poll indicated many people would be willing to see nurses for some basic services instead of a doctor "if they thought it would lower health-care costs," says Pamela Maraldo, the nursing league's chief executive officer. People are particularly interested in getting nurses to provide more care at home to avert nursing home admissions for the elderly.

But even when nurses provide such services, usually doctors must bill Medicare and many other insurers for them. "There's no reason why Medicare should pay physicians to give nursing care when nurses provide the care," argues Ms. Maraldo. The poll, she says, supports her profession's quest for status to bill Medicare directly.

It's an uphill fight. For one thing, policy makers worry that opening the Medicare spigot to another provider group could cause an immediate runup in spending. Then there's another poll that nurses lost decisively. In June, the American Medical Association voted to oppose moves to give more clinical and financial autonomy to nurses and other non-physician providers.

1991, p. 36). In the 1992 presidential campaign, candidates presented various plans for health care reform. Some experts predict that there will be a form of national health insurance in the United States by 1995.

In addition to presidential candidates and major political parties, nonpartisan groups also call for health care reform. These include nursing organizations, the American Association of Retired Persons (AARP), labor unions, the American College of Physicians, the National Leadership Coalition for Health Care Reform, and several members of the U.S. Congress. Most have put forward specific plans for reform, including "Nursing's Agenda for Health Care Reform," discussed in Chapter 4. Details of proposals vary and conflict. Some propose a variation on Canada's National Health Service. Others prefer to reform the current system. Recommended funding mechanisms also vary widely. All agree that reforming health care in America is needed and will probably be very expensive.

Guidelines for Evaluating Reform Proposals

In spite of wide-ranging differences of opinion about the specifics of health care reform proposals, there *are* areas of general agreement. Some general guidelines to look for in evaluating such proposals are:

1. Is there a uniform minimum set of benefits for all citizens, otherwise known as universal care?
2. Are coverage and benefits continuous and not dependent on where people live or work?
3. Are there mechanisms for controlling costs, especially administrative expenses?
4. Are provisions made for care to be provided by the most cost-effective personnel?
5. Are the issues of adequate facilities and personnel to ensure access for all addressed?
6. Is there an emphasis on quality care?
7. Are there incentives for healthy life-styles and preventive care?

A point of particular interest to nurses is the issue of cost-effectiveness of personnel. If care is to be provided by the most cost-effective personnel, it will mean an expansion of the role of nurses as primary care providers. Studies have shown that nurses are very cost-effective care givers and are well accepted by the public (Holzemer 1990; Lampe 1987; Winslow 1990). Organized medicine, however, actively opposes moves to give clinical autonomy to almost all non-physician providers (Winslow 1990). This is a conflict that must be resolved for true reform to occur, and nurses themselves must be active in its resolution.

CHAPTER SUMMARY

How health care is financed in the United States has changed dramatically during the past 50 years from a system dominated by personal payment to one dominated by third-party payment. This change created basic economic disequilibrium in health care. People who do not pay directly for health care are not sensitive to the price of care. Medicare and Medicaid programs, begun in 1965, created a serious financial drain on federal and state budgets. In response, cost containment efforts were begun by the federal government in the 1970s. Initial efforts were unsuccessful, so in 1982 more sweeping reforms were initiated. Retrospective payment was replaced by prospective payment. In a prospective payment system, health care providers are reimbursed a set fee, depending on the patient's diagnosis. They receive the same fee regardless of how much it actually costs to treat the patient. Since prospective payment has the potential to encourage providers to undertreat patients to reduce costs, quality management initiatives were implemented to protect consumers. The entire health care system, including nurses and nursing services, has been profoundly affected by these changes. Further changes are on the horizon. Some experts expect that a form of national health insurance will be instituted before 1995.

REVIEW/DISCUSSION QUESTIONS

1. In your view, is access to health care a basic right? Be prepared to defend your opinion.
2. List the basic health care services that should be provided to all citizens. Compare your list with classmates' lists and discuss the reasons for your priorities.
3. Should there be a limit on the percentage of national resources expended on health care? If so, how should the limit be established?
4. What process should be used to determine how health care resources are allocated? List criteria you would suggest to determine whether or not a person should receive a kidney transplant.
5. Should people with healthy life-styles pay the same for care or insurance as those whose habits result in a greater likelihood of illness? How could such a differentiation be determined?
6. Should there be rationing of extremely expensive procedures, such as heart transplants, even if the patient is able to pay? Give a rationale for your answer.

REFERENCES

Ables, J. (1992). Personal communication.

Arthur Andersen & Company and American College of Healthcare Executives. (1991). *The future of healthcare: Physician and hospital relationships.* Author.

Anderson, K. (1992). Pay more now to save more later? *USA TODAY,* January 23, 1992, 11-A.

Black, C. (1989). Think your hospital care has changed? It has! *Accent on Living,* 33(2), 46–48.

Black, H. C. (1988). *Black's law dictionary.* St. Paul, MN: West Publishing.

Bocchino, C. A. (1990). An interview with Kathryn M. Mershon. *Nursing Economics,* 8(4), 219–228.

Castro, J. (1991). Condition: Critical. *Time,* November 25, 1991, 34–42.

Cuniff, J. (1991). Soaring health costs need brake. *Chattanooga News–Free Press,* January 31, 1991, B5.

DiVestea, N. (1985). The changing health care system: An overview. In F. A. Shaffer (Ed.), *Costing out nursing: Pricing our product.* New York: National League for Nursing.

Dougherty, C. J. (1989). Cost containment, DRGs, and the ethics of health care. *Hastings Center Report,* 19(1), 5–7.

Eason, F. R., Lee, B. T., and Spickerman, S. (1988). Analyzing cost: A learning module. *Nurse Educator,* 13(4), 9–10, 13.

Health care expenditures and other data: An international compendium from the Organization for Economic Cooperation and Development. (1989). *Health Care Financing Review*, annual supplement, 111–195.

Holzemer, W. L. (1990). Quality and cost of nursing care: Is anybody out there listening? *Nursing and Health Care*, 11(8), 412–415.

Horine, M. (1990). Assuring access to quality care. *Pension World*, 26(9), 26–28.

Johnson, P. A. (1990). A national health insurance program: A nursing perspective. *Nursing and Health Care*, 11(8), 416–429.

Kerr, P. (1991). Workers' comp fraud blamed for inflating cost of health care. *Chattanooga Times*, December 30, 1991, A1.

Lampe, S. (1987). *Costing hospital nursing services: A review of the literature.* Washington, D.C.: U.S. Department of Health and Human Services.

McKibben, R. C. (1985). *DRGs and nursing care.* Kansas City: American Nurses Association Center for Research.

Robertson, C. (1992). Personal communication.

Silver, A. (1987). We'd like to be more optimistic about 1987—but. *Rate Controls*, 2(2a),1.

Ward, D. (1990). National health insurance: Where do nurses fit in? *Nursing Outlook*, 38(5), 206–207.

Ward, G. (1992). Personal communication.

Ward, J. W. (1988). *An introduction to health care financial management.* Owings Mills, MD: Rynd Communications for National Health Publishing.

Winslow, R. (1990). Nurses get public's vote as best bet to cut costs. *The Wall Street Journal*, September 21, 1990, B-1.

SUGGESTED READINGS

AMA recommends health care plan. (1990). *New York Times*, March 8, 1990, B-9.

Beyers, M. (1988). Quality: The banner of the 1980s. *Nursing Clinics of North America*, 23, 617–623.

Curtin, L. Determining costs of nursing services per DRG. *Nursing Management*, 14(4), 16–20.

Fagin, C. M. (1986). Opening the door on nursing's cost advantage. *Nursing and Health Care*, 7(7), 353.

Omachonu, V. K., and Nanda, R. (1988). A conceptual framework for hospital nursing unit productivity measurement. *I(ndustrial) E(ngineering)*, May 1988, 56–67.

Tolchin, M. (1989). Sudden support for national health care. *New York Times*, September 24, 1989, E4.

Chapter

Nursing Care Delivery Systems

Nancy L. Davis

CHAPTER OBJECTIVES

What students should be able to do after studying this chapter:

1. Differentiate among four nursing care delivery systems.

2. Discuss the advantages and disadvantages of the various delivery systems.

3. Explain differentiated practice and why it is an important challenge for nursing.

4. Recognize the responsibilities of registered nurses in supervising nonlicensed (ancillary) workers.

VOCABULARY BUILDING

Terms to know:

accountability	case management nursing	functional nursing
acuity level	collaboration	primary nursing
ancillary workers	delegation	supervision
autonomy	differentiated practice	team nursing

*C*hapter 13 covered aspects of the health care delivery system, discussed the organizational structure of hospitals, and reviewed the various roles of nurses in hospitals. This chapter will take a closer look at hospital nursing and review four common ways of organizing at the unit level to facilitate the delivery of nursing care to patients.

Scenes from the Hall

To set the stage for this discussion, let us pretend that you are a brand-new nursing student arriving at the hospital for your first clinical day. You arrive early to familiarize yourself with the hospital. As you walk down various halls, you pay particular attention to the activities going on in patients' rooms.

In one room you see a nursing assistant making an unoccupied bed, while a registered nurse (R.N.) is talking to the patient. She seems to be showing him something in a booklet she is holding. The nursing assistant is performing one task for the patient; the registered nurse is performing another for the same patient.

As you walk down another hall, you pass a registered nurse wearing street clothes. He is conducting a tour for a family of two adults and a child. He is taking them all around the hospital, showing them the equipment and explaining the procedures. They even look into the surgical suite and postanesthesia care unit. They seem to be discussing what will happen when the child is admitted for surgery.

As you pass a conference room, you see an R.N. sitting at a table with a group of other health care personnel. She is talking to them about the status of her patient's progress toward his weekly goals. Others also discuss how the patient is progressing from their perspectives.

On another unit you see a registered nurse and a social worker walking down the hall with a patient. Together, they are assisting the patient to identify community resources she may need once she is discharged to her home. You hear the patient tell the R.N. that she is afraid to use the stove at home because she cannot stand for long periods of time.

As you wait in the main lobby before meeting your instructor, it occurs to you that the registered nurses you have seen were all doing different things. They seemed to be providing nursing care in very different ways. You might wonder, "Is there more than one way to deliver nursing care to patients?" As a matter of fact, there is. You have seen four different types of delivery systems.

Types of Nursing Care Delivery Systems

As seen in Chapter 1, pre–World War I nurses cared for the sick in the patients' homes. As hospital care improved and nursing education evolved, more and more sick people were treated in hospitals. Transferring the case method as it was used in home settings to the hospital would have created prohibitively high costs. Nurses had to change from the case method, where one nurse took care of all the needs of one patient around the clock, to another method wherein groups of patients received nursing care in the same setting—a hospital unit.

Providing care to groups of patients rather than individuals required nurses to be more efficient and use their time more effectively. Various types of care delivery systems were designed to meet the goals of efficient and effective nursing care. There are several types of patient care delivery systems in use today. Four systems—functional nursing, team nursing, primary nursing, and case management nursing—will be reviewed.

Functional Nursing

By the 1930s, advances in medical technology had evolved to a point where hospital treatment surpassed that which could be provided at home. As more patients were admitted to hospitals, more nurses were employed to care for them.

The functional approach to nursing care grew out of a need to provide care to large numbers of patients. It focused on organizing and distributing tasks, or functions, among the personnel. Trained nurses provided care that required higher skill levels, and untrained workers with little skill or education performed many less complex tasks.

In **functional nursing**, personnel worked in isolation, each performing his or her tasks. The goal of functional nursing was efficient management of time, tasks, and energy. Although this practice saved hospitals money, patient care was fragmented, and patients had to relate to numerous personnel. There was no one person they could call, "My nurse."

Today, functional nursing is still used in some settings. It is particularly useful when there are few personnel available, such as at night, on weekends, and on holidays. It often is combined with another method, however, and is rarely used as the sole care delivery method (Bernhard and Walsh 1990).

Case Study: Functional Nursing

A registered nurse on the evening shift at a local nursing home has been assigned to administer special skin care treatments to bed-bound patients, change dressings, and give all medications. A licensed practical nurse (L.P.N.) will monitor all patient temperatures and blood pressures, weigh patients, record the amount they eat and drink, and monitor the blood sugar of diabetic patients. The nursing assistants have each been assigned a different group of patients for whom they are responsible during the shift. They will help these patients with personal hygiene; see that they receive their meals and snacks; and assist them with eating, toileting, and other tasks. Since it is evening, the head nurse is not there. In her place is a "charge nurse" who will sign all charts, indicating

---

Box 15–1 Advantages and Disadvantages of Functional Nursing

ADVANTAGES

Efficient—can complete many tasks in a reasonable time frame

Workers do only tasks they are educated to do

Promotes organizational skills—each worker must organize his or her own work

Promotes worker autonomy

DISADVANTAGES

Care is fragmented—emphasis on task, not person

Patients do not know who their nurse is

R.N.s have little time to talk with patient or render personal care

---

that care was administered; talk with physicians and family members; and order supplies and medications.

As they go about their work, there is little interaction among the personnel. Often they can be heard telling a patient who asks for something, "I'm not assigned to do that tonight. I'll tell the other aide you need something."

Box 15–1 shows some advantages and disadvantages of functional nursing.

INTERVIEW WITH A FUNCTIONAL NURSE

Dot Joiner (1992) is an R.N. who delivered functional nursing care during her four years as shift supervisor in a long-term care facility.

Q: What did you like most about functional nursing?
A: The interaction you have with so many patients and families. You see all the patients on the unit.
Q: What did you like least about the functional nurse's role?
A: I always felt like I never had enough time. I was constantly on the go. It's frustrating to say to patients, "Just a minute, please, and I will get someone else to help you."
Q: What, in your opinion, is the biggest advantage to the functional method of delivering nursing care?
A: The functional approach allows each person to utilize the skills he or she does best. For nurses, those are communication with patients and families, management of other personnel, and clinical skills.

Team Nursing

In response to the frustration some nurses felt when using the functional approach to patient care, Lambertson (1953) designed **team nursing**. She envisioned nursing teams as democratic work groups with different skill levels represented by different team members. They were assigned as a team to a group of patients.

Team nursing is widely used in hospitals today. The members of the team are often an R.N., who serves as team leader, an L.P.N., and one or more certified nursing assistants.

The team leader is ultimately responsible for all the care provided but delegates (assigns responsibility for) certain patients to each team member. Each member of the team provides the level of care for which they are best prepared. The least skilled and experienced members care for the patients who require the least complex care, and the most skilled and experienced members care for the sickest patients who require the most complex care.

Team nursing allows the team leader to shift, match, and redistribute patient assignments to team members according to their level of education and expertise. For example, due to the acuity level (extent of illness) of a group of patients, a team leader may "trade" **another team** leader a nursing assistant for an additional R.N. The nursing assistant will work on the team with less acutely ill patients, and the team with the sickest patients will have an extra R.N.

Team nursing enables the registered nurse team leader to supervise, coordinate, and manage the care given to all the team's patients. The team leader also reports to the head nurse.

Case Study: Team Nursing

The team leader for 12 patients on a medical/surgical unit during the night shift has one L.P.N. and one certified nursing assistant (C.N.A.) on his team. First, the R.N. team leader makes visits to all patients' rooms to assess their conditions.

Based on those assessments, he assigns the L.P.N. to five patients. Three patients had surgery within the past three or four days and are recovering without complication. The other two have routine conditions.

The nursing assistant is assigned to two patients who are ready for discharge tomorrow, two more who are within two days of discharge, and one newly admitted patient who will have surgery tomorrow.

One patient has had surgery that day and has intravenous fluids as well as a lot of pain. There is a family member spending the night with him. The team leader takes this patient himself but doesn't overload himself with patients because he needs the flexibility to assist where needed and to supervise the other team members. During the night the team leader will also develop and update nursing care plans.

Box 15–2   Advantages and Disadvantages of Team Nursing

ADVANTAGES

Potential for building team spirit

Provides comprehensive care

Each worker's abilities are used to the fullest

Promotes job satisfaction

Decreases nonprofessional duties of R.N.s

DISADVANTAGES

Constant need to communicate among team members is time-consuming

All must promote teamwork

Team composition varies from day to day, which can be confusing and disruptive

---

In team nursing, the R.N. team leader oversees all care, makes assessments, and documents responses to care. The L.P.N. team member provides direct care by performing treatments and procedures and reports patient responses to the team leader. The C.N.A. provides simple, direct, personal care.

Like functional nursing, team nursing has both advantages and disadvantages. Box 15–2 lists some of these.

INTERVIEW WITH A TEAM NURSE

Ruth Ebert (1992) functioned as a team leader on a 40-bed medical-surgical unit in a small, rural Texas hospital.

Q: What did you like most about your professional role as a team leader?
A: My team consisted of two R.N.s, three L.P.N.s, and four C.N.A.s. We had 36 post–intensive care beds and 4 semi–intensive care beds for patients with burns and other severe problems. What I liked most was the feeling of being part of a cooperative effort—we used true teamwork, and at the end of the day, we all felt really good about what we had accomplished.
Q: What did you like least about team nursing?
A: The major drawback was the tendency people had to become rather compartmentalized in their focus. In other words, they became so good at a particular level of care that they didn't always stretch themselves. I think a good team leader needs to challenge people to always grow and develop.
Q: What is the biggest advantage to the team nursing method of delivery of care?

A: I improved greatly in my use of organizational skills. Team nursing develops your management skills, teaches you when and how to delegate to others, helps you learn to prioritize, and increases teamwork.

Primary Nursing

Developed by Manthey et al. (1970), **primary nursing** was designed to promote the concept of having an identified nurse for every patient. The goal of primary nursing is to deliver consistent, comprehensive care. Although it is impossible to have one nurse totally responsible for each patient's care around the clock, primary nursing focuses on care given by a nurse who has a consistent relationship with the patient (Mayer et al. 1990).

In primary nursing, each newly admitted patient is assigned by the head nurse to a primary nurse. Primary nurses assess their patients, plan their care, and write the plan of care. They care for their patients when they are at work and delegate responsibility to associate nurses when they are off duty. Associate nurses may be other R.N.s or L.P.N.s.

Patients are divided among primary nurses in such a manner that each nurse is responsible for the care of a group of patients 24 hours a day. Unless there is a compelling reason to transfer a patient, the primary nurse will care for the patient from admission to discharge. These nurses know their patients well and can enjoy a feeling of accomplishment and completion when the patients leave the hospital.

Primary nursing is like practice in other professions because there is a continuing relationship between the professional nurse and the patient. It promotes both **autonomy** and **accountability** because one nurse is responsible for everything that happens to the patient. Although there was initial concern that a nearly all-R.N. staff would be prohibitively expensive, primary nursing has been demonstrated to be a cost-effective method of delivering care (McClelland, Kolesar, and Bailey 1987).

Case Study: Primary Nursing

A primary nurse in a rehabilitation hospital is assigned a new patient. He is a 25-year-old man who sustained a neck injury in a diving accident. He has been in a trauma intensive care unit, and now that his condition has stabilized, he has been transferred. He is paralyzed from the shoulders down.

In addition to providing direct care and writing the care plan, the primary nurse assesses that his wife of two months has few sources of emotional support and is growing anxious about the future. In addition, she feels guilty about her anger and frustration over this dramatic change in their life plans.

The primary nurse acknowledges and discusses her feelings. She explains that patients and family members often have angry feelings under similar circumstances. She refers

---

Box 15-3   Advantages and Disadvantages of Primary Nursing

ADVANTAGES

High patient and family satisfaction

Promotes R.N. responsibility and authority

Patient knows nurse well, and nurse knows patient well

Cost-effective

Promotes professionalism

Promotes job satisfaction and sense of accomplishment for nurses

DISADVANTAGES

Difficulty hiring all R.N. staff

Nurses don't know other patients—cannot "cover" for each other

Stress of round-the-clock responsibility

Heavy responsibility, especially for new nurses

---

the couple to a rehabilitation psychologist who works with
them in replanning and reprioritizing their life goals.

Primary nursing has several advantages. A major advantage is that owing to the amount of time they spend with patients, primary nurses are in a position to deal with the entire person—physical, emotional, social, and spiritual. Other advantages and disadvantages of primary nursing are listed in Box 15-3.

INTERVIEW WITH A PRIMARY NURSE

Ketha Kollman (1992) has practiced primary nursing more than five years, both in acute care and physical rehabilitation settings. Ketha says, "You can't beat primary nursing! It's the best way to deliver care!"

Q: What do you like best about primary nursing?
A: I know everything about my patients. I have a broad knowledge of their conditions, past histories, and I understand their potential.
Q: What do you like least about primary nursing?
A: It makes you rather indispensable. Only you have all the facts and details. When you are not on duty, pieces are missing. It can foster dependence of the patient on one nurse.
Q: What is the biggest advantage of primary nursing?
A: It allows the nurse to provide consistent, comprehensive care.

This chapter's research note compares primary nursing and team nursing.

Research Note

Kathryn Gardner studied primary and team nursing in eight medical units of a hospital over a four-year period. She examined three different areas: quality of nursing care, nurse retention and stress, and cost. She conducted the study before the implementation of primary and team nursing on the units, 12 months following implementation, and again 30 months after implementation.

Gardner found that scores on a standardized scale measuring quality of nursing care were higher for primary than for team nursing. There was no significant difference between primary and team nursing in terms of nurses' stress. Retention on primary care units, however, was better with lower turnover. Primary nurses interviewed were not willing to change to team nursing

and had higher levels of both autonomy and competence than the team nurses. Costs per patient per day were as much as $6.48 lower with primary nursing.

This study seems to confirm previous studies showing that primary nursing produces high-quality nursing care, favorable conditions for nurses, and cost reductions. Gardner cautioned that since the study was conducted in only one hospital and since "research in a natural clinical setting cannot be carefully controlled" (p. 116), generalizing these findings to other settings should be done with caution.

(Abstracted from Gardner, K. (1991). A summary of findings of a five-year comparison study of primary and team nursing. *Nursing Research*, 40(2), 113–117.)

Case Management Nursing

The most recent innovation in nursing care delivery systems is **case management nursing**. Begun in the late 1980s as yet another attempt to improve the cost-effectiveness of hospital nursing, case management ensures that patients receive the services they need in an efficient manner while holding costs down (Fagin 1990).

Case managers are involved with patients from the time of their admission to the health care system until they return home again. They may stay involved in their patients' care beyond the immediate posthospital period. The goals of case management are to promote **collaboration** with all health care providers who can contribute to the patient's care, to promote continuity of care during the entire episode of illness, to promote appropriate use of community resources, and ultimately to promote independent living for patients and families.

Case managers involve patients and families in every phase of care. This includes introductions at time of admission, giving patients and families verbal and written educational materials, involving patient and family members in planning, posthospitalization follow-up phone calls to check on progress, arranging transportation to physician and physical therapy appointments, and many other activities. The relationship of the case manager and the patient does

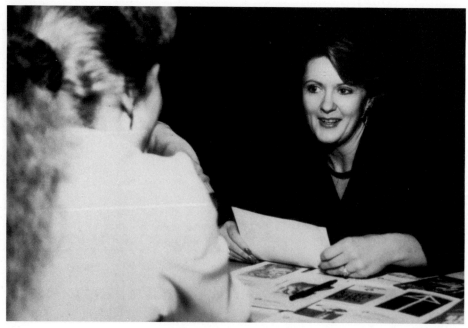

The nurse case manager works with the patient following discharge from the hospital. (Courtesy of Memorial Hospital, Chattanooga, TN.)

not end until there is no longer a need or the patient's care has been transferred to another health provider, such as a home care agency.

Some case managers have attained certification in their specialty areas or have advanced degrees. For example, a nurse with years of rehabilitation nursing expertise who is a certified rehabilitation registered nurse (C.R.R.N.) may be a case manager for all spinal cord—injured patients in her facility.

Case Study: Case Management Nursing

A registered nurse case manager is working with a patient scheduled for a modified mastectomy the following day. He explains the sequence of events to the patient and family and tells them what to expect. He gives the patient and family a tour of the hospital, especially the surgical suite and post-anesthesia care unit.

As her case manager, he will care for the patient after surgery, providing direct nursing care. He will make sure a "Reach to Recovery" volunteer from the American Cancer Society is called in to see his patient before she leaves the hospital and that she has a follow-up home visit planned with the volunteer. He will talk with the patient's family

---

Box 15–4   Advantages and Disadvantages of Case Management

ADVANTAGES

Nurse has increased responsibility

Promotes collaboration with other health professionals

Cost-effective

Eases patient's transition from hospital to community services

DISADVANTAGES

Requires additional training

Requires nurses to be off unit for periods of time

Time consuming

---

members, especially her spouse, to help them understand their own feelings and those of the patient.

Prior to discharge, he will provide any discharge planning or teaching she may need. He will make sure she has a follow-up appointment scheduled with the surgeon and that she has transportation to the appointment. After discharge, he will call the patient to check on her progress and report back to the physician.

Advantages and disadvantages of case management nursing are shown in Box 15–4.

INTERVIEW WITH A NURSE CASE MANAGER

Irene Foster (1992), case manager for medical patients at a 250-bed hospital in the Southwest, thoroughly enjoys the challenges of her role.

Q: What do you like most about your professional role as a case manager?
A: I enjoy the collaboration with so many people—other health care professionals and people in the community. I also like the fact that I am empowering people to care for themselves. And it's a joy to be able to offer support to patients and families.
Q: What do you like least about case management?
A: It can be a very time-consuming process. Sometimes it can take several months to coordinate and document all the care a patient needs. Often you are coordinating care and services long after the patient is discharged from the hospital.
Q: What's the biggest advantage to case management?
A: It's an ongoing process. It keeps you in touch with patients, families, and

physicians. You see real progress over an extended period of time. With team or primary nursing you never really know what happens to your patients after discharge.

Challenges in Nursing Care Delivery

A variety of nursing care delivery models may be used in the same hospital. For example, primary nursing may be used in critical care units and team nursing on a medical/surgical unit. A 1989 survey by the American Hospital Association (1991) revealed that team nursing was the system used to care for the most inpatients in the nation's hospitals. Nearly 39 percent of inpatients in 1989 were cared for using team nursing. The number of patients cared for using primary nursing, 13.6 percent, was down 3 percent from the previous year. This may be due to the difficulty many hospitals have experienced in obtaining the number of registered nurses required by primary nursing. Case management, which was not in use at the time of earlier surveys, was reportedly used by 2 percent of the hospitals in caring for 6 percent of hospitalized patients. It was expected to rise in the future. Functional nursing had decreased by 47 percent since the 1983 survey. In 1989 only 6.6 percent of inpatients were cared for using functional nursing. Table 15–1 shows the percentage of hospital inpatients cared for by type of nursing delivery system in 1989.

Many hospitals use creative blends of care delivery systems to retain the advantages while eliminating the disadvantages. One trend that is safe to predict is that as cost becomes a greater issue, more "nurse extenders" will be used. Two issues related to the use of varying levels of nursing personnel will present challenges for nurses in the future. These are differentiating levels of practice, and legal issues.

Table 15–1   Mean Percent of Hospital Inpatients Cared for by Type of Nursing Delivery System, 1989

Type of Delivery System	Percent
Functional	6.6
Team	38.7
Primary	13.6
Case management	6.0
Other	35.1
Total	100.0

(Data from American Hospital Association. (1991). *Hospital nursing in the '90s: The effect on patient care.* Chicago: Author.)

■

Box 15–5 Comparison of Selected A.D.N. and B.S.N. Competencies

	A.D.N.	B.S.N.
Clients:	Individuals and family members	Individuals; families; aggregate and community groups
Level of responsibility:	For a specified work period	From admission to post discharge
Type of setting:	Structured; other personnel available	Unstructured; other personnel may not be available

(Data from Primm, P. (1987). Differentiated practice for ADN and BSN prepared nurses. *Journal of Professional Nursing*, 3(4), 218–225.)

Differentiating Levels of Practice

A growing issue in the delivery of nursing care is differentiating among the levels of nursing practice. Historically, nurses with different levels of education were used interchangeably in hospitals. Even today, all nursing graduates qualify for the same license, and in many hospitals, diploma, associate degree, and baccalaureate nurses all function under the same job description. This sometimes creates a discrepancy between the competencies nurse managers expect of new graduates and their actual competencies.

The goal of **differentiated practice** is to define two levels of practice. This implies that there are also two levels of education and two levels of licensure. This is a difficult issue that nurses have been struggling with for years.

Differentiated practice can provide a common understanding of nursing practice in terms of technical skills needed to provide care, interpersonal skills needed for care, and leadership skills to manage care. In the mid-1980s, the W. K. Kellogg Foundation funded the South Dakota Statewide Project for Nursing and Nursing Education. This project lasted for two years. The project participants described the differentiated associate degree in nursing (A.D.N.) and bachelor of science in nursing (B.S.N.) competencies as follows:

> The B.S.N. cares for focal clients who are identified as individuals, families, aggregate, and community groups. The level of responsibility of the B.S.N. is from admission to postdischarge. The unstructured setting is a geographical and/or situational environment that may not have established policies, procedures, and protocols and has the potential for variation requiring independent nursing decisions. The A.D.N. cares for focal clients who are identified as individuals and

members of a family. The level of responsibility of the A.D.N. is for a specified work period and is consistent with the identified goals of care. The A.D.N. is prepared to function in a structured health care setting. The structured setting is a geographical and/or situational environment where the policies, procedures, and protocols for the provision of health care are established and there is recourse to assistance and support from the full scope of nursing expertise (Primm 1988, p. 2). Box 15–5 compares selected competencies of A.D.N. and B.S.N. nurses.

To deliver high-quality care in the future, it will be necessary to differentiate among nurses with regard to the level of care they are best prepared to provide. This issue will become an increasing focus of attention by professional nursing associations in the future.

Legal Issues in the Delivery of Nursing Care

As the need for nurses and **ancillary workers** such as nursing assistants increases, nurses will be asked to supervise more and more unlicensed health care workers. In making assignments and delegating tasks to these workers, nurses must determine what the workers can safely and effectively do. Nurses should consider the following questions: What can I legally delegate to ancillary personnel? What is my responsibility to them, to the patient, and to the facility?

Licensed nurses are responsible and accountable for actions that require nursing assessment and judgment. These actions are clearly identified in each state's nurse practice act. It is not currently the responsibility of ancillary workers to recognize that they should or should not perform a patient care activity. In the future, boards of nursing may choose to prosecute nonlicensed health care workers for their actions; but at present, they clearly hold registered nurses responsible for the actions of unlicensed personnel.

The *Administrative Rules* of the Tennessee Board of Nursing (1988) state that "failing to supervise persons to whom nursing functions are delegated or assigned" constitutes negligence on the part of registered nurses. **Supervision**, the initial direction and periodic inspection of the actual accomplishment of a task, is a very important activity for professional nurses and is closely related to **delegation**. If nurses delegate responsibility to other health care personnel, they are legally responsible for providing adequate supervision as well. Delegation to another does not absolve R.N.s from accountability for the nursing care of all patients under their care.

CHAPTER SUMMARY

There are a number of systems of nursing care delivery, each of which has advantages and disadvantages. Functional nursing, team nursing, primary nursing, and case management nursing were reviewed in this chapter. Each was presented in its theoretical or pure form, but in reality, there are many variations in use today.

As seen in the comments of the interviewed nurses, either satisfaction or frustration can result from the match between nurses' expectations and the system of care delivery on a given hospital unit. When interviewing for a position in hospital-based nursing, nurses must assess the delivery system carefully to make sure it is congruent with their values about nursing practice. In addition, nurses must understand the laws regulating delegation of nursing tasks and supervision of ancillary workers.

REVIEW/DISCUSSION QUESTIONS

1. Compare and contrast the four types of nursing care delivery systems from the viewpoint of the patient. If you were a consumer of nursing care, which system would you prefer? Why?
2. Look at the same question from the standpoint of the nurse. Which system would you find most satisfying in terms of your practice? Which would you like least?
3. Talk to a practicing nurse and find out which system(s) he or she has used to deliver care. What were the strong and weak points?
4. Obtain your state's nurse practice act and read the passage relating to registered nurses' responsibilities for unlicensed personnel. Initiate a class discussion of the implications for professional nurses.

REFERENCES

American Hospital Association. (1991). *Hospital nursing in the '90s: The effect on patient care.* Chicago: Author.

Bernhard, L. A., and Walsh, M. (1990). *Leadership: The key to the professionalization of nursing* (2nd ed.). St. Louis, MO: C.V. Mosby.

Ebert, A. R. (1992). Personal communication.

Fagin, C. M. (1990). Nursing's value proves itself. *American Journal of Nursing, 90*(10), 17–30.

Foster, I. (1992). Personal communication.

Gardner, K. (1991). A summary of findings of a five-year comparison study of primary and team nursing. *Nursing Research, 40*(2), 113–117.

Joiner, D. (1992). Personal communication.

Kollman, K. (1992). Personal communication.

Lambertson, E. (1953). *Nursing team organization and functioning.* New York: Columbia University.

Manthey, M., et al. (1970). Primary nursing: A return to the concept of "my nurse" and "my patient." *Nursing Forum, 9,* 65–83.

Mayer, G. G., et al. (1990). *Patient care delivery models.* Rockville, MD: Aspen.

McClelland, M. R., Kolesar, M. J., and Bailey, M. A. (1987). From team to primary nursing. *Nursing Management, 18*(10), 69–71.

Primm, P. L. (1987). Differentiated practice for ADN and BSN prepared nurses. *Journal of Professional Nursing, 3*(4), 218–225.

Primm, P. (1988). Differentiated nursing care management patient care delivery system. *Kansas Nurse*, April 1988, 2.

Tennessee Board of Nursing. (1988). *Administrative rules.* Nashville, TN: Author.

SUGGESTED READINGS

Burkholz, G. (1989). Supervising unlicensed technicians in critical care. *Dimensions of Critical Care Nursing*, 8(5), 317–323.

Cooper, R. G., and Leja, J. A. (1990). An investigation of managed health care case managers. *Journal of Allied Health*, 19, 219–225.

Dittmar, S. (1989). *Rehabilitation nursing: Process and application.* St. Louis: C.V. Mosby.

Koerner, J. G., et al. (1989). Implementing differentiated practice: The Sioux Valley Hospital experience. *Journal of Nursing Administration,* 19(2), 13–22.

Morse, G. G. (1990). Resurgence of nurse assistants in acute care. *Nursing Management,* 21(3), 34–36.

Zander, K. (1988). Nursing case management: Strategic management of cost and quality outcomes. *American Journal of Nursing,* 18(5), 23–30.

Chapter

The Scientific Method

Kay K. Chitty

CHAPTER OBJECTIVES

What students should be able to do after studying this chapter:

1. Differentiate between pure and applied science.

2. Describe the historical development of the scientific method.

3. Give examples of inductive and deductive reasoning.

4. Explain the steps of the scientific method.

5. Discuss the limitations of the scientific method when applied to nursing.

VOCABULARY BUILDING

Terms to know:

applied science	hypothesis	scientific method
data	inductive reasoning	valid
deductive reasoning	Newton	
Galileo	pure science	

A recurring theme in this book is the interrelatedness of nursing theory, research, and practice. Chapter 11 described how nurses are learning to use theoretical models as frameworks for professional practice. Chapter 12 presented the ideas that clinical research questions can best be formulated by nurses in practice and that research findings should be tested by nurses in clinical practice.

Chapters 13, 14, and 15 presented systems in which nurses practice, some of the roles and care delivery models nurses use, and how health care is financed. The purposes of Chapters 16 and 17 are to examine the basis for a method of problem solving that nurses use in their day-to-day professional lives and to examine that problem-solving method itself.

In the 1960s the nursing profession was poised on the threshold of a higher level of development. There was recognition that the mature professions had strong scientific bases, which were lacking in nursing. Nursing scholars realized that nursing could achieve its potential and desired professional status only to the extent that the discipline was based on a scientifically derived body of knowledge unique to nursing. As a result of that recognition, nursing researchers set about developing knowledge, and nursing theorists began developing theories and testing them.

At the same time, nurses realized that a similar professionalization of patient care practices was needed. Using traditional methods to deal with familiar patient problems and trial and error or intuition to deal with unfamiliar ones was no longer seen as an acceptable way to care for patients and move the profession toward science-based practice. Practitioners of nursing, therefore, also developed a more scientific approach to patient care that is an adaptation of the classic scientific method. This problem-solving approach is called "the nursing process." An understanding of the scientific method is helpful in appreciating the nursing process.

The **scientific method** is an orderly, systematic way of thinking about and solving problems. It has been used by scientists for centuries to discover and test facts and principles. The scientific method is the same, regardless of the discipline using it; any subject studied by using the scientific method or other methods of reasoning can be considered "science."

Pure and Applied Science

Scientists divide scientific knowledge into two categories: pure and applied. **Pure science**, sometimes called basic science, summarizes and explains the universe without regard for whether the information is immediately useful. When Joseph Priestly discovered oxygen in 1774, he did not have an immediate use for that information. Therefore, that discovery could be classified as "pure science," that is, information gathered solely for the sake of obtaining new knowledge. **Applied science**, on the other hand, seeks to use scientific theory and laws in some practical way. The use of oxygen with premature infants is an example of applied science. From this example it can be seen that today's pure science can become tomorrow's applied science. Nursing makes use of applied scientific principles.

History of the Scientific Method

Until the time of Hippocrates, the Greek physician who lived around 460–377 B.C., illness was believed to be caused by evil spirits. Gradually, over the years and through the efforts of many scientists, humankind has learned a great deal about the human body, health, and illness. Most of this knowledge was developed after the scientific method came into widespread use.

A period of great intellectual activity, known as the "Age of Reason," began in the 1600s and lasted until the late 1700s. During that time, scientists made unparalleled advances in understanding the laws by which nature operates by using reason and experimentation. **Galileo** (1564–1642), the Italian physicist and astronomer, and Sir Isaac **Newton** (1642–1727), the English philosopher and mathematician, are usually credited with developing and refining the scientific method. A scientific revolution and technological explosion resulted from the use of the scientific method. In the area of health care alone, profound and far-reaching scientific discoveries have changed human life dramatically. Some important scientific discoveries related to health are listed in Box 16–1.

Inductive and Deductive Reasoning

The scientific method requires the use of two types of logic: inductive and deductive reasoning. In **inductive reasoning**, the process begins with a particular experience and proceeds to generalizations. Repeated observations of an experiment or event enable the observer to draw general conclusions. For example, the statement "All the St. Bernard dogs I have encountered are gentle; therefore, St. Bernards are gentle" is an example of inductive reasoning. It is obvious from this example that this type of logic leads to probabilities—not certainties—unless the world's entire population of St. Bernard dogs is observed.

Scientists also use **deductive reasoning**, a process through which conclusions are drawn by logical inference from given premises. It proceeds from the general case to the specific. For example, if the premises "All schoolchildren like chocolate" and "Missie is a schoolchild" are accepted, the conclusion "Missie likes chocolate" can be drawn. It may be entirely possible, however, that Missie, although a schoolchild, does not like chocolate at all. In deductive reasoning, the premises used must be correct or the conclusions will not be. Conclusions drawn through deductive processes are called *valid* rather than *true*. **Valid** is a term meaning "soundly founded," whereas *true* means "in accordance with fact or reality" (Flexner, Stein, and Su 1980). It is possible for a conclusion to be solidly founded without it being fact. There is a subtle, but real, difference in the two terms.

As seen by these examples, neither inductive nor deductive processes alone are adequate. If scientists used only deductive logic, experience would be ignored. If they used only inductive logic, relationships among facts and principles would be ignored. A combination of both types of reasoning processes in science unifies the theoretical and the practical, which is the basis for the scientific method.

Box 16−1   Important Health-Related Events in the Evolution of Science

ca. 400 B.C.	Hippocrates taught that diseases have natural, not supernatural, causes.
A.D. 100	Galen laid the foundation for the study of anatomy and physiology.
ca. 1500	Leonardo da Vinci recognized the importance of observation and experimentation in learning.
1543	Andreas Vesalius published a book on human anatomy, based on observation.
1628	William Harvey published his theory on the circulation of blood.
1774	Joseph Priestly discovered oxygen.
ca. 1796	Edward Jenner discovered a method of smallpox vaccination.
1839	Matthias Schleiden and Theodor Schwann developed the theory that all living things are composed of cells.
1866	Gregor Mendel demonstrated the laws of heredity.
ca.1876	Louis Pasteur demonstrated that microorganisms cause fermentation and disease.
1882	Robert Koch isolated the bacterium that causes tuberculosis.
1895	Wilhelm K. Roentgen discovered X rays.
1898	Marie and Pierre Curie isolated the element radium.
ca. 1900	Paul Ehrlich originated chemotherapy, the treatment of diseases with chemicals (drugs).
1928	Alexander Fleming discovered penicillin.
1953	Jonas Salk developed the first effective polio vaccine.
1957	Arthur Karnberg grew DNA (deoxyribonucleic acid), the basic chemical of genes, in a test tube.
1978	The world's first "test tube baby" was delivered.
1982	William DeVries implanted the world's first artificial heart.
1989	The first authorized use of genetic engineering involved injecting genetically altered cells into patients with malignant melanoma.
1992	A team of international scientists reported the discovery of the gene that causes *fragile X syndrome*, a common inherited form of mental retardation.

(Data from: Kuhn, T.S. (1970). The structure of scientific revolutions. In O. Neurath, (Ed.), *International encyclopedia of unified science* (2nd ed., vol. 2). Chicago: University of Chicago Press; and Ware, C.F., Panikkar, K.M., and Romein, J.M. (1966). *The twentieth century. History of mankind, cultural and scientific development* (vol. 6). New York: Harper & Row; and other sources.)

Steps in the Scientific Method

There are five steps in the scientific method. The following steps will remind you of the steps in the research process you studied in Chapter 12. They are:

1. Stating a problem.
2. Stating hypotheses (possible explanations).
3. Experimenting and observing.
4. Interpreting data.
5. Drawing conclusions from the observed results.

1. *Stating a problem.* This step is sometimes referred to as "defining the problem." Human beings are curious about how and why things are the way they are. Identifying problems to study is easy and natural. Children are particularly good at identifying problems. They ask, "Why is the sky blue?" and "Where does the wind come from?" These questions can be developed into excellent problem statements and subjected to the scientific method. Although it is easy and natural, it is absolutely essential to clearly understand and define a problem before attempting to solve it or investigate it further.

A problem of interest to all health professionals is why people continue to smoke even though smoking is known to be destructive to health. Most problems have many causes, and this one is no exception. Several problem statements may be contained in such a complex problem: What factors influence the desire to smoke? When are people most likely to stop smoking? How does advertising affect young people in relation to smoking? A variety of problems can be identified, but one must be singled out in order to define the problem precisely enough to investigate.

2. *Stating hypotheses.* The next step is to think about the problem and ask, "What could possibly explain this?" A hunch that could possibly explain the problem is known as a **hypothesis**. There may be more than one possible explanation or hypothesis for a single problem.

The past education and experience of the scientist will shape each hypothesis. A psychologist, for example, will probably have a different hypothesis about smoking than a biochemist. If the problem statement is, "What factors influence the desire to smoke?" a psychologist may state as a hypothesis, "Smokers smoke more cigarettes per hour when under stress than when not under stress." The hypothesis—that stress makes people smoke more—is a statement that can be either validated or refuted. The biochemist, on the other hand, may state as a hypothesis, "When a smoker's blood level of nicotine falls below 0.02 mEq/liter, the desire to smoke is triggered." This hypothesis can also be validated or refuted.

3. *Experimenting and observing.* In this phase of the scientific method, the scientist devises an experiment to help prove or disprove the hypothesis and observes the results of the experiment. In the smoking example, this might include keeping careful records for several days about the number of cigarettes a group of people smoke; then subjecting them to a stressor, such as having them perform mathematical calculations in shorter and shorter periods of time; and finally observing to see if the number of cigarettes smoked increases, decreases,

---

Box 16–2   Steps in the Scientific Method

- Stating a problem.
- Stating hypotheses.
- Experimenting and observing.

- Interpreting data.
- Drawing conclusions.

---

or remains the same as before the stress was applied. There could be a control group of smokers who are not subjected to the experimental conditions but whose smoking is also monitored. In this example, the scientist would use observation before, during, and after the experiment.

4. *Interpreting data.*   Next the information (**data**) gathered is analyzed. Cigarette consumption during the experiment would be compared with preexperiment baseline data. Let's suppose that data interpretation revealed that cigarette consumption by the experimental group *did* increase during the experiment when compared with the preexperiment baseline, whereas the control group's smoking remained the same. The researcher would determine how much smoking behavior increased in the experimental group and perhaps subject the numbers to statistical analyses to determine whether the change could have simply been caused by chance.

5. *Drawing conclusions.*   In this phase of the scientific method, conclusions are drawn about whether the hypothesis has been upheld or refuted by the experiment. The scientist would interpret the smoking data as supporting or not supporting the hypothesis "Smokers smoke more cigarettes per hour when under stress than when not under stress." In this step, solutions are often suggested or recommendations made. If they are, a sixth step of the method would be to evaluate, or test, the solutions.

In practice, these steps are not always rigidly followed in the order listed because the human mind does not always function in a completely linear fashion. An observation may lead to a hypothesis, and then the problem statement may be generated. All steps must be completed, however, and when one writes about the scientific method, the report is organized around the steps in the order listed. Box 16–2 contains the steps in the scientific method.

Limitations of the Scientific Method in Nursing

Polit and Hungler (1978, p. 26) believe that the scientific method is the "highest form of attaining human knowledge that human beings have devised." Many authorities believe that using any other method is less than scientific and thus to be avoided. However, there are at least four reasons why the scientific method has limitations when applied to nursing.

The first and most obvious drawback is that health care settings are not comparable to laboratories. There are realities and priorities operating in health care settings that must take precedence over laboratory protocols. The safety and security of human patients are of the utmost importance and cannot be jeopardized.

Second, human beings are far more than collections of parts that can be dissected and subjected to examination or experimentation. A strength of nursing is that nurses view patients holistically, whereas the scientific method is based on dividing a problem into manageable problem statements, each of which can be tested. Since humans are complex organisms with interrelated parts and systems, the classic scientific method loses some of its usefulness.

A third limitation of the scientific method as the only approach to solving patient problems is the fact that it is so objective; it fails to take the meaning of patients' own experiences, that is, their subjective view of reality, into consideration. Nurses are keenly aware that patients' perceptions of their experiences, or subjective data, are just as important as objective data.

Finally, there are definite ethical implications involved in experimenting with humans that make reliance on the scientific method impractical. The rights of human subjects in research are paramount, as discussed in Chapter 12.

Where, then, does that leave nurses in relation to using the scientific method to increase the body of nursing knowledge? Ever resourceful, nurses have developed a modification of the scientific method, known as the nursing process. This method of clinical problem solving is taught in nursing curricula across the nation, and many states have included it in their nurse practice acts.

A challenge to the universal acceptance and use of the nursing process is the fact that many nurses who are now in practice were educated prior to the development of the nursing process and its inclusion in school curricula. They have had to learn how to use this process "on the job." Regardless of how some individuals may view it, the nursing process is now so widely accepted that the Joint Commission on the Accreditation of Healthcare Organizations expects nurses to use the nursing process as the basis for clinical decision making. The universal use of the nursing process, which is based on the scientific method, gives credence to nursing's claim of being an applied science.

CHAPTER SUMMARY

The scientific method is the name given to a systematic, orderly process of solving problems. It has been used for centuries and is applicable in many different situations. Knowledge can be categorized as either pure knowledge— that is, knowledge that is not immediately useful—and applied knowledge— that is, knowledge that can be used in a practical way.

Much of the scientific knowledge we take for granted today was discovered through use of the scientific method. This method has been particularly useful in the fields of medicine and health care, and human existence has been profoundly affected by discoveries made through its use.

The scientific method uses two types of logic: inductive and deductive reasoning. A combination of both types of reasoning is necessary to combine the theoretical and the practical aspects of the scientific method.

There are five steps in the scientific method: stating a problem, stating hypotheses, experimenting and observing, interpreting data, and drawing conclusions from the observed results. Although there are limitations on the use of the scientific method with human beings, nurses have developed a modification called the nursing process. The nursing process is used as a problem-solving technique in clinical nursing practice.

REVIEW/DISCUSSION QUESTIONS

1. Why is nursing called an applied science? Tell why you agree or disagree with this description.
2. Name and describe the two types of reasoning that are used in the scientific method. Explain why neither alone is adequate to advance knowledge.
3. List and discuss each step of the scientific process.
4. Explain why a purely experimental model is an inadequate one for nursing.

REFERENCES

Flexner, S. B., Stein, J., and Su, P.Y. (Eds.), (1980). *The Random House Dictionary*. New York: Random House.

Kuhn, T. S. (1970). The structure of scientific revolutions. In O. Neurath (Ed.), *International encyclopedia of unified science* (2nd ed., vol. 2). Chicago: University of Chicago Press.

Polit, D., and Hungler, B. (1978). *Nursing research: Principles and methods*. Philadelphia: J.B. Lippincott.

Ware, C. F., Panikkar, K. M., and Romein, J. M. (1966). *The twentieth century*. History of mankind, cultural and scientific development (vol. 6). New York: Harper & Row.

SUGGESTED READINGS

Andreoli, K. G., and Thompson, C. E. (1977). The nature of science in nursing. *Image*, 9, 32–37.

Bargagliotti, L. A. (1983). The scientific method and phenomenology: Toward their peaceful coexistence in nursing. *Western Journal of Nursing Research*, 5(4), 409–411.

Kidd, P., and Morrison, E. F. (1988). The progression of knowledge in nursing: A search for meaning. *Image*, 20(4), 222–224.

Watson, J. (1981). Nursing's scientific quest. *Nursing Outlook*, 29(7), 413–416.

Winstead-Fry, P. (1980). The scientific method and its impact on holistic health. *Advances in Nursing Science*, 2(4), 1–7.

Chapter

17

The Nursing Process

Barbara R. Norwood

CHAPTER OBJECTIVES

What students should be able to do after studying this chapter:

1. Define the nursing process including the steps involved.
2. Explain the difference between subjective and objective patient data.
3. Discuss three methods used to obtain patient data.
4. Discuss two frameworks for prioritizing nursing diagnoses.
5. List the components of short-term and long-term patient goals.
6. Differentiate between nursing orders and medical orders.
7. Explain the differences between independent, interdependent, and dependent nursing actions.
8. Describe evaluation and its importance in the nursing process.

VOCABULARY BUILDING

Terms to know:

affective goal	consultation	independent
analysis	dependent	intervention
assessment	intervention	interdependent
cognitive goal	evaluation	intervention

intervention
long-term goals
North American
   Nursing Diagnosis
   Association
   (NANDA)
nursing diagnosis

nursing orders
nursing process
objective data
outcome criteria
patient interview
physical examination
planning

primary source
psychomotor goal
secondary goals
secondary source
short-term goals
subjective data
tertiary source

*A*daily decision that most people face is how to dress for the day. Before putting on their clothes, there are several factors people need to consider. What is the temperature expected to be? Will it be clear, raining, or snowing? How much time will be spent outdoors? Are there any activities planned that require special dress? Next, they probably look at the possible clothing choices. Some clothes may be out of season, others need repairs, and some don't fit quite right. After considering the environmental factors, the day's activities, and mood, people select the day's clothing. After dressing, many people look in a mirror to evaluate how they look. They may then add a scarf or change shoes based on the image in the mirror. At this point, they have solved the problem of clothing themselves. They have identified a problem, considered various factors related to the problem, identified possible actions, selected the best alternative, evaluated the success of the alternative selected, and made adjustments to the solution based on the evaluation. This is the same general framework nurses use in solving patient problems.

The **nursing process** is a method used by nurses in solving patient problems in professional practice. It is an outgrowth of the scientific method and can be used as a framework for approaching almost any problem. Yura and Walsh (1983) defined the nursing process as "a designated series of actions intended to fulfill the purposes of nursing—to maintain the patient's wellness—and, if this state changes, to provide the amount and quality of nursing care the situation demands to direct the patient back to wellness." They went on, "if wellness cannot be achieved, then [the purpose of the nursing process is] to contribute to the patient's quality of life, maximizing his resources as long as life is a reality" (p. 71).

Steps in the Nursing Process

As in the scientific method, a series of steps is involved in the nursing process. This chapter will discuss each of the steps and give an example of the use of the nursing process in a clinical situation.

Assessment

The first step in the nursing process is **assessment**. Assessment is defined as the collecting of information about the patient. Nurses must have information about patients in order to determine if a problem exists, how severe the problem is, and what the patient's resources are for solving the problem. Patient resources include physical, mental, emotional, spiritual, and financial supplies. This problem- and resource-related information is commonly called "patient data."

SUBJECTIVE DATA

There are two different types of data that nurses obtain from patients: subjective and objective data. **Subjective data** are obtained from patients as they describe their needs, feelings, strengths, and perceptions of the problem. Subjective data are frequently referred to as "symptoms." Examples of subjective data are statements such as "I am in pain" and "I don't have much energy." The source for these data can only be the patient. Subjective data should include both physical and emotional information. For nurses to be successful in obtaining subjective data, some of which are quite private, patients must view nurses as trustworthy. You will learn more about establishing trust in nurse-patient relationships in Chapter 19.

OBJECTIVE DATA

The second type of patient data is **objective data**. These are data that the nurse obtains through observation, examination, and/or consultation with other health care providers. These data are factual, not colored by patients' perceptions, and include patient behaviors observed by the nurse. Objective data can also be called "signs." Examples of objective data include blood pressure readings, laboratory findings, and facial expressions.

SOURCES OF PATIENT DATA

Patient data can be obtained from many sources. When they come directly from the patient, the patient is considered a "**primary source**." Sources of data such as the nurse's own observations or perceptions of family and friends of the patient are considered "**secondary sources**." "**Tertiary sources**" of data include the medical record and other health care providers such as physical therapists, doctors, or dietitians.

METHODS OF COLLECTING PATIENT DATA

A number of methods are used when collecting patient data. A very important one is the **patient interview**. This usually involves a face-to-face interaction with the patient and requires the nurse to use the skills of interviewing, observation, and listening. The environment in which the interaction occurs or other internal/external factors can influence the amount and the type of data obtained. For example, when interviewing a patient who is in considerable pain, data may be limited. If the interview room is cold, noisy, or lacks privacy, the data obtained may be affected.

A second method of obtaining data is through **consultation**. Consultation is discussing patient needs with other health care workers involved in the care of

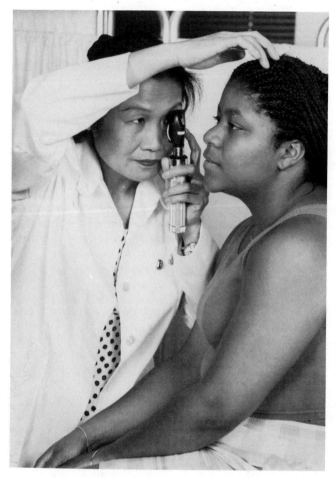

Physical examination as a method of obtaining patient data.

that patient. Nurses consult with patients' families to obtain background information and their perceptions about the patients' needs. They also consult with physicians and other health care workers.

Physical examination is the third method for obtaining data. Nurses use sight, smell, touch, and hearing to obtain these data. Special instruments such as scales, thermometers, stethoscopes, and blood pressure cuffs are used by nurses in obtaining these data.

ORGANIZING PATIENT DATA

Once patient data have been collected, they must be sorted or organized. A number of methods have been developed to assist nurses in organizing patient data. Nurses choose different methods of organizing patient data depending on personal preference and the method used in the agency where they are employed.

An early data classification system developed by Faye Abdellah (1959) resulted in what she termed "21 nursing problems." She believed that all patient problems could be classified under one of the 21 problems.

A few years later, Virginia Henderson (1966) advocated using 14 components of basic nursing care activities as a method of classifying patient data. Henderson's 14 problems are listed in Box 11–1.

In 1978, Helen Yura and Mary Walsh began developing what they termed "a human needs approach" to classifying patient data. Still later, Marjory Gordon (1982) designed an approach that utilized 11 functional health patterns.

Many other renowned nursing leaders including Martha Rogers (1979), Sister Callista Roy (1976), Dorothea Orem (1980), and others continue to work toward developing frameworks for sorting and organizing patient data. These frameworks, or theoretical models, were discussed in Chapter 11.

Once collected from primary, secondary, and tertiary sources and organized according to a classification system, patient data are entered in the patient's record or chart. A number of forms have been devised to assist nurses in recording patient data efficiently. These forms vary from hospital to hospital but are generally similar. Figure 17–1 shows an example of one such form.

Analysis

Once patient data are collected, sorted, and recorded, they must be analyzed. **Analysis** is the second step in the nursing process. Knowledge from biological sciences, social sciences, and nursing enables nurses to analyze relationships among various pieces of patient data. The outcome of that analysis is one or more nursing diagnoses. (Students should be aware that the singular form of the term is *diagnosis*. When speaking of more than one diagnosis, the plural form, *diagnoses*, is correct.)

NURSING DIAGNOSIS

Nursing diagnosis was defined by Marjory Gordon (1976) as "actual or potential health problems which nurses, by virtue of their education and experience, are capable and licensed to treat" (p. 1299). Nursing diagnosis is a process of describing a patient's response to health problems that either already exist or may occur in the future. Nurses diagnose patient problems by comparing patient data obtained in the assessment phase of the nursing process with accepted norms. Each patient usually has several nursing diagnoses.

An important difference between nursing diagnosis and medical diagnosis is that nursing diagnoses cover patient problems for which nurses can legally order treatment. It would do little good for nursing diagnoses to include "appendicitis" since appendicitis is a medical diagnosis requiring surgery, and it is not legal for nurses to perform surgery. An appropriate nursing diagnosis for a patient with appendicitis might be: "ineffective airway clearance related to incisional

ADMISSION INFORMATION

Date _____

ADDRESSOGRAPH

PATIENT DATA COLLECTION	PATIENT DATA COLLECTION LPN / RN

A. Date _____ Time _____ Correct I.D. Band _____ Yes

___Ambulatory   Admitted From:

___Wheelchair   ___Direct   ___E.R.   ___PACU

___Stretcher   ___Doctor's Office

        ___Other _____

B. VITAL SIGNS:

Ht. _____ Wt. _____ Reported Wt. _____   B/P ____

Temp _____   ___Oral   ___Rectal   ___Axillary   _____RA

Pulse _____   ___Regular   ___Irregular   _____LA

Resp _____   ___Regular   ___Irregular   _____RL

        _____LL

C. VALUABLES:

List: _____

Disposition of Valuables:

___Sent Home   ___Sent to Cashier's Office   ___Patient Kept

D. ORIENTATION TO HOSPITAL:

Received Hospital Information Packet: ___Yes ___No

Oriented to: ___Patient   ___Significant Other   ___N/A

___Visiting Hours   ___Emergency Light BR/Shower

___Bed Rail   ___Activity Level

___Smoking Policy   ___Bed Mechanics

___Call Light   ___Television Control

___Telephone   ___Patient ED TV Channel 5

___Pastoral Services

PATIENT/FAMILY VERBALIZES UNDERSTANDING: ___Yes ___No

_____
(Signature/Title)

PATIENT DATA COLLECTION   LPN / RN

A. REASON FOR ADMISSION:

Patient's own words include signs and symptoms:

_____

_____

Organ Donor   ___Yes   ___No

Living Will   ___Yes   ___No

B. ALLERGIES: Chart Flagged: ___Yes

Food: ___Yes ___No Name: _____

Reaction: _____

Drugs: ___Yes ___No Name: _____

Reaction: _____

Previous Blood Transfusion: ___Yes ___No

Reaction: _____

C. MEDICAL PROBLEMS/SURGERIES:

___No Problems   ___Cancer   ___Hypertension   ___Heart Disease

___Lung Diseases ___Diabetes ___GI Problems   ___Seizures

___Hepatitis   ___CVA   Other_____

Surgeries/Year: _____

D. MEDICATION TAKEN AT HOME: NONE

NAME	DOSE	TIME

Disposition of Home Meds: ___Sent Home

        ___Stored in Pharmacy

Other _____

E. COMMUNICATION/HEARING & VISION STATUS:

Visual Impairment: ___None   ___Wears Glasses

___Contacts: ___Right   ___Left

___Blind: ___Right   ___Left

___Cataract: ___Right   ___Left

Hearing Impairment: ___None   ___Hard of Hearing

___Deaf: ___Right   ___Left

___Uses Hearing Aid: ___Right   ___Left

Speech Impairment:

___None   ___Cannot Express

___Slurred   ___Cannot Understand

___Mute   ___Tracheostomy

___Stutters   ___Laryngectomy

Language Barrier: ___Yes   ___No

Describe: _____

F. NUTRITIONAL HABITS:

How is appetite: _____

Special diet and reason: _____

Dietitian notified for Diet Instruction   ___Yes   ___No

        Time: _____

Dentures (U) ___Yes ___No Partial Plate (U) ___Yes ___No

        (L) ___Yes ___No   (L) ___Yes ___No

Difficulty:

Swallowing liquid?   ___No   ___Yes

Swallowing solid food?   ___No   ___Yes

Chewing?   ___No   ___Yes

NS-141   Page 1A

Figure 17–1 Patient data form. (Courtesy of Memorial Hospital, a division of Sisters of Charity of Nazareth Health Corporation, Chattanooga, TN.)

PATIENT DATA COLLECTION LPN / RN	RN BIOPHYSICAL ASSESSMENT

G. ACTIVITY/EXERCISE

Mobility Status: ____Ambulatory   ____Ambulatory with Assist
____Bedrest   ____Transfer with Assist
Assistive Devices: ____None   ____Cane   ____Wheelchair
____Walker   ____Crutches   ____Prosthesis
____Other: _____

Limitations: ____None   ____Weakness   ____Fatigue
____Dizziness   ____Unsteady Gait   Other: _____

Do you have enough energy for desired activity?   ____Yes   ____No
Describe: _____

Activities of Daily Living:
I = Independent   A = Assist   D = Dependent
____Feeding   ____Bathing   ____Grooming
____Toileting   ____Dressing   ____Other
Describe: _____
Functional Level: _____
Level O: Full self-care
Level I: Requires use of equipment or device
Level II: Requires assistance or supervision from another person
Level III: Is dependent and does not participate

H. REPRODUCTIVE STATUS:

Male: ____NA
____Penile Discharge   ____Scrotal Mass
____Tenderness   ____Inguinal Mass
____Pain   ____Other: _____
Female: ____NA
LMP _____   Itching ——   PMS ____
Last Pap Smear _____   Abnormal Bleeding ____
Discharge ____   Pregnant ____
Contraceptive _____   Breast Lumps ____
Pain: Menstruation ____   Other: _____

I. PSYCHOSOCIAL STATUS:

Level of Education: ____Grade School   ____High School   ____Other
Employment: ____Yes ____No ____Retired Occupation: _____
Home Situation: ____Stairs ____Heat (type) _____
Sleep: ____No problem   ____Does not feel rested after sleep
____Difficulty falling asleep ____Other _____
____Difficulty staying asleep
What helps you sleep? _____
Who lives with you? _____
Support System (Close friend/family member) _____

Experienced any recent major changes in your life? _____

Will being here interfere with any religious practices?   ____Yes ____No
Concerns due to Hospitalization/Illness: ____None
____Family/Child Care ____Employment ____Financial/Insurance
____Other _____
Habits: Tobacco ____Yes ____No _____ per day
Alcohol ____Yes ____No _____ per day

J. LEARNING NEEDS:

What do you know about your present illness? _____

What information do you want or need about your illness?
_____
_____

_____
(Signature/Title)

____Unable to obtain history due to patient's condition/not
accompanied by family or friend.

NS-141   Page 1B

A. INTEGUMENTARY STATUS:

Color: ____WNL   ____Pale   ____Cyanotic   ____Jaundiced
Temp: ____Warm   ____Cool   Turgor: ____WNL ____Poor
Edema: ____No   ____Yes, Where? _____
Lesions: ____No ____Yes Complete Pressure Sore Assessment sheet

B. RESPIRATORY STATUS: Breath Sounds:

Quality of respirations ____WNL   ____Clear all lobes
Abnormals: _____   ____Equal and Bilateral
Explain: _____   ____Rales
_____   ____Rhonchi
_____   ____Wheezes

C. CARDIOVASCULAR STATUS: Pulses classification

Pulses: N/A _____	Right	Left	0 = Completely absent
Radial			+ 1 = Markedly impaired
Femoral			+ 2 = Moderately impaired
Post Tibial			+ 3 = Slightly impaired
Dorsalis Pedis			+ 4 = Normal
Popliteal			

Pacemaker: ____Yes ____No
Pedal Edema: ____Yes ____No

D. GASTROINTESTINAL STATUS:

Bowel Pattern _____ Last B.M. _____
Bowel Sounds ____N/A ____Present ____Absent
Abdominal Distention ____No ____Yes

Explain: _____
_____

E. NEUROLOGICAL STATUS:

____Headache/Pain   Pupil Size: Level of Consciousness:
____Motor Disturbances   ____PERL   ____Alert
____Seizures   ____Other   ____Stuporous
____Numbness   ____Semicomatose
____Tingling   ____Comatose

Oriented to: ____Person ____Place ____Time ____Event

F. MUSCOSKELETAL STATUS:

Motor Function: ____All extremities WNL for strength, ROM and
coordination.
Abnormals: RA _____
LA _____
RL _____
LL _____
Recent history of falls ____Yes____No
Fall risk category: ____Low   ____Moderate   ____High

G. GENITOURINARY STATUS:

Pain _____   ____Bladder Distention
Frequency _____ Urgency _____   ____Foley Catheter
Burning _____ Nocturia _____   ____Suprapubic Catheter
Comments _____   ____Urostomy
_____   ____Dialysis Access
_____

Is there anything else the nursing staff should know to plan
your care? _____
_____
_____

_____
(RN Signature)

*COMPLETE ADMISSION DISCHARGE PLANNING ASSESSMENT

Box 17–1   NANDA Approved Nursing Diagnoses, 1990

Activity intolerance
Activity intolerance, high risk for
Adjustment, impaired
Airway clearance, ineffective
Anxiety
Aspiration, high risk for
Body image disturbance
Body temperature, high risk for altered
Breastfeeding, effective
Breastfeeding, ineffective
Breathing pattern, ineffective
Communication, impaired verbal
Constipation
Constipation, colonic
Constipation, perceived
Decisional conflict (specify)
Decreased cardiac output
Defensive coping
Denial, ineffective
Diarrhea
Disuse syndrome, high risk for
Diversional activity deficit
Dysreflexia
Family coping, compromised, ineffective
Family coping, disabling, ineffective
Family coping: potential for growth
Family processes, altered
Fatigue
Fear
Fluid volume deficit
Fluid volume deficit, high risk for
Fluid volume excess
Gas exchange, impaired
Grieving, anticipatory
Grieving, dysfunctional
Growth and development, altered
Health maintenance, altered
Health-seeking behaviors (specify)
Home maintenance management, impaired
Hopelessness

Hyperthermia
Hypothermia
Incontinence, bowel
Incontinence, functional
Incontinence, reflex
Incontinence, stress
Incontinence, total
Incontinence, urge
Individual coping, ineffective
Infection, high risk for
Injury, high risk for
Knowledge deficit (specify)
Noncompliance (specify)
Nutrition: less than body requirements, altered
Nutrition: more than body requirements, altered
Nutrition: potential for more than body requirements, altered
Oral mucous membrane, altered
Pain
Pain, chronic
Parental role conflict
Parenting, altered
Parenting, high risk for altered
Personal identity disturbance
Physical mobility, impaired
Poisoning, high risk for
Posttrauma response
Powerlessness
Protection, altered
Rape-trauma syndrome
Rape-trauma syndrome: compound reaction
Rape-trauma syndrome: silent reaction
Role performance, altered
Self-care deficit, bathing/hygiene
Self-care deficit, feeding
Self-care deficit, dressing/grooming
Self-care deficit, toileting
Self-esteem, chronic low
Self-esteem, situational low

Self-esteem disturbance	Thermoregulation, ineffective
Sensory/perceptual alterations (specify) (visual, auditory, kinesthetic, gustatory, tactile, olfactory)	Thought processes, altered
	Tissue integrity, impaired
	Tissue perfusion, altered (specify type)
Sexual dysfunction	(renal, cerebral, cardiopulmonary,
Sexuality patterns, altered	gastrointestinal, peripheral)
Skin integrity, impaired	Trauma, high risk for
Skin integrity, high risk for impaired	Unilateral neglect
Sleep pattern disturbance	Urinary elimination, altered
Social interaction, impaired	Urinary retention
Social isolation	Violence, high risk for: self-directed or
Spiritual distress (distress of the human spirit)	directed at others
Suffocation, high risk for	(From the Proceedings of the Ninth National Conference of the North American Nursing Diagnosis Association, March 1990.)
Swallowing, impaired	

pain." Since it is legal in all states for nurses to provide comfort measures and to assist patients to cough and deep breathe, this would be both an appropriate and a legal nursing diagnosis.

NANDA DIAGNOSES

The North American Nursing Diagnosis Association (NANDA) has worked for two decades to develop a comprehensive list of nursing diagnoses. Box 17–1 contains the 1990 list of NANDA nursing diagnoses. NANDA is a group of nursing educators, theorists, and practitioners from the United States and Canada who first met in 1973 to develop standard terminology, content, and format for nursing diagnoses. The group has continued to meet every two years to revise the original list of approved diagnoses. Following each revision, new diagnoses are tested by nurses in practice settings to evaluate their appropriateness and usefulness. This is a continuing process. NANDA membership is open to all nurses interested in advancing nursing diagnosis.

PRIORITIZING NURSING DIAGNOSES

After diagnoses are identified, the nurse must put them in order of priority. There are two common frameworks used to establish priorities. One of these considers the relative danger to the patient. Using this framework, diagnoses that are life-threatening are the nurse's first priority. Next come those that have the potential to cause harm or injury. Last in priority are those that are related to the overall general health of the patient. Thus, a diagnosis of "ineffective airway clearance" would be dealt with before "sleep pattern disturbance," and "sleep pattern disturbance" would have priority over "knowledge deficit."

Another framework that may be used to prioritize diagnoses is Maslow's (1970) hierarchy of needs, seen in Figure 10–3. When this framework is used, there is an inverse relationship between high-priority nursing diagnoses and high-level needs. In other words, highest priority is given to diagnoses related to basic physiologic needs. Diagnoses related to safety and security needs would have second priority. And those diagnoses related to higher-level needs such as love and belonging or self-esteem would have lower priority.

Except in life-threatening situations, nurses should take care to involve patients in identifying priority diagnoses. If patients' priorities and the nurses' priorities are in opposition to each other, very little will be accomplished toward solving patient problems. This involvement of patients in planning their own care is called "collaboration."

Planning

Planning is the third step in the nursing process. Planning begins with the identification of patient goals. These are goals that are used by the patient and the nurse to guide the selection of interventions and to evaluate patient progress. Each nursing diagnosis has at least one patient goal.

Just as nursing diagnoses are written in collaboration with the patient, goals should also be agreed upon by both nurse and patient unless collaboration is impossible, such as when the patient is unconscious. In that event, family members can collaborate with the nurse. Goals give the patient, family, and nurse direction and make them active partners.

WRITING PATIENT GOALS/OUTCOME CRITERIA

Patient goals are also called **outcome criteria**. These goals should be written in terms of the patient rather than the nurse; in other words, the goals generally involve action on the part of the patient. Goals should be measurable and contain an action verb that tells specifically what the patient is to do or how the nurse can evaluate whether the goal has been met.

Effective goals also tell under what conditions and within what time frame the patient is to act. A sample goal might be: "Using a walker, patient will walk ten feet within two days." It is easy to see that this goal is written in terms of patient action, is measurable (ten feet), contains an action verb (walk), tells under what conditions (with a walker), and has a specified time frame for accomplishment (in two days). Box 17-2 lists the essential elements of an effective goal.

TYPES OF PATIENT GOALS

There are three types of patient goals: psychomotor, cognitive, and affective goals. The walker example just given is a **psychomotor goal** because it requires motor skills or actions by the patient. **Cognitive goals** deal with a desired change in a patient's knowledge level. An example of a cognitive goal might be: "The patient will list three effects of a high cholesterol level on the heart prior to

---

Box 17–2   Essential Elements of an Effective Patient Goal

- Stated as a patient goal, not a nursing goal.
- Contains an action verb.

- Describes conditions under which the action is to take place.
- Contains a realistic time frame.

---

discharge from the hospital." **Affective goals** involve a change in values or belief systems. An example of an affective goal is: "The patient will express an increased sense of well-being after participating in an exercise program for one month." A single patient may have a combination of psychomotor, cognitive, and affective goals.

ESTABLISHING TIME FRAMES FOR PATIENT GOALS

One aspect of goal setting not yet discussed is the estimated length of time needed to accomplish the goal. **Short-term goals** may be attainable within hours or days. They are usually very specific and are small steps leading to the achievement of broader, **long-term goals**. For example, "The patient will lose two pounds" is a short-term goal, and the time limit can be brief, perhaps a week or ten days.

Long-term goals are usually major changes that may take months or even years to accomplish. A goal such as "The patient will lose 75 pounds" may take months or perhaps even years to accomplish, and the time frame should be set accordingly.

It is extremely important to assist patients to set realistic goals for themselves. Setting their sights too high causes frustration and discouragement in patients, families, and nurses.

NURSING ORDERS

After short- and/or long-term goals are identified through collaboration between nurse and patient, the nurse writes **nursing orders**. Nursing orders are actions designed to assist the patient in achieving a stated patient goal. Every goal has specific nursing orders. Nursing orders may be carried out by a registered nurse (R.N.) or delegated to other members of the nursing staff.

Nursing orders and medical orders differ. Nursing orders are those interventions that are designed to treat the patient's response to an illness or medical treatment, whereas medical orders are designed to treat the actual illness or disease. An example of a nursing order is: "Teach turning, coughing, and deep-breathing exercises prior to surgery." These activities are designed to prevent postoperative respiratory problems due to immobility. They are appropriate nursing orders because prevention of complications due to immobility *is* a nursing responsibility. Nursing orders may include instructions regarding consultation with other health care providers such as the dietitian, physical therapist, or pharmacist.

Implementation/Intervention

When nursing orders are actually carried out, the fourth step of the nursing process, **intervention**, begins. Most people think of nursing as "doing something" for or to a patient. Notice, however, that in using the nursing process, nurses must do a great deal of thinking, processing, and planning before the first actual nursing action takes place.

Nurses who skip the essential first three steps of the nursing process and jump immediately into action are not behaving in a responsible, professional manner. Patients feel a greater sense of trust in a nursing staff if both physicians' orders and nurses' orders are carried out in an orderly, planned, and competent manner.

It is difficult to make general statements about this step in the nursing process because interventions vary widely, depending on the nursing diagnosis and patient goals. Typical nursing interventions include such actions as monitoring patients' responses to medications, patient teaching, and performing certain procedures, such as changing dressings on a wound.

Very sick patients require intense nursing care. As patients improve, however, they are gradually able to assume responsibility for self-care. It is important for nurses to allow patients to do as much for themselves as their illnesses allow. Patient independence is an important step in recovery.

TYPES OF NURSING INTERVENTIONS

Nursing interventions are of three basic types: independent, dependent, or interdependent.

Independent Interventions. **Independent interventions** are those for which the nurse's intervention requires no supervision or direction by physicians. Nurses are expected to possess the knowledge and skills to carry out independent actions safely. An example of an independent nursing intervention is teaching a patient how to examine her breasts for lumps. The nurse practice act of each state usually specifies types of independent nursing actions.

Dependent Interventions. **Dependent interventions** do require instructions, written orders, or supervision of another health professional, usually a physician. These actions require knowledge and skills on the part of the nurse but may not be done without explicit directions. An example of a dependent nursing intervention is the administration of medications. While a physician must order most medications, it is the responsibility of the nurse to know how to administer them safely and monitor their effectiveness.

Interdependent Interventions. The third type of intervention, **interdependent**, is the type of action in which the nurse must collaborate or consult with another health professional prior to carrying out the action. One example of this type of action is when the nurse implements orders that have been written by a physician in a protocol. Protocols define under what conditions and circumstances the nurse is allowed to treat the patient as well as what treatments are permissible. They are often used in situations where nurses can take immediate action without consulting with a physician.

Evaluation

The final step in the nursing process is **evaluation**. In this step the nurse examines the patient's progress to determine if a problem is solved, is in the process of being solved, or is unsolved. Evaluation may reveal that data, diagnosis, goals, and nursing interventions were all on target and that the problem is solved.

Evaluation may also indicate a need for a change in the care plan. Perhaps inadequate patient data were the basis for the plan, and further assessment has uncovered additional needs. The nursing diagnoses may have been incorrect or placed in the wrong order of priority. Patient goals may have been inappropriate or unattainable within the designated time frame. It is possible that nursing actions were incorrectly implemented.

Evaluation is a critical step in the nursing process and one that is often slighted. It is not enough to continue to do the "right things" if the patient is not improving in the expected manner. If, upon evaluation, the problem has not been resolved, the nursing care plan must be revised to reflect the necessary changes, and the process must begin again.

The Cyclic Nature of the Nursing Process

Although the steps in the nursing process are discussed separately here, in practice they are not so clearly delineated. Nor do they always proceed from one to another in a linear fashion. The nursing process is cyclic in nature, meaning that nurses are continuously going from one step to another and then beginning the process again. Often a nurse will perform two steps at the same time, for instance, observing a wound for signs of infection (assessment) while changing the dressing on the wound (intervention).

Now that you understand the steps in the nursing process, let us look back at the situation at the beginning of the chapter and compare the nursing process to the opening scenario. The problem that was identified was the necessity to don appropriate clothing. Data, both objective (the temperature outdoors) and subjective (the mood one is in), were gathered. A selection was made and implemented, and an evaluation of the implementation was carried out by looking into the mirror. This comparison reveals that problem solving is something each person does every day. The use of the nursing process simply provides professional nurses with a patient-oriented framework with which to solve clinical problems.

Box 17–3   A Nursing Process Case Study

The following case study identifies how the nurse used the nursing process in caring for patients.

At 7:30 A.M., before entering Mrs. Casey's room, Sally Barnes, R.N., recalled the night shift nurses' comments. They said that since admission the patient had complained about everything. Miss Barnes noted from the chart that Mrs. Casey had come to the nursing unit following emergency abdominal surgery at midnight the previous night. She also noted that Mrs. Casey had not had any pain medication since being admitted to the unit.

As Miss Barnes entered the room, she noticed that the patient was alone, lying on her right side in bed with her legs curled up toward her chest, and was rocking back and forth. When asked how she was feeling, she began to cry, then said, "I am in such terrible pain," and gestured toward the incision area with her hand.

Based on subjective and objective data, Miss Barnes realized that a priority nursing diagnosis was "pain." She told Mrs. Casey that she would immediately bring back some medication that would relieve her pain. While she was preparing the medication, she planned other pain-relieving nursing measures, such as repositioning the patient and giving her a back rub.

After returning to Mrs. Casey's room and giving her the medication for pain, Miss Barnes rubbed her back and positioned her with extra pillows. She told the patient that she would return shortly to check on her. When she returned 30 minutes later, she found the patient lying quietly with her eyes closed and breathing evenly. Miss Barnes concluded that her actions were both appropriate and effective.

ASSESSMENT

Subjective Data

1. Numerous verbal complaints
2. "I am in such terrible pain."

Objective Data

1. First postoperative day following abdominal surgery.
2. Patient has received no pain medication since admission.
3. In curled-up position, rocking back and forth.
4. Crying.

ANALYSIS

Pain related to abdominal incision.

PLAN

Short-term Goal

Patient will have decreased pain within one hour as evidenced by verbal expression.

Long-term Goal

Patient will rate pain as "2" on a scale of "1" = no pain to "10" = unbearable pain within 48 hours and be able to actively participate in activities of daily living (bathing, grooming, toileting, walking).

IMPLEMENTATION

Administer pain medication, reposition with pillows to splint the incision, and administer back rub.

EVALUATION

Short-term Goal

Achieved, as evidenced by patient lying quietly, with eyes closed and breathing slowly and evenly. Patient stated, "I feel better now."

Long-term Goal

Will be evaluated in 48 hours.

An example of using the nursing process in a clinical situation is found in Box 17–3. This situation demonstrates how the nursing process becomes so ingrained that experienced nurses go through the steps almost automatically.

CHAPTER SUMMARY

The nursing process is a systematic problem-solving process that is based on the scientific method. It is used by nurses when delivering patient care. The steps in this process are assessment, analysis, planning, implementation, and evaluation.

The activities of each step were outlined and discussed. The nursing process is cyclic and dynamic, or ever changing. Like any new behavior, nurses initially find that using the nursing process feels awkward or slow. After practice, however, most find it becomes a very natural way to approach patient care.

When all nurses use the nursing process, patient care is consistent, comprehensive, and coordinated. Through the use of the nursing process, nurses are able to work toward resolving patient problems in a systematic manner, thus advancing both the scientific base of nursing and professionalism.

Steps in the Nursing Process

Assessment

Analysis/Nursing diagnosis

Planning

Implementation

Evaluation

REVIEW/DISCUSSION QUESTIONS

1. Describe the steps in the nursing process and the activities of each step.

2. Describe a recent problem you needed to solve. Identify the steps that you used to solve the problem. Which of your steps resemble those in the nursing process?

3. Think of a recent conversation you have had and give examples of subjective and objective data from that conversation.

4. List a short-term personal goal and a long-term personal goal using all the essential elements of effective goals.

5. Compare the nursing process with the scientific method and state how they are similar and how they differ.

REFERENCES

Abdellah, F. (1959). Improving the teaching of nursing through research in patient care. In L. E. Heidgerken (Ed.), *Improvement of nursing through research* (pp. 83–88). Washington, D.C.: Catholic University Press.

Gordon, M. (1976). Nursing diagnosis and the diagnostic process. *American Journal of Nursing, 76*(5), 1298–1300.

Gordon, M. (1982). *Manual of nursing diagnosis.* New York: McGraw-Hill.

Henderson, V. (1966). *The nature of nursing.* New York: Macmillan.

Maslow, A. (1970). *Motivation and personality.* New York: Harper & Row.

North American Nursing Diagnosis Association. (1990). *Proceedings of the ninth national conference.* St. Louis: C.V. Mosby.

Orem, D. (1980). *Nursing: Concepts of practice.* New York: McGraw-Hill.

Rogers, M. (1979). *An introduction to the theoretical basis of nursing.* Philadelphia: F.A. Davis.

Roy, C. (1976). *Introduction to nursing: An adaptation model.* Englewood Cliffs, N.J.: Prentice-Hall.

Yura, H., and Walsh, M. B. (1978). *Human needs and the nursing process.* New York: Appleton-Century-Crofts.

Yura, H., and Walsh, M. B. (1983). *The nursing process: Assessing, planning, implementing, evaluating.* Norwalk, CT: Appleton-Century-Crofts.

SUGGESTED READINGS

Carpenito, L. J. (1989). *Nursing diagnosis: Application to clinical practice.* Philadelphia: J.B. Lippincott.

Gordon, M. (1987). *Nursing diagnosis: Process and application.* 2nd ed. New York: McGraw-Hill.

Chapter

Illness and Its Impact on Patients and Families

Carolyn Maynard

CHAPTER OBJECTIVES

What students should be able to do after studying this chapter:

1. Describe three stages of illness.
2. Describe behavioral responses to illness.
3. Identify internal and external influences on illness behaviors.
4. Discuss the influence of culture on illness behaviors.
5. Characterize four levels of anxiety.
6. Describe the physical, emotional, and cognitive effects of stress.
7. Give examples of three types of crises.
8. Discuss the effect of balancing factors in a stressful event.
9. Discuss how family functioning is altered during illness.

VOCABULARY BUILDING

Terms to know:

acceptance stage	dependency	situational crisis
anxiety	disease	social crisis
convalescence stage	hardiness	stress
crisis	illness	stressor
culture	maturational crisis	transition stage

*N*urses are involved in prevention and health maintenance activities, but many of their interactions center around illness and people who are ill. A unique characteristic of nursing is the emphasis on viewing patients holistically. Nurses recognize that human beings are complex organisms with physical, mental, emotional, social, and cultural components, all of which affect how a person responds when ill. The effective nurse takes each of these dimensions into consideration when planning nursing care. This chapter explores the stages of illness, illness behaviors, internal and external influences on illness behaviors, and the impact of illness on patients and families.

Illness

Benner and Wrubel (1989) described **illness** as the experience of a loss or dysfunction. They defined **disease** as an alteration at the tissue or organ level. Even though disease may be present, individuals are not considered "ill" until they become aware of the disease process through symptoms.

A person's perception of a change or loss is the major factor in whether illness exists and how serious it is. For example, a minor injury to the face of a fashion model may be perceived as very serious, whereas the same injury to a boxer would go virtually unnoticed. Because illness is relative and is experienced differently by different people, it must be defined in terms of each individual's reactions.

Stages of Illness

Although the behaviors are different for each person, people who are ill tend to progress through certain recognizable stages. These have been labeled transition, acceptance, and convalescence. Nurses encounter patients in each stage, so it is important to have some understanding of the types of behaviors that are associated with each.

TRANSITION STAGE

Moving from a state of wellness into illness is difficult for most people. According to Stuart and Sundeen (1991), the first stage of illness, the **transition stage**, begins when a person recognizes changes occurring in the body. Each person evaluates the changes, compares them to what is "normal" or usual, and makes a decision about whether or not these changes signal illness. Once people identify the presence of symptoms, they begin to be aware of themselves as ill. For many people, there is a gradual recognition of illness. They note minor changes over time, and their awareness of illness is cumulative. For those who experience an acute illness or an accident, the transition stage is abrupt.

Denial is a defense mechanism that people sometimes use to try to avoid the anxiety associated with becoming ill. People who pride themselves on their vigor and health may deny that the symptoms are significant. If this occurs, these individuals may attempt inappropriate self-treatment or completely avoid treatment. Extended denial may have serious results. Left untreated, some illnesses may become too advanced for effective treatment.

ACCEPTANCE STAGE

In the **acceptance stage**, people come to acknowledge the presence of an illness. They experience a multitude of feelings during this stage, depending on the body part affected, the severity of the illness, their personality type, and activity limitations imposed by the illness. Generally, once the presence of illness is accepted, the individual begins to behave in ways that lead toward recovery. At this point, if self-care has been unsuccessful, treatment will be sought from health care providers.

CONVALESCENCE STAGE

The **convalescence stage** is the final stage of illness for most people. According to Norris (1990), recovering people are expected to be grateful, cheerful, and eager to get back into the usual way of life. In reality, people who are recovering from illness tend to be upset and anxious, particularly if the illness was severe or extended. They are frustrated with the limitations on their functioning and with the expectations of others that they may feel unable to meet. Just as there are anxieties and problems with making the transition to the illness state, there are similar feelings and difficulties with making the changes back to the preillness state.

Not all sick people go through each stage, nor do they necessarily go through them at the same rate or in the same way. People who experience a sudden illness may not progress in the same way as those who develop a gradual illness. Because of individual differences, people will have more or less difficulty at each stage. Nevertheless, these stages represent a useful model to keep in mind when working with those who are ill.

Illness Behavior and the Sick Role

Some hospitalized patients who are restricted to bed may insist on getting up and doing everything for themselves against medical advice. Others in the same situation may ask that the nurses do things for them that they are capable of doing for themselves. Both types of patients are responding to the experience of illness and hospitalization—but in very different ways. Although there are many different factors that influence the way individuals respond to illness, an important influence is the societal expectation about how people who are ill *should* behave.

Each society generally requires that certain criteria be met before people can qualify as "sick." Talcott Parsons (1951), a sociologist, identified five attributes and expectations of the sick role that guided the view of illness in American society for some time. According to Parsons, the sick person:

1. Is exempt from social responsibilities.
2. Cannot be expected to care for himself or herself.
3. Should want to get well.
4. Should seek medical advice.
5. Should cooperate with the medical experts.

Although the current expectation is that people should accept responsibility for their own care rather than turn themselves completely over to health care providers, there continues to be some presumption that ill people should want to get well and should behave in a way that will lead to wellness. The individual who does not do so will probably not be seen as legitimately ill. In addition, there must be an inability to get well just by choosing to do so. Those who call themselves sick and who refuse to accept treatment may be seen as malingering, or faking illness, in order to avoid responsibilities.

Illness carries both privileges and obligations. The ill person is often allowed to evade some troubling situations or to escape the necessity of having to live up to others' expectations. Frequently, the ill person is entitled to be taken care of for some period and to give up some or all of the usual duties. The degree of exemption from responsibilities usually depends on the extent and severity of the illness.

While there are benefits from being ill, there are also obligations. One obligation is to seek and accept competent help. People who are ill generally must accept help with the duties they are unable to perform. For instance, the housewife who prides herself on doing everything for her family must accept help with cooking the meals and cleaning the house while she is restricted to bed.

The expectation that ill persons should want to get well and return to their normal duties as quickly as possible usually means that they should cooperate in the treatment process and, to a great extent, become submissive and compliant, placing themselves in the hands of the caretakers. Persons who refuse to take medications as ordered or who refuse to perform prescribed activities, such as adhering to an exercise program or therapeutic diet, are viewed in a negative light. Others may become irritated at their lack of participation in getting well again.

Influences on Illness Behavior

While there are some behaviors expected of sick people, there is also a wide variation of responses. Each person who is newly diagnosed with diabetes will behave somewhat differently from other people with the same condition. Both internal and external variables affect how an individual acts when ill. The personality of the ill individual has a great deal of influence on his or her response to illness. Past experiences with illness and cultural background also influence illness behaviors.

INTERNAL INFLUENCES

The personality structure of an individual is an internal variable that determines, to a large extent, how one manages illness. Two personality characteristics the nurse should consider when assessing the ill person are **dependency** and **hardiness**.

Dependency.   Patients have greater or lesser needs to be dependent that are unrelated to the severity of their illnesses. Some patients who are ill adopt a passive attitude and rely completely on others to take care of them. Others may deny that they are ill or have problems with being dependent and try to continue to do what they did before becoming sick.

We have all known sick people who have said something like, "I don't ask any questions—I know that my doctor and nurses know what is best for me, and I do what they tell me." Perhaps you also know someone who reacted to illness by saying, "They don't know what they are talking about. I don't need to be in bed, and I don't need to take that medicine." These two sentiments are at the opposite ends of the dependency continuum.

People who perceive themselves as helpless may be more willing to turn themselves over to health care personnel and do what they are told. Those who are used to being in charge and see themselves as being independent may resent the enforced dependency of hospitalization and illness. These two different attitudes are illustrated in the clinical vignettes below.

Clinical Vignette: Dependency

Mrs. Johnson has been in the hospital for several days following abdominal surgery. Even after she progressed to the point that she could feed herself, turn over in bed, and get up to the bathroom unaided, she continued to call for assistance when she needed to turn or to get out of bed. She now calls the nurse every few minutes, making some small request that she is quite capable of performing for herself. She is communicating to the nurse that she needs a great deal of assistance and is demonstrating overly dependent behavior.

Now consider the behavior of another patient.

Clinical Vignette: Independence

Mr. Thomas is just back to his room from surgery. The nurse found him trying to get out of bed by himself. He does not call to ask for medication, says that he is used to doing things for himself, and feels uncomfortable asking the nurses for help. Mr. Thomas is demonstrating behavior that is too independent for his current physical status.

Both overly dependent and overly independent behavior can be frustrating to nurses. They sometimes become angry with patients who request help with

activities they are capable of doing for themselves. The patient who is too dependent requires assistance to gradually assume more responsibility for the self. The
patient who needs to be "in charge" may have problems turning enough control
over to caregivers and will often be too independent. This patient will require
help with accepting assistance when activity is limited.

Hardiness.   Hardiness is a personality characteristic that affects how a person reacts to being ill. Stuart and Sundeen (1991) described three components of
hardiness. They state that people who exhibit hardiness tend to:

1. View change as a challenge rather than a threat.
2. Feel a sense of commitment to people or a cause.
3. Feel a sense of control over their lives.

The person with greater hardiness is believed to be better able to manage the
changes associated with illness and to have less physical illness resulting from
stress. Hardy people are likely to perceive themselves as having some control
over what happens to them, even when ill. This sense of being able to exert some
control over the situation can affect an ill person's sense of well-being (Lambert
et al. 1989).

EXTERNAL INFLUENCES

External factors that bear on illness behaviors include past experiences and
cultural group. Both directly influence how one perceives and responds to illness. The values that guide one's feelings about illness and steer one toward
particular methods of treatment are acquired primarily in the family of origin
and in the culture.

Past Experiences.   Adults who were pampered during childhood illnesses
may accept being ill fairly easily. Relying on others to care for them may not
concern them, and they may settle into the sick role easily.

On the other hand, there are adults who received childhood messages such
as "It is weak to be ill" or "One must keep going even when not feeling well."
They may have difficulty accepting the restrictions that often go with illness.

Still other adults who were hospitalized as small children or threatened with
injections for misbehaving may see hospitals and nurses as threatening. Clearly
these adults will behave very differently when ill.

Nurses should determine patients' past experiences with illness and the
health care system during a careful admission assessment. They can then use
these findings to individualize care.

Culture.   "Culture is the pattern of all learned behavior and values shared
by members of a particular group. It is transmitted by members of the group
from one generation to the next" (Cook and Fontaine 1991, pp. 156–157).
Culture is learned behavior that is reinforced through social interactions (Johnson 1989).

Culture exerts considerable influence over most of an individual's life experiences, including illness. Meanings attached to illness and perceptions of treat-

ment are affected to a large degree by one's culture. Culture determines when one seeks help and the type of practitioner consulted. It also prescribes customs of responding to the sick. Culture determines whether illness is seen as a punishment for misdeeds or as the result of inadequate personal health practices. It influences whether one goes to an acupuncturist, an herbalist, or a physician.

Knowledge of the patient's culture assists the nurse in understanding behaviors and provides direction for appropriate approaches to patient problems. Because culture may guide the patient's response to health care providers and to the care provided, it is necessary for the nurse to be knowledgeable about cultural influences. Failing to understand the cultural background of the patient limits the nurse's ability to provide the best care. Understanding a patient's cultural background can facilitate communication and assist in establishing an effective nurse-patient relationship.

The shared values and beliefs in a culture enable its members to predict each other's actions. They also influence how members react to each other's behavior. When nurses work with patients from cultures about which little is known, they lack familiar guidelines for predicting behavior. This can cause anxiety and feelings of distrust for both patient and nurse.

In an effort to predict behavior, the nurse may resort to stereotyping patients from different cultures. It is important that nurses refrain from overgeneralizing and stereotyping members of cultures or ethnic groups that are different from their own. Individual assessment is always the best basis for care, whatever the patient's culture or ethnic group.

Patterns of communication are strongly influenced by culture. The Asian patient who smiles and nods may be communicating politeness and respect rather than agreeing or indicating understanding. Americans tend to value a direct approach to problems, but in other cultures, subtlety and indirectness may be valued.

The amount of personal space needed is another factor that varies depending on cultural experience. Some cultures utilize touch as a major form of communication; in others, touching between persons who are not considered family is disrespectful. While Western culture values direct eye contact, some cultures view this as impolite, particularly direct eye contact between men and women.

Culture also has a primary influence on the type of stress its members experience at various points in their lives. Every society places stress on its members at one or more stages of development. For instance, American adolescents are typically under great stress as they struggle with independence issues. Amish adolescents tend to experience less stress because their behavior during this period is more rigidly prescribed by their culture.

Values held by the nurse may come into conflict with patients' cultural values. In the Navajo culture, for example, great value is placed on keeping pain and discomfort to oneself. Letting others know how you feel is seen as weak. The nurse who expects patients to complain and ask for medication when in pain may assume that the Navajo patient is comfortable when he is not. On the other hand, a nurse who values suffering in silence may underrate the discomfort of a patient who comes from a culture that proclaims pain loudly.

Box 18–1   Sociocultural Self-Assessment

Directions: Use your answers to these questions to better understand your own social and cultural beliefs and expectations.

- To what groups do I belong? What is my cultural heritage? My socioeconomic status? My age-group? My religious affiliation?
- How do I describe myself? What parts of the description come from the groups I belong to?
- What kinds of contact have I had with persons from different groups?

- What about my different groups do I feel proud of? What would I change if I could?
- Have I ever experienced the feeling of being rejected by another group?
- When I was growing up, what messages did I get from parents and friends about people from groups different from mine?
- What are the major stereotypes I hold about people from different groups?
- In order to work effectively with people from different groups, what do I need to change about myself?

The role expectations of nurses vary from culture to culture. A common white, middle-class American view of nurses is that they treat people as equals, are passive, and take direction from physicians. These patients feel free to ask questions of their nurses. Asians, however, may expect nurses to be authoritative, to provide directives, and to be expert practitioners who take charge. Out of respect for authority they may not speak until spoken to and may verbally agree with anything nurses propose (Cook and Fontaine 1991). The following patient vignette illustrates a cultural difference between patient and nurse in regard to expressing pain.

> Mrs. L., a 42-year-old Asian woman, became ill and required surgery while visiting her daughter in the United States. Following surgery, she was placed on a patient-controlled analgesia pump (PCA). The nurse explained how she should self-administer medication when she felt pain. Mrs. L. smiled and nodded her head when asked if she understood the instructions. Much later the nurse noticed that this patient appeared to be in great pain. On talking with her daughter, the nurse realized that Mrs. L. had not understood how to use the equipment but felt that she should not ask for additional instructions or complain of pain.

Nurses respond to sick people based not only on their formal education but also on the socialization and culture in their own background (Piper 1987). The nurse who identifies personal beliefs and expectations and how they influence care will be more able to recognize and deal with any factors that may impede patient care. Cultural assessment, therefore, begins with self-assessment.

To begin a cultural self-assessment, ask what your own values are. What behavior do you expect from people who are ill? Toward what groups do you have prejudices or biases? The nurse who is frustrated at the difficulty of caring for a patient from a different culture may benefit from taking a few minutes to imagine what it would be like to be hospitalized in a foreign country. Candidly answering the questions in Box 18–1 will help you begin this important process.

The nurse who does not take cultural differences into consideration may misinterpret patient behavior and fail to recognize problems that need to be managed. Cultural norms must be included in the care plan in order to achieve the desired goals. Being knowledgeable about other cultures can promote feelings of respect and enhance understandings of attitudes, behaviors, and the impact of illness.

Impact of Illness on Patient and Family

Illness results in a number of changes for both patients and families. Common experiences include behavioral and emotional changes, changes in roles, and disturbed family dynamics. Typical emotional responses to illness include stress and anxiety.

Severe illnesses that profoundly affect physical appearance and functioning are more likely to result in high levels of anxiety and extensive behavioral changes than are short-term, non–life-threatening illnesses. When planning care, the nurse must consider how illness impacts both the individual and the family.

Impact of Illness on the Patient

Illness creates a variety of emotional responses. Two of the most common responses are anxiety and stress. Both of these responses will be discussed.

ANXIETY

A student nurse is assigned to give a report in front of his class. On the morning the report is due he asks to meet with the instructor and tells her that he has sweaty palms, "butterflies" in his stomach, a rapid heart rate and did not sleep well the night before. He mentions that he has always had problems with speaking in front of groups. This student is experiencing anxiety.

Anxiety is a common and universal experience. It is also a common emotional response to illness and hospitalization. **Anxiety** is defined as a diffuse, vague feeling of apprehension and uncertainty. According to Stuart and Sundeen (1991), anxiety occurs as a result of some threat to an individual's selfhood, self-esteem, or identity. It is experienced when "the values a person identifies with his existence are threatened" (p. 319).

A number of threats are associated with illness. Illness may alter the way people view themselves. Some illnesses result in a change in physical appearance. Often there is some change in the ability to function, creating alterations in relationships, work performance, and abilities to meet others' expectations. In addition to potential changes caused by illness, there may be concern about pain and discomfort associated with illness or treatment. Because of real and poten-

---

Box 18–2   Symptoms of Anxiety

PHYSIOLOGICAL SYMPTOMS

Increased heart rate, faster respirations, increased blood pressure, insomnia, nausea and vomiting, fatigue, sweaty palms, tremors.

COGNITIVE SYMPTOMS

Inability to concentrate, forgetfulness, inattention to surroundings, preoccupation.

EMOTIONAL SYMPTOMS

Restlessness, irritability, feelings of helplessness, crying, depression.

---

tial threats and changes arising from illness, nurses must develop skills that will enable them to help patients recognize and manage anxiety.

Although the responses are similar, there is general agreement that anxiety and fear are different. Fear results from specific, known causes, whereas with anxiety the cause of the feelings is unknown (Haber et al. 1992). For example, if you are home alone at night and you hear an unusual noise outside, your heartbeat and respirations increase, your stomach tightens, and you perspire. The emotion in this situation is fear. If you begin to have the same feelings but have heard no noises and cannot identify a source of fear, then you are experiencing anxiety. Both emotions may be present at the same time. The patient who is in the hospital for an operation may experience anxiety about the unknown consequences of the surgery and fear of the procedure itself.

Symptoms of Anxiety.   Nurses should be familiar with the numerous symptoms of anxiety. They are classified as physiological, emotional, and cognitive. Physiological symptoms include increased heart rate, respirations, and blood pressure; insomnia; nausea and vomiting; fatigue; sweaty palms; and tremors. Emotional responses include restlessness, irritability, feelings of helplessness, crying, and depression. Cognitive symptoms include inability to concentrate, forgetfulness, inattention to surroundings, and preoccupation. Box 18–2 summarizes the physiological, emotional, and cognitive symptoms of anxiety.

Responses to Anxiety.   Responses to anxiety occur on a continuum. Peplau (1963) described four levels: mild, moderate, severe, and panic. In the mild level, there is increased alertness and ability to focus attention and concentrate. There is an expanded capacity for learning at this stage.

At the moderate level the person is able to concentrate on only one thing at a time. Frequently, there is increased body movement and more rapid speech. There is subjective awareness of discomfort.

Box 18–3 Levels of Anxiety

MILD ANXIETY

Increased alertness, increased ability to focus, concentration good, expanded capacity for learning.

MODERATE ANXIETY

Concentration limited to one thing, increased body movement, rapid speech, subjective awareness of discomfort.

SEVERE ANXIETY

Scattered thoughts, difficulty with verbal communication, considerable discomfort, purposeless movements.

PANIC

Complete disorganization, difficulty differentiating reality from unreality, constant random movements, unable to function without assistance.

At the severe level thoughts become scattered. The severely anxious person may not be able to communicate verbally, and there is considerable discomfort accompanied by purposeless movements such as handwringing and pacing.

At the panic level the person becomes completely disorganized and loses the ability to differentiate reality and unreality. There are constant random and purposeless movements. The individual experiencing the panic level of anxiety is unable to function without assistance. Panic levels of anxiety cannot be continued indefinitely because the body will become exhausted, and death may occur if anxiety is not reduced. Box 18–3 contains the characteristics of each level of anxiety.

Because anxiety is such a common response to illness and hospitalization, nurses often encounter patients who are experiencing mild or moderate anxiety. Occasionally, patients who are severely anxious are seen. When interacting with an anxious patient, the nurse should carefully assess the level of anxiety before attempting to develop the plan of care.

According to Peplau (1963), anxiety is communicated interpersonally. In other words, it is "contagious." For this reason it is crucial that the nurse be aware of and manage personal anxiety so that it is not inadvertently transferred to patients. Self-awareness is also essential to prevent absorbing patients' anxiety.

STRESS

Stress is another internal variable that impacts patients. Stress is both a response to illness as well as an important factor in the development of illness. Because illness and hospitalization involve so many alterations in life-style, they tend to cause a great deal of stress.

Stress is a part of life. It is unavoidable and essential. "Throughout life a person must cope with demands and change to survive and grow" (Beare and Myers 1990, p. 43). The stress related to examinations, for example, motivates most students to grow by studying and learning. Although stress is unavoidable, and even sometimes desirable, some control can be exerted over the number and types of **stressors** encountered, and responses to the stressors can often be managed.

Hospitalized patients are removed from their usual support systems. They lose much of their control because nurses and other care providers make decisions for them. Being ill often means that they are no longer able to perform activities as they did before the illness occurred. Stress is a common response to all these changes.

Differentiating Between Stress and Anxiety. Stress and anxiety have some characteristics in common. The physiological responses are certainly similar. But whereas anxiety is a response to some real or perceived threat to the individual, stress is an interaction between the individual and the environment. Stress includes all the responses the body makes while striving to maintain equilibrium and deal with demands. The following situation provides an example of both stress and anxiety:

> Mary S. is a 32-year-old single mother and a lawyer who was recently hired as the first woman in an established law firm. One morning as she prepares to take her 2-year-old daughter to the child care center, she receives a call saying that the woman who has provided child care was in an accident and will be closing the center indefinitely. Miss S. experiences both stress and anxiety in this situation. She has a number of demands placed on her from her workplace and from her family that lead to stress. The additional demands caused by the sudden change in her plans results in even higher levels of stress. In addition, Miss S. has placed the expectation on herself that she will perform her job exactly like the men in the firm do. Being late or missing work due to having to make new arrangements for child care conflicts with her self-expectations and poses a threat to her self-esteem. This threat leads to feelings of anxiety.

Internal, External, and Interpersonal Stressors. Selye (1956) defined stress as the nonspecific response of the body to any demand made upon it. He named the general adaptation syndrome (GAS) and identified three stages through which the body progresses while responding to stress.

Stressors trigger the body's stress response. Stressors are agents, or stimuli, that an individual perceives as demanding (Stuart and Sundeen 1991). Stressors may come from external, interpersonal, or internal sources. External stressors include such things as noise, heat, cold, malfunctioning equipment (such as a car that won't run), or organizational rules and expectations. Interpersonal sources of stress include the demands made by others and conflicts with others. Placing unrealistic expectations on oneself is an example of an internal stressor. In the example of Mary S., an internal stressor is her expectation that she will perform just like the men in the firm. It is an unrealistic expectation for any single parent of a small child to expect that the child's needs will never interfere with work.

Responses to Stress. Outward responses to stress are determined by the individual's evaluation of it. Cognitive appraisal, or the way one thinks about a specific situation, determines whether that situation is stressful for that particular individual (Stuart and Sundeen 1991). For example, loud music at a rock concert may be perceived as considerably less stressful by an adolescent than by his parents.

Another factor related to the assessment of threat is whether the individual feels capable of handling the threat, that is, whether the person exhibits hardiness. The person who feels capable of dealing with whatever problem arises can be expected to feel less stress than the person who does not generally feel competent.

Stress affects the physical, emotional, and cognitive areas of functioning just as anxiety does. Physically, there is a feeling of fatigue; muscles feel tight and tense. There is an increase in heart rate and respiration. The person who is under prolonged stress may be unable to sleep or eat, or there may be excessive sleeping or eating in an attempt to avoid or cope with the stress.

Emotionally, stressed people feel drained and unable to care for themselves or others. This can result in social isolation and distancing from others. There is difficulty with enjoying life. There may be feelings of hopelessness and of being out of control. Irritability and impatience often occur.

Cognitively, stress causes decreased mental capacity and problem-solving skills are reduced. Therefore, there is a tendency to have difficulty making decisions.

Stress and Illness. It has been known for some time that stress plays a major role in the development of illness. More recent research has provided better understanding of the links between prolonged stress and body functioning.

The person who is under stress for long periods of time is at risk for a number of physical problems. The exhaustion that results from excessive, unmanaged stress leads to physiological breakdowns and predisposition to a number of problems. Disorders such as peptic ulcers, hypertension, and rheumatoid arthritis are called "stress-related" diseases because they frequently occur in individuals who have been severely stressed.

Stress has been found to be related to a reduction in the immune response, which can delay healing and result in greater susceptibility to infectious disorders such as colds and flu. Holmes and Rahe conducted long-term studies of persons with medical illness and found that the more stress people experienced in a given year, the more likely they were to develop physical illness (Barry 1989). Refer to Chapter 10 for Holmes and Rahe's Social Readjustment Rating Scale.

Coping with Stress. Nurses have a role in helping patients modify their stressors. Nurses should assess patients' abilities to recognize symptoms of stress and their usual methods of coping.

Box 18–4   Breathing Exercises

Lie or sit in a comfortable position. Uncross your legs and arms; close your eyes, if
    comfortable. Place one hand on your chest and the other on your abdomen,
    below the rib cage. Inhale, allowing the hand on the abdomen to rise. The hand
    on the chest remains still. Exhale, letting the abdomen fall. Repeat. Notice with
    each breath that the abdomen rises and the chest remains quiet.
Continue the breathing. In a slow, rhythmic voice, begin to count mentally with
    each breath saying:
In—Two . . . Hold—Two . . . Out—Two—Three—Four—Relax
In—Two . . . Hold—Two . . . Out—Two—Three—Four—Relax
Repeat this process for 10 minutes. When other thoughts come in to interrupt, say,
    "Back to center—breathe" and begin the count again (In—Two, etc.).

(From McFarland, G. K., and Thomas, M. D. (1991). *Psychiatric mental health nursing.* Philadelphia: J.B. Lippincott. Used by permission.)

Coping with stress can be direct or indirect. In using direct action, nurses
assist patients to identify those situations that can be changed and take responsibility for changing them. The focus is on using problem-solving skills and planning to eliminate or avoid as many stressors as possible. It is important to realize
that completely eliminating stress from one's life is neither possible nor desirable.

In helping patients use indirect coping, nurses' actions are aimed at reducing
the affective (feelings) and physiological (bodily) disturbances resulting from
stress. Patients are taught techniques such as deep breathing, muscle relaxation,
and imagery, which help them cope more effectively with stress. Boxes 18–4
and 18–5 contain breathing and progressive relaxation exercises that you can
use yourself and teach patients to use to reduce the consequences of stress.

In order to assist patients to manage stress, it is important that nurses be
skilled in assessing and managing their own personal stress. Nurses who are
feeling stressed themselves will probably have difficulty assisting patients to deal
with similar problems. Identifying your own sources of stress is an important
first step. The questions in Box 18–6 will help you begin the process of becoming
self-aware and thereby effective in helping patients deal with stress.

CRISIS

A person who is ill and experiencing high levels of stress may, if unable to cope
with the stress, develop a **crisis** situation. Everyone experiences stress, and as
long as the stress is managed, harmful consequences may be avoided. Any
stressful situation can, however, precipitate a crisis if the individual becomes
overwhelmed. Stress produces a crisis only if the usual methods of coping fail.

Box 18–5   Active Progressive Relaxation Exercise

Get yourself into a comfortable position and begin to focus on slow, deep breathing. Allow your eyes to close. Let go of any thoughts from the day. Remember to continue to breathe calmly and regularly throughout the exercise, releasing tension each time you exhale. Follow the instructions below for each muscle group listed in the "Sequence of Muscle Groups" section:

STEPS IN EXERCISE

• Slowly tense the muscle.
• Hold the tension.
• Focus on the tension, noticing how it feels and where you feel it.
• Release the tension.
• Notice the difference between tension and no tension.
• At each step, check for residual tension in the rest of your body; check your breathing to make sure it is slow and regular; allow the tension to drain out of the body with each exhalation.

SEQUENCE OF MUSCLE GROUPS

• Right toes and foot; left
• Right lower leg; left
• Right upper leg; left
• Buttocks
• Lower back
• Abdomen
• Upper back and shoulders
• Right forearm; left
• Right upper arm; left
• Neck
• Forehead
• Jaw and mouth (exaggerate a smile)
• Eyes (squeeze shut)

(From McFarland, G. K., and Thomas, M. D. (1991). *Psychiatric mental health nursing.* Philadelphia: J.B. Lippincott. Used by permission.)

Crises can occur in anyone's life if particularly difficult situations are encountered. Caplan (1961) stated that a crisis exists when a problem or situation exists that poses a threat to the individual and is not solved by the usual coping methods. He identified the following developmental phases in a crisis:

1. There is an initial rise in tension as the usual problem-solving methods are tried.
2. There is a lack of success in coping as the stimulus continues and more discomfort is felt.
3. There is a further rise in tension, and emergency problem-solving methods are tried.
4. If the problem continues and can neither be solved nor avoided, tension increases and a major disorganization occurs.

According to Caplan, *crisis* refers to the individual's emotional response to an event rather than to the event itself. Just as with stress, the same event will not result in a crisis for everyone. The loss of a job may precipitate a crisis for one person, whereas another may see it as an opportunity to find an even better job. Although all persons facing the same event will not be in a crisis, there are some

Box 18–6   Stress Self-Test

Directions: Answer yes or no to the following questions:

DO YOU FREQUENTLY: YES   NO

1. Neglect your diet
2. Fail to exercise regularly
3. Ignore self-examinations
4. Ignore symptoms of stress
5. Procrastinate
6. Fail to see humor in situations
7. Fail to use some time each day for relaxation
8. Try to do everything yourself
9. Set unrealistic goals
10. Look to others to make things happen for you
11. Have difficulty making decisions
12. Keep everything inside
13. Feel disorganized
14. Get too little rest
15. Race through the day
16. Make a "big deal" of everything
17. Feel your life is out of control
18. Find yourself getting angry because others are not doing
    what is expected
19. Find yourself worrying about the past or future
20. Say yes to everything

Score 1 for each "yes" answer. The closer your score is to 20, the higher your stress index. A score of 14 or above indicates the need for stress management strategies.

(Adapted from Slaby, A. E. (1988). *60 Ways to Make Stress Work for You*. Summit, NJ: PIA Press. Used by permission.)

situations, such as the death of a loved one or loss of a body part, that nurses can expect will result in some degree of crisis for most people.

Balancing Factors.   When a stressful event occurs, there are certain factors that can help the person to return to a state of equilibrium and avoid a crisis. Aguilera (1990) identified three factors as critical in determining whether a crisis develops in a particular situation:

1. The person's perception of the situation.
2. The person's situational supports.
3. The person's coping mechanisms.

If these balancing factors are operating, a crisis may not develop. If one or more of the factors are absent, the resolution of the problem may be blocked, and a crisis is more likely to occur.

A crisis is likely to be avoided if the person perceives the situation realistically rather than distorting it. A realistic perception of the problem situation makes it more likely that problem solving can be used. Similarly, if situational supports are adequate, there is a greater likelihood that the person will have the necessary resources to respond adequately and will feel that others are present who can be depended upon. Having adequate coping mechanisms means that the person has a number of possible responses to the situation that have been effective methods of dealing with stresses in the past. Figure 18–1 contains a diagram that explains the effect of balancing factors on the outcome of a stressful event.

Resolution of Crisis.   Crises are self-limiting. This means that they are generally resolved, either positively or negatively, within a period of approximately six weeks (Haber et al. 1992). During a crisis the normal methods of coping with stress are not working, and the person actively desires to be helped by others. According to crisis theorists, this makes the person in crisis more accepting of assistance and to developing new methods of coping (Aguilera 1990).

A crisis period, then, may end with the individual continuing to use maladaptive behavior or using improved coping skills. The Chinese symbol for crisis is a combination of two others that mean "danger" and "opportunity" (Dixon 1987). This ancient symbol validates the modern belief that crisis is a turning point at which the person can either gain strength and learn new coping skills or regress to a level of functioning below that which existed prior to the crisis.

Types of Crisis.   Hoff (1989) described three types of crises: maturational, situational, and unanticipated social. **Maturational**, or developmental, **crises** occur as a response to the stresses associated with predictable events occurring in the lives of most people. Examples of maturational crises are adolescence, adulthood, marriage, parenthood, and job changes. Maturational crises arise gradually. They are also resolved gradually. Most people manage maturational crises without professional assistance.

The second type of crisis is **situational**. These crises occur as a result of unanticipated events. Examples of situational crises are loss of a job, failure at school, loss of a loved one, or a geographic move. Because situational crises are unexpected, they are more hazardous than the maturational type. In addition,

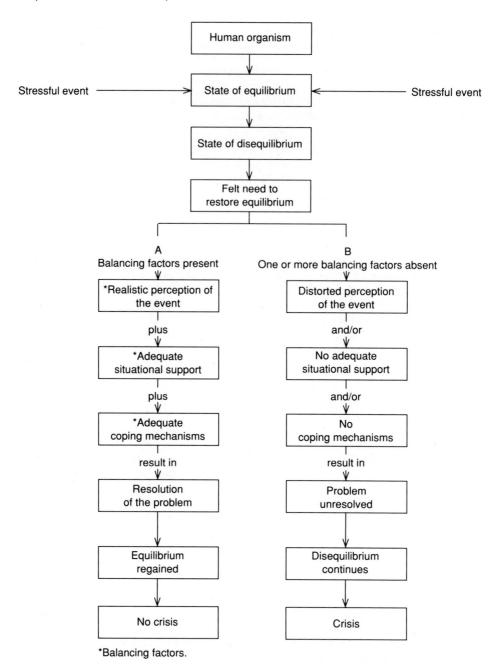

Figure 18–1   The effect of balancing factors in a stressful event. (From Aguilera, D. (1990). *Crisis intervention: Theory and methodology* (6th ed.). Baltimore: C.V. Mosby. Used by permission.)

the nature of situational crises means that many areas of a person's life may be affected. People experiencing situational crises may require counseling.

The third type of crisis, unanticipated **social crises**, are unexpected and uncommon events that do not occur in the everyday lives of most people. Examples of social crises are earthquakes, violent crimes (such as mass murders), nuclear accidents, hurricanes, and floods. Social crises generally affect large numbers of people. Victims of social crises usually can benefit from professional counseling.

Nurses frequently work with people who are experiencing crisis situations. They need to recognize when crises are occurring and assist patients to regain emotional equilibrium (Johnson 1989). The goal is for patients to return to at least their precrisis levels of functioning.

Impact of Illness on the Family

While anxiety, stress, and crisis situations are factors that may affect an ill person, it is important to remember that the entire family system is affected by a member's illness. Illness and hospitalization are situations that can drastically increase stress in a family and disrupt family functioning (Barry 1989).

Stress is one of the greatest threats to the healthy functioning of a family. The most important factor in how a family tolerates stress is the coping abilities of the members. Families already experiencing difficulties may find that their problems are worsened by having an ill member.

Families are seen as systems, which means that change in one member will change the functioning of the total family. When a member of a family becomes ill, the sick member has to give up responsibility to other family members. The family must continue to fulfill its usual functions while dealing with the alterations imposed by the illness or absence of a member. Flexible family members who are able to shift and assume different roles, who can share their feelings, and who seek assistance as needed will adjust to these changes better (Cook and Fontaine 1991).

Resentment is an emotion that may be experienced in families with a sick member. Those family members who must take over the sick person's responsibilities may be angry and then feel guilty about the anger. Family members who are unable to deal with feelings of anger may displace them onto the nursing staff by becoming critical and demanding.

Similarly, patients may feel guilty about creating hardships for loved ones. They may become convinced that they are no longer essential because family members are capably taking over their roles (Barry 1989).

Family members sometimes withdraw from each other because they fear that their negative feelings may not be understood and accepted. This mutual withdrawal leads to feelings of isolation for both patients and family members.

Families are often confused or uncertain about how to treat the sick member. They may have problems accepting and responding appropriately to the patients' dependency needs. As discussed earlier in the chapter, patients may react to illness with either overly dependent or overly independent behaviors. Nurses need to monitor whether family members foster dependence thereby keeping the patient from becoming more independent. Nurses should also be aware that some families are uncomfortable with the ill person being in a dependent role and will not allow the necessary dependency for recovery. For example, if a man who is very much in control in a family has a heart attack and is in the coronary care unit, family members may have difficulty seeing the usually strong father in a helpless position. They may continue to bring family problems to him.

Typically, family members experience considerable anxiety and fear about the outcome of their loved one's illness. They also experience discomfort with the strange environment of the hospital. Their anxiety may be communicated to the patient. It can also be expressed in angry outbursts directed at members of the nursing staff. The wise nurse will not take these outbursts personally.

The nurse needs to recognize the anxiety in the family and take steps to reduce it. Talking with members, explaining what is happening and what to expect, and teaching them how to participate in their loved one's care can help the family considerably.

The nurse should assess the family functioning and the ability of the family to provide support for the patient. The nurse needs to determine the level of knowledge of the family members and assist them to identify concerns and make realistic plans. Providing information and including the family in the planning can result in increased support for the patient and more effective care.

CHAPTER SUMMARY

Illness involves a perception of loss. Sick people tend to progress through transition, acceptance, and convalescence stages. Societal expectations of sick people are that they want to get well, will seek appropriate care, and will cooperate in treatment. In return, they are exempted from some of their usual responsibilities during their illnesses.

While society has expectations about how sick people should behave, there are several factors that influence actual behavior. Previous experience and personality characteristics of dependency or hardiness are factors that affect individuals' responses to illness.

Because of the stress and anxiety involved with illness, it is important for the individual to have methods of handling them. A crisis situation occurs when stress is not adequately managed. Three types of crises have been identified: maturational, situational, and social.

Providing holistic care means that nurses must consider their patients' families. The family is a system in which a change in one member affects all the other members. Illness causes alterations in usual family functioning that can result in feelings of anger and guilt. The nurse needs to assess both how the family is influencing the patient and how they are being influenced by the member who is ill.

An understanding of the factors that affect behaviors associated with illness can provide a better framework for the delivery of nursing care that is satisfying to both patient and nurse. As nurses view responses to illness in the context of the person's total life, they are better able to understand and accept the unique ways in which individuals and families react to illness and hospitalization.

REVIEW/DISCUSSION QUESTIONS

1. Think of your most recent illness. Can you identify any benefits you gained from being ill?
2. If you or someone close to you has been hospitalized, how did the nurses encourage or discourage dependent behaviors?
3. How much do you value your independence? Would it be easy or hard to allow yourself to be bathed and have other intimate needs met by nurses?
4. Identify your own cultural group's response to illness. What are your family's characteristic responses to illness of a member?
5. Interview someone from another cultural background to learn how he or she perceives illness.
6. Speculate about the potential changes in the family of a husband and father of four small children who has experienced a severe illness and will be unable to work for an extended period. What stresses is this family likely to encounter? How would these stresses change if the wife/mother were the sick family member?

REFERENCES

Aguilera, D. C. (1990). *Crisis intervention: Theory and methodology* (6th ed.). Baltimore: C.V. Mosby.

Barry, P. (1989). *Psychosocial nursing assessment and intervention* (2nd ed.). Philadelphia: J.B. Lippincott.

Beare, P., and Myers, J. (1990). *Principles and practice of adult health nursing.* Baltimore: C.V. Mosby.

Benner, P., and Wrubel, J. (1989). *The primacy of caring: Stress and coping in health and illness.* Menlo Park, CA.: Addison-Wesley.

Caplan, G. (1961). *An approach to community mental health.* New York: Grune & Stratton.

Cook, J., and Fontaine, K. (1991). *Essentials of mental health nursing* (2nd ed.). New York: Addison-Wesley.

Dixon, F. (1987). *Working with people in crisis: Theory and practice* (2nd ed.). St. Louis: C.V. Mosby.

Haber, J., et al. (1992). *Comprehensive psychiatric nursing* (4th ed.). New York: McGraw-Hill.

Hoff, L. A. (1989). *People in crisis* (3rd ed.). Reading, MA: Addison-Wesley.

Johnson, B. (1989). *Psychiatric mental health nursing: Adaptation and growth* (2nd ed.). New York: J.B. Lippincott.

Lambert, V., et al. (1989). Social support, hardiness and psychological well-being in women with arthritis. *Image, 21,* 128–131.

McFarland, G. K., and Thomas, M. D. (1991). *Psychiatric mental health nursing.* Philadelphia: J.B. Lippincott.

Norris, C. M. (1990). The work of getting well. *American Journal of Nursing, 90,* 47.

Parsons, T. (1951). *The social system.* New York: Free Press.

Peplau, H. (1963). A working definition of anxiety. In S. F. Burd and M. A. Marshall (Eds.), *Some clinical approaches to psychiatric nursing.* New York: Macmillan.

Piper, L. R. (1987). The sick role. *Nursing Management,* 18(9), 108.

Selye, H. (1956). *The stress of life.* New York: McGraw-Hill.

Slaby, A. E. (1988). *60 Ways to Make Stress Work for You.* Summit, NJ: PIA Press.

Stuart, G., and Sundeen, S. (1991). *Principles and practice of psychiatric nursing* (4th ed.). Boston: C.V. Mosby.

Chapter

19 *Therapeutic Use of Self Through Communication*

CHAPTER OBJECTIVES

What students should be able to do after studying this chapter:

1. Describe "therapeutic use of self."

2. Explore the role self-awareness plays in the ability to use nonjudgmental acceptance as a helping technique.

3. Discuss factors creating successful or unsuccessful communication.

4. Evaluate interactions according to criteria for successful communication: feedback, appropriateness, efficiency, and flexibility.

5. Differentiate between therapeutic and social relationships.

6. Identify and describe the phases of the nurse-patient relationship.

7. Recognize own helpful and unhelpful communication patterns.

VOCABULARY BUILDING

Terms to know:

acceptance
action language
active listening
appropriateness
clarification
communication
congruent
context
contract
efficiency
empathy
evaluation
false reassurance
feedback

flexibility
incongruent
irrational belief
message
nonjudgmental
  acceptance
nonverbal
  communication
nurse-patient
  relationship
open-ended question
open posture
orientation phase
perception

receiver
reflection
self-awareness
sender
somatic language
stereotypes
termination phase
transmission
ventilation
verbal communication
working phase

*T*he interpersonal aspect of the **nurse-patient relationship** is an extremely important one. Patients must feel comfortable with their nurses and must trust them to be knowledgeable providers of care. If comfort and trust are not present, providing effective nursing care is impeded.

Aspects of the Therapeutic Use of Self

As mentioned in Chapter 11, Hildegard Peplau first focused on the importance of the nurse-patient relationship in her 1952 book *Interpersonal Relations in Nursing.* She called using one's personality and communication skills to help patients improve their health status "therapeutic use of self."

The ability to use oneself therapeutically can be developed. Nurses develop this ability by acquiring certain knowledge, attitudes, and skills that assist them in relating effectively to patients, patients' families, coworkers, and other health care professionals. This chapter includes information that enhances the development of self-awareness, nonjudgmental acceptance of others, communication skills, and knowledge of the phases of the nurse-patient relationship, all of which are essential components of effective interpersonal relationships in nursing.

Developing Self-Awareness

Awareness of oneself, called **self-awareness**, is basic to effective interpersonal relationships. Robert Burns (1955), the eighteenth-century Scottish poet, described the desire for self-awareness in his poem *To a Louse*: "Oh wad some Power the giftie gie us/To see oursels as ithers see us!"

Few people have the innate capacity to recognize their own emotional needs, biases, blind spots, and their impact on others. With practice, however, most can become more effective in doing so, thus improving self-awareness.

An important guideline in professional nursing is that nurses should get their own emotional needs met outside of the nurse-patient relationship. When nurses' strong unmet needs for acceptance, approval, friendship, or even love enter into their relationships with patients, professionalism is lost, and relationships become social in nature. Becoming aware of one's needs and making conscious efforts to meet those needs in one's private life make professional, therapeutic relationships with patients possible.

Nurses care for a widely diverse array of patients whose values, beliefs, and life-styles may challenge nurses' own. Patients sometimes are attractive or repellant to nurses. Sometimes nurses find themselves meeting their own needs to be liked or needed through relationships with patients. Nurses who have emotional reactions to patients, positive or negative, sometimes feel disturbed or guilty about these feelings. Part of self-awareness is recognizing one's feelings and understanding that while feelings cannot be controlled, behaviors can. Effective nurses control their behaviors to prevent their own prejudices, beliefs, and needs from intruding into nurse-patient relationships.

Avoiding Stereotypes

Stereotypes and prejudices are attitudes developed through interactions with family, friends, and others in each individual's social and cultural system. It is not uncommon for even well-educated professionals to have stereotyped expectations about groups of people different from themselves. These stereotypes are established through childhood experiences and affect relationships with people in the stereotyped group. Since stereotypes and prejudices tend to persist in spite of contrary experiences, they are **irrational**, or illogical, **beliefs.**

The subtle intrusion of stereotyped expectations into the nurse-patient relationship can cause disturbed patterns of relating. For example, the expectation that all elderly people are irritable and demanding may cause the nurse to avoid all elderly patients or treat their complaints as unimportant.

Professional nurses deliver high-quality care to all patients regardless of ethnicity, age, gender, religion, life-style, or diagnosis. The *Code for Nurses* (Box 4–1) calls upon nurses to do this. Nurses are not without stereotypes and prejudices, however, and must strive to be aware of their own irrational feeling responses toward patients. Every professional nurse's goal is to accept all patients as individuals of dignity and worth who deserve the best nursing care possible.

Becoming Nonjudgmental

Acceptance is not always easy because prejudices are strong, and judging others as "good" or "bad" is often automatic. It is important to remember that acceptance conveys neither approval nor disapproval of patients, their personal beliefs, habits, expressions of feelings, or chosen life-styles. **Nonjudgmental**

Research Note

Concern about registered nurses' attitudes toward older people led Barbara W. McCabe to conduct a study of 318 randomly selected nurses in a midwestern state. She wanted to answer three research questions:

1. What are the attitudes of registered nurses (R.N.s) toward older people?
2. Is there a relationship between ego defensiveness (self-protection to avoid anxiety or threat) and the attitudes of R.N.s toward older people?
3. Is there a relationship between certain demographic variables (age, education) and the attitude of R.N.s toward older people?

McCabe's study had a response rate of 80.1 percent, or 255 people. Their mean (average) age was 38 years, and they received their basic nursing education in diploma, associate degree, and baccalaureate nursing programs.

Using two validated instruments, the Marlowe-Crowne Social Desirability Scale and the Kogan's Attitudes Toward Old People Scale, McCabe found primarily positive attitudes. The scores on ego defensiveness, however, suggested that many of the respondents tended to present themselves in an idealized image. In other words, they may have reduced the expression of negative attitudes in order to conform with an idealized nursing image. Those with higher educational levels were more likely to have positive attitudes, as were those in administrative positions. It can be speculated that administrators do not have to deal with elderly patients on a day-to-day basis and therefore may tend to be more positive about them.

McCabe suggested that nursing students and practicing nurses should be taught that it is helpful to express feelings, even when they are negative, in order to keep unexpressed feelings from interfering with nursing care.

(From McCabe, B. W. (1989). Ego defensiveness and its relationship to attitudes of registered nurses toward older people. *Research in Nursing and Health*, 12(2), 85–91.)

---

acceptance means that nurses acknowledge all patients' rights to be different and to express their "differentness."

Therapeutic use of self begins with the ability to convey acceptance to patients and requires self-awareness and nonjudgmental attitudes on the part of nurses. Ongoing examination of attitudes toward others is both a lifelong process and an essential part of self-awareness and interpersonal growth.

Communication Theory

Communication is the exchange of thoughts, ideas, or information and is at the heart of nurse-patient relationships. Communication is a dynamic process that is the primary instrument through which change is effected in nursing situations. Nurses use their communication skills in all phases of the nursing process. These skills are vital to effective nursing care.

Jurgen Ruesch (1972, p. 16), a communications theorist, defined communication as "all the modes of behavior that one individual employs, conscious or unconscious, to affect another: not only the spoken and written word, but also gestures, body movements, somatic signals, and symbolism in the arts."

Communication begins the moment two people become aware of one another's presence. It is impossible *not* to communicate when in the presence of another person, even if no words are spoken. Even when alone, people routinely engage in "self-talk," which is an internal form of communication.

Levels of Communication

Communication exists on at least two levels: verbal and nonverbal. **Verbal communication** consists of all speech and represents only a small part of communication. The majority of communication is **nonverbal communication**, which consists of grooming, clothing, gestures, posture, facial expressions, tone and volume of voice, and actions, among other things. Because individuals tend to exercise less conscious control over their nonverbal communication than the verbal, nonverbal is considered a more reliable expression of feeling.

Consider, for example, a young woman who is angry with her boyfriend. She may "clam up," pout, or otherwise show her displeasure nonverbally but when asked, "What's wrong?" may reply, "Nothing. Nothing at all!" The wise suitor will pay more attention to her nonverbal communication than to the spoken word. If he pays attention only to her words, she may become even more annoyed at his lack of perceptiveness. His job in evaluating her intent is made more difficult by the incongruence between her verbal and nonverbal messages.

When **congruent** communication occurs, the verbal and nonverbal aspects match and reinforce each other. For example, the words "I'm glad to see you!" spoken in a pleasant tone and accompanied by a smile and a proffered hand represent congruence between verbal and nonverbal behavior. The same words spoken listlessly, in a monotone, and without eye contact convey **incongruent** communication. Incongruent communication creates confusion in receivers, who are unsure to which level of communication they should respond.

Elements of the Communication Process

Ruesch identified five major elements that must be present in order for communication to take place: a sender, a message, a receiver, feedback, and context. The **sender** is the person sending the message, the **message** is what is actually said plus accompanying nonverbal communication, and the **receiver** is the person receiving the message. A response to a message is termed **feedback**. The setting in which an interaction occurs—the mood, relationship between sender and receiver, and other factors—is known as the **context**. All these elements are necessary for communication to occur.

Consider the classroom situation for a moment. During a lecture, the professor is the sender, the lecture is the message, and students are the receivers. The

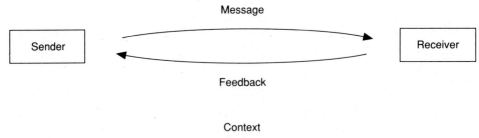

Figure 19–1 The communication process.

professor (sender) receives feedback from the students (receivers) through their facial expressions, alertness, posture, and attentiveness. The atmosphere in the classroom is the context. If the atmosphere is a relaxed one of give and take between students and professor, the feedback will be quite different from feedback in a more formal context. Figure 19–1 shows the relationships among the five elements of communication.

Operations in the Communication Process

In addition to the five elements of communication, Ruesch also identified three major operations in communication. They are perception, evaluation, and transmission.

PERCEPTION

Perception is the selection, organization, and interpretation of incoming signals into meaningful messages. In the classroom situation just given, students select, organize, and interpret various pieces of the professor's message or lecture. Different students perceive the information differently, based on factors such as personal experience, previous knowledge, alertness, sensitivity to subtleties of meaning, and sociocultural background.

EVALUATION

Evaluation is the analysis of information received. Is the content of the professor's lecture useful? Is it important or relevant to the students' needs? Is it likely to be on the next test? Again, each student will evaluate the message in a different manner.

TRANSMISSION

Transmission refers to the expression of information, verbally or nonverbally. While the professor is transmitting his verbal message to the students, his nonverbal behavior of excitement with his subject also transmits a message to the class.

INFLUENCES ON PERCEPTION, EVALUATION, AND TRANSMISSION

Perception, evaluation, and transmission are influenced by many factors. The attractiveness of the sender; the interest and mood of the receiver; the value, clarity, and length of the message; the presence or absence of feedback; and the atmosphere in the context all are powerful influences. Also involved are individuals' needs, values, self-concepts, sensory and intellectual abilities or deficits, and sociocultural conditioning. Given the variety of factors involved, it is clear that communication is a complex human activity worthy of nurses' attention.

How Communication Develops

People learn to use language (and therefore to communicate verbally) through a certain developmental sequence, which begins in infancy. Infants use **somatic language** to signal their needs to caretakers. Somatic language consists of crying; reddening of the skin; fast, shallow breathing; facial expressions; and jerking of the limbs. The sequence progresses to **action language** in older infants. Action language consists of reaching out for or crawling toward a desired object, or closing the lips and turning the head when an undesired food is offered. Last to develop is verbal language, beginning with repetitive noises and sounds and progressing to words, phrases, and complete sentences.

If a child's development is normal, any one or combination of these forms of communication can be used. Somatic language usually decreases with maturity, but since it is not under conscious control, some somatic language may persist past childhood. A familiar example is facial blushing when embarrassed or angry.

The development of communication is determined by inborn and environmental factors. The amount of verbal stimulation an infant receives can enhance or retard the development of language skills. The extent of a caretaker's vocabulary and verbal ability is therefore influential. Some families engage in lengthy discussions of a variety of all kinds of issues, thus providing intense verbal stimulation, whereas others are quiet.

Nonverbal communication development is similarly influenced by environment. Some families communicate through nonverbal gestures such as touch or facial expressions, which children learn to "read" at very young ages. Other families ascribe to the adage, "Children should be seen and not heard," thus discouraging verbal expression and increasing dependence on nonverbal cues for communicating.

The ability to communicate effectively is dependent on a number of factors. Primary among these are the quantity and quality of verbal and nonverbal stimulation received during early developmental periods.

Criteria for Successful Communication

Everyone has had the experience of being the sender or receiver of unsuccessful communication. An example is arriving for an appointment with a friend at the wrong time or wrong place because of a communication mixup. Unsuccessful communication creates little harm when done under social circumstances. In nursing situations, however, accurate, complete communication is vitally important. Nurses can achieve successful communication on most occasions if they plan their communication to meet four major criteria: feedback, appropriateness, efficiency, and flexibility. Each of these criteria will be examined.

Feedback

When a receiver relays back to a sender the effect that the sender's message has had, feedback has occurred. Feedback was identified as one of Ruesch's five elements necessary for communication (Fig. 19–1). It is also a criterion for successful communication. In making the social appointment mentioned above, if the receiver of the message had said, "Let's make sure I understand you. We'll meet at 12:30 on Tuesday at Cafe Al Fresco," that feedback could have led to successful communication.

In a nurse-patient interaction, a nurse can give feedback to a patient by saying, "If I understand you correctly, you have pain in your lower abdomen every time you stand up." The patient can then either agree or correct what the nurse has said: "No, the pain is there only when I arise in the morning." Effective nurses do not assume that they fully understand what their patients are telling them until they feed the statement back to the patient and receive confirmation.

Appropriateness

When a reply fits the circumstances and matches the message, and the amount is neither too great nor too little, **appropriateness** has been achieved. In day-to-day conversation among acquaintances passing on the street, most people recognize the question, "How are you?" as a social nicety, not a genuine question. The individual who launches into a detailed description of how his morning has gone has communicated inappropriately. The reply doesn't fit the circumstances, and the quantity is too great. An appropriate response is, "Fine, and how are you?"

If a nurse inquires of a patient, "You called for a nurse, Mrs. Todd?" and the patient replies, "Next Tuesday my daughter is coming," the nurse will be alert to other inappropriate responses by this patient that may signal a variety of problems. In this instance the inappropriate reply doesn't match the message.

Efficiency

Using simple, clear words that are timed at a pace suitable to participants meets the criterion of **efficiency**. Explaining to an adult that she will have "an angioplasty" tomorrow morning probably will not create successful communication. Telling her she will have "a procedure where a small balloon is threaded into an artery and inflated to open up the vessel so more blood can flow through" will more likely ensure her understanding. This message would not be an efficient one for a small child, however. Messages must be adapted to each patient's age, verbal level, and level of understanding.

Some examples of patients who require special assistance in evaluating and responding to messages are young children, depressed people, some people with neurological impairments, and those recovering from anesthesia. For efficient communication to occur, nurses must recognize patients' needs and adjust messages accordingly.

Flexibility

The fourth criterion for successful communication is **flexibility**. The flexible communicator bases messages on the immediate situation rather than preconceived expectations. When a student nurse who plans to teach a patient about diabetic diets enters the patient's room and finds her crying, the nurse must be flexible enough to change gears and deal with the feelings the patient is expressing. Pressing on with the lesson plan in the face of the patient's distress shows a lack of compassion as well as inflexibility in communicating.

Nurses can learn to use these four measures of successful communication to enhance their effectiveness with patients. The continuing absence or malfunction of any of these four criteria can create disturbed communication and hamper the implementation of the nursing process.

Becoming a Better Communicator

People are not born being good communicators. Communication skills can be developed if you are willing to put forth a moderate amount of time and energy. Becoming a better listener, learning a few basic helpful responding styles, and avoiding common causes of communication breakdown can put you on the path to becoming a better communicator.

Listening

A requirement of successful verbal communication in any setting is listening. **Active listening** is a method of communicating interest and attention. Using such signals as good eye contact, nodding, use of "mumbles" (mmhmm), and encouraging the speaker ("Go on" or "Tell me more about this") all help to communicate interest. Facing the speaker squarely and using an **open posture** (arms uncrossed) also communicate interest.

Having someone listen to concerns, even if no problem solving takes place, is considered therapeutic. **Ventilation** is the term used to describe the verbal "letting off steam" that occurs when talking about concerns or frustrations. The experience of feeling "listened to" is becoming so rare in contemporary American society that a columnist in the *Christian Science Monitor* was prompted to write about it (see "Where Did All The Listeners Go?", p. 350).

Nurses may have difficulty listening for a variety of reasons. They may be intent on accomplishing a task and be frustrated by the time it takes to be a good listener. They may be planning their own next response and not hear what the patient is saying. And, like other people, nurses have their own personal and professional problems that sometimes preoccupy them and interfere with effec-

News Note   Where Did All the Listeners Go?

When everybody learned how to tune out their machines—blabbing-off radio and television ads, hanging up on computer phone calls, and so on—they also learned how to tune out other people.

During the talkiest era ever, nobody listens. Or so it is assumed. In his new novel, "A Tenured Professor," Harvard economist John Kenneth Galbraith puts it nicely:

"By long custom, social discourse in Cambridge is intended to impart and only rarely to obtain information. People talk; it is not expected that anyone will listen. A respectful show of attention is all that is required until the listener takes over in his or her turn."

But wait. Just as it seems that the glazed-over eye and the numbed ear typify the Age of the Non-Listener, there is heartening news.

In Milwaukee, the Roman Catholic Archdiocese is sponsoring six "listening sessions" to give Catholic women a chance to express their feelings about abortion.

The first session, held last month in a college gymnasium in Fond du Lac, Wis., drew 100 women. While participants gathered in small groups to discuss the volatile issue, Archbishop Rembert Weakland, who organized the event, moved from table to table, listening and reportedly saying little.

Archbishop Weakland, considered one of the more liberal Catholic leaders, has been criticized within his church for his gesture. But as he explained to a reporter. "The polarization about this issue has become so great that I had to admit we needed dialogue about it within the Catholic community."

It is one thing for equals to listen to equals, or for subordinates to listen to those in authority. But it is a high tribute when individuals in power listen to those below them.

Once upon a time, being a "good listener" was considered a social grace. At least 51 percent of the world were "good listeners." They were also called women. A young woman learned by example that her gender role was to listen to what others—especially men—were saying. Her mouth was primarily for smiling at what she heard, with an occasional rhythmic "uh-huh."

Today that "uh-huh" is increasingly likely to come from a stranger. Lending an ear has become a paid profession. As if to signify a national hunger for "listening sessions," an entire industry has sprung up.

Eight-year-olds phone latchkey hotlines for after-school comfort and conversation while Mom—the original "good listener"—is off at work. Bereaved dog and cat owners call on pet grief counselors for animal-loving shoulders to cry on. Even technology offers an ear, this one electronic, as answering machines and voice mailboxes do more and more of the listening.

Then of course there is the biggest listening post of all, the talk show. What does it say about the desperate yearning for an audience, any audience, that guests are willing to bare their souls and share their most intimate secrets not with close friends but with Oprah, Phil, Geraldo—and millions of TV viewers?

Is this what it takes to get a word in edgewise in the late 20th century?

Outside the TV studio, other cameras reveal that finding a "good listener"—or any listener at all—can be a tricky business in classrooms as well, especially for women.

Catherine Krupnick, a researcher

at the Harvard Graduate School of Education, videotaped thousands of hours of college classes. She discovered that even when male students made up just one-tenth of a class, the men would do one-quarter of the talking. Other studies over the past two decades confirm Ms. Krupnick's findings, showing that professors are more likely to call on men.

The philosopher Mortimer Adler has called listening "the untaught skill." Those like Archbishop Weakland may be thought of as pioneers in retraining. But the changeover from mouth to ear won't come easily. The thing about listening is that it takes more time and, in fact, more thought than merely talking.

When a reporter, after one of the "listening sessions" in Wisconsin, asked the Archbishop what he thought, he gave the right answer: "I'm still listening."

—Marilyn Gardner

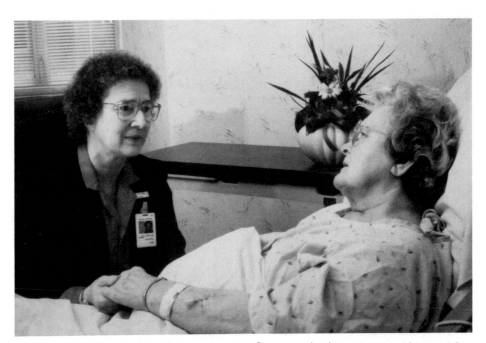

Being an active listener is an important part of communication. (Courtesy of Memorial Hospital, Chattanooga, TN.)

tive listening. Nurses must remember that no verbal message can be received if the receiver (the nurse) isn't listening.

Three common listening faults include interrupting, finishing sentences for others, and lack of interest. It is important for nurses to remember that what the patient is saying is just as important as what the nurse wishes to say.

Being listened to meets the patient's emotional need to be respected and valued by the nurse. Listening can help avert problems by letting people ventilate about the pressures they feel. Hospitalized patients particularly may feel that their lives are out of control and may need to discuss those feelings with someone who will listen without becoming defensive.

Nurses at all levels find listening a useful skill. Nurse managers often use listening as a tool for dealing with staff members' problems and concerns and find that no other intervention is required. Listening is a talent that can be developed; properly used, it can be an important part of a nurse's communication repertoire.

Using Helpful Responding Techniques

There are many helpful responding techniques nurses can use to demonstrate respect and encourage patients to communicate openly. Helpful responses that have already been discussed in this chapter include being nonjudgmental, observing body language, and active listening. Other useful responses include empathy, open-ended questions, giving information, reflection, and silence.

EMPATHY

Empathy consists of awareness of, sensitivity to, and identification with the feelings of another person. Nurses can empathize with patients even if they have not experienced an event in their own lives exactly like the patient is experiencing. If nurses have had a similar or parallel experience, empathy is possible. For example, the feeling of loss is familiar to most nurses, even though they may not personally have lost a close family member.

Empathy is different from sympathy in that the sympathizing nurse enters into the feeling with the patient, whereas the empathizing person appreciates the patient's feelings but is not swept along with the feelings. "You seem upset about this procedure" is an example of a nursing statement that demonstrates empathy to the patient's feelings.

OPEN-ENDED QUESTIONS

An **open-ended question** is one that causes the patient to answer fully, giving more than a yes or no answer. Open-ended questions are very useful in data gathering and in the opening stages of any nurse-patient interaction. For example, asking a patient, "Are you uncomfortable?" may elicit only a confirmation. Saying to him, "Tell me about your discomfort" is more likely to elicit information about the site, type, intensity, and duration of his discomfort and therefore makes the nurse-patient interaction more meaningful.

GIVING INFORMATION

An essential part of nursing is providing information to patients. Giving information includes sharing knowledge with patients that they are not expected to know. Nurses provide information when they tell patients what to expect during diagnostic procedures, inform them of their rights as patients, or teach them about their medications.

An important distinction every nurse needs to make is the difference between providing information and giving opinions. While providing information to patients is a helpful response, giving opinions is considered unhelpful. Patients should be encouraged to consider their own opinions as primary in importance. The nurse's opinion is irrelevant.

REFLECTION

The nurse using **reflection** is serving as a mirror for the patient. Reflection is a method of encouraging patients to think through problems for themselves by directing patient questions back to the patient. Reflection implies respect because the nurse believes the patient has adequate resources to solve the problem without outside assistance. In response to the patient's question, "Do you think I should go through with this surgery?" the nurse can reflect the question: "*Your* thinking on this question is most important. Do *you* think you should have the surgery?"

USING SILENCE

Although silent periods in social conversations are considered uncomfortable, using silence in nurse-patient relationships is often a helpful response. Using silence means allowing periods of reflection during an interaction without feeling pressure to "fill the gap" with conversation or activity. For example, when a patient has just been given upsetting news, sitting quietly without making any demands for conversation may be the most therapeutic response a nurse can make at that time. "Being with" patients is often just as valuable as "doing for" them. Professional nurses learn to do both.

There are many more helpful responding styles nurses can use in their interactions with patients. The five discussed here can be a foundation upon which to build.

Avoiding Common Causes of Communication Breakdown

Just as there are many factors influencing successful communication, unsuccessful communication can occur for many reasons. A sender may send an incomplete or confusing message. A message may not be received, or it may be misunderstood or distorted by the receiver. And incongruent messages may cause confusion in the receiver. In nursing situations there are several common causes of communication breakdown. They include failing to see each patient as unique, failure to recognize levels of meaning, using value statements, using false reassurance, and failure to clarify unclear messages.

FAILING TO SEE THE UNIQUENESS OF THE INDIVIDUAL

Failing to see the uniqueness of each individual patient is a frequent cause of communication breakdown. This failure is caused by preconceived ideas, prejudices, and stereotypes on the part of the nurse. This problem is illustrated by the following interchange between patient and nurse:

P: My back is really hurting today. I can hardly turn over in bed.
N: I guess we have to expect these little problems when we get older.

This nurse has pigeonholed her patient in her mental group "old people" and therefore does not react to the patient as an individual. The nurse could have promoted continued communication by responding to the patient as an individual:

N: Tell me exactly how your back hurts, Mrs. Jameson.

FAILING TO RECOGNIZE LEVELS OF MEANING

When nurses recognize no level of meaning other than the obvious ones, communication breakdown can occur. Patients often give verbal cues to meanings that lie under the surface content of their verbalizations:

P: It's getting awfully warm in here.
N: (*Responding only to surface meaning*) I'll adjust the air conditioning for you.

This response is not very helpful in helping the patient express himself fully. A different type of response focuses on the symbolic level of meaning.

N: Perhaps the questions I am asking are making you uncomfortable.

While it takes a lot of experience to know when and how to respond to symbolic communication, nurses should be aware of its existence.

USING VALUE STATEMENTS AND CLICHÉS

Using value statements and clichés is another communication problem. The use of clichés, which are trite, stereotyped expressions, is common in social conversation. Consider the prevalence of the cliché "Have a good day." This statement has come to have very little real meaning.

This common error can cut off communication by showing the patient that the nurse doesn't really understand the patient's feelings.

P: My mother is coming to see me today.
N: How nice. Do you want to put on a fresh gown?

This nurse has failed to verify that the patient actually wishes to see her mother. In fact, the patient and her mother may have a difficult relationship, and the patient may dread the impending visit. By assuming otherwise, the nurse has contributed to communication breakdown. This patient probably won't attempt to discuss her relationship with her mother any further with this nurse. A more helpful response would be:

N: How do you feel about her visit?

This would allow the patient to ventilate her feelings about her mother's visit, whether positive or negative. The nurse would have conveyed a genuine interest in the patient's true feelings.

USING FALSE REASSURANCE

Using **false reassurance** is another communication pitfall. It may help the nurse feel better but will not facilitate communication and help the patient.

> P: I'm so afraid the biopsy will be cancer.
> N: Don't worry. You have the best doctor in town. Besides, cancer treatment is really good these days.

For a fearful patient, this type of glib reassurance does not help. This nurse has no way of knowing that the patient's concerns are not legitimate. She may indeed *have* cancer. A more sensitive response would be:

> N: Why don't we talk about your concerns?

This kind of response keeps the lines of communication open between patient and nurse.

FAILING TO CLARIFY

Failing to clarify the patient's unclear statements is a fifth common communication pitfall.

> P: I've got to get out of the hospital. They have found out I'm here and may come after me.
> N: No one will harm you here.

This nurse has responded as if the patient's meaning was clear. A more clarifying response might be:

> N: Who are "they," Mrs. Johnson?

Confused patients or those with psychiatric illnesses often communicate in ways that are difficult to understand. It is reassuring to patients to know that nurses are trying to understand them, even if they are not always successful. Communication is facilitated by **clarification** responses.

Practicing Helpful Responses

Nurses can practice using helpful responses and avoiding common communication pitfalls with family members and friends as well as in patient contacts. Being a good communicator takes practice and usually feels unnatural at first. Any new behavior takes time to integrate into habitual patterns. By continuing to practice, nurses soon find themselves feeling more natural. They find that these newly acquired skills are beneficial both professionally and personally.

Box 19–1 compares different responses in a nurse-patient interaction and will help you understand these techniques.

Box 19–1 Case Study: Helpful and Unhelpful Responding Techniques

Instructions: Critique both interactions, identifying the helpful and unhelpful responses used by the nurse. Describe how you imagine the patient might feel at the close of each interaction. Itemize what the nurse has accomplished in each instance.

Mr. Goodman has been admitted to the hospital for coronary bypass surgery. During the admission process the following interactions might take place.

INTERACTION #1

N: Mr. Goodman, I am Mrs. Scott. Can I get some information about you now?

P: Okay.

N: You're here for bypass surgery?

P: Yes, that's what they tell me.

N: (Taking blood pressure) Do you have any allergies to foods or medications?

P: Not that I know of. I've never been in a hospital before.

N: Well, your blood pressure looks good. (*Silence while patient has thermometer in mouth*) This is a really nice room—just remodeled. I know you'll be comfortable here. Will your wife be coming to see you tonight? (*Removes thermometer*)

P: My wife is sick. She hasn't been able to leave home for two years. I don't know what will happen to her while I am here.

N: Gosh, I'm so sorry to hear that. I guess having you back home healthy is what she wants though, isn't it? And you've got a great surgeon. Well, I've got to run now. Check on you later.

INTERACTION #2

N: Good afternoon, Mr. Goodman. I'm Mrs. Scott, and I'll be your nurse this evening. If this is a good time, I'd like to ask you some questions and complete your admission process.

P: Okay

N: First, I'll get your temperature and blood pressure, and then we'll talk. (*Silence while nurse takes vital signs*) Everything looks good. Do you have any allergies to foods or medications?

P: Not that I know of. I've never been in a hospital before.

N: Hospitals can be a little overwhelming, especially when you've never been a patient before. Now, would you please tell me in your own words why you are here?

P: Well, the doc tells me I have a clogged artery, and I need a bypass. I guess they'll open up my heart.

N: What exactly do you know about the surgery?

P: Not too much, really. He told me yesterday that I need it right away— and here I am.

N: It sounds like you need some more information about what will happen. Later this evening I will come back, and we'll talk some more. Are you expecting to have visitors tonight?

P: No, my wife can't leave home. I don't know what she will do without me while I'm here. This came up so suddenly.

N: I can see that this is a serious concern for you. We can explore some possibilities when I come back this evening. I'll plan to come around 7:15, if that suits you.

P: Sure, I can use all the help I can get.

The Nurse-Patient Relationship

The nursing process begins after nurse and patient establish a beginning therapeutic relationship. Awareness of the three identifiable phases of the nurse-patient relationship helps nurses be realistic in their expectations of this important relationship. The three phases—orientation, working, and termination—are sequential and build on previous phases.

The Orientation Phase

The **orientation,** or introductory, **phase** is the period often described as "getting to know you" in social settings. Relationships between nurses and their patients have much in common with other relationships. The chief similarity is that there must be trust between the two parties for the relationship to develop. Nurses cannot expect patients to automatically trust them and reveal their thoughts and feelings.

During the orientation phase, nurse and patient assess one another. Early impressions made by the nurse are important ones. Many people have difficulty accepting help of any kind, including nursing care. Putting the patient at ease with a pleasant, unhurried approach is important during the early part of any nurse-patient relationship.

During the orientation phase the patient has a right to expect to learn the nurse's name, credentials, and extent of responsibility. The use of simple orienting statements is one way to begin:

> N: Good morning, Mr. Davis. I am Jennifer Harkey, and I am your nurse until noon today. I am responsible for your total care while I am here.

DEVELOPING TRUST

The orientation phase includes the beginning development of trust. Notice the use of the term *beginning development*. Full development of trust is slow and may take months. A reality of contemporary nursing practice is that an interaction with a patient may be brief, sometimes lasting only minutes. Even in the briefest contacts nurses must orient patients and help them feel comfortable and as trusting as possible.

Certain nursing behaviors help patients develop the feeling that the nurse can be trusted. A straightforward and nondefensive manner are important ingredients of trust. Answering all questions as fully as possible and admitting not knowing everything also facilitate trust. Promise to find out the answer and report the information to the patient as soon as possible. Be there at the designated time or make arrangements to let the patient know of a change in plans. Use active listening behaviors and accept the patient's thoughts and feelings without judgment.

Box 19–2 Communication Patterns Self-Assessment

Answer the following true/false questions as honestly as possible. Then review your answers and draw at least two conclusions about your habitual communication patterns. Check your conclusions for accuracy with a friend who knows your style of communicating well.

_____ 1. I usually listen about as much as I talk.
_____ 2. I rarely interrupt others.
_____ 3. I pay close attention to what others say.
_____ 4. I usually make eye contact with the person I am talking with.

_____ 5. I can usually tell if someone is angry or upset.
_____ 6. I would hesitate to interrupt someone to ask for clarification.
_____ 7. People often tell me personal things about themselves.
_____ 8. I find it is best to change the subject if someone gets too emotional.
_____ 9. If I can't "make things better" for a friend with a problem, I feel uncomfortable.
_____ 10. I am comfortable talking with people much older or much younger than myself.

Congruence between verbal and nonverbal communication is a key factor in the development of trust. Communicating in a congruent manner requires that nurses be aware of their own thoughts and feelings and be able to share those with others in a nonthreatening manner. The communication patterns self-assessment in Box 19–2 is the type of activity that can help improve self-awareness.

Developing a beginning understanding of the patient's problem or needs also starts in the orientation phase. Because patients themselves often do not clearly understand their problems or may be reluctant to discuss them, nurses must use their communication skills to elicit the information needed in order to make a nursing diagnosis.

TASKS OF THE ORIENTATION PHASE

By the end of a successful orientation phase, regardless of its length, several things will have happened. First, the patient will have developed enough trust in the nurse to continue the relationship. Second, the patient and nurse will see each other as individuals, unique from all others and worthy of one another's respect. Third, the patient's perception of major problems and needs will have been identified. And fourth, the approximate length of the relationship will have been estimated, and the nurse and patient will have agreed to work together on some aspect of the identified problems. This agreement is sometimes called a "**contract**." Contracts in the nurse-patient relationship are usually unwritten. An example of a contract that might emerge from the orientation phase of the nurse-patient relationship is an agreement to work together during a newly diagnosed diabetic patient's hospitalization on his ability to calculate and inject his own daily insulin requirement.

The Working Phase

The second phase of the nurse-patient relationship is called the **working phase** because it is during this time that the nurse and patient tackle tasks outlined in the previous phase. Because the participants now know each other to some extent, there may be a sense of interpersonal comfort in the relationship that did not exist earlier.

Nurses should recognize that in the working phase patients may exhibit alternating periods of intense effort and periods of resistance to change. Using the diabetic patient example, the nurse can anticipate that he will experience some degree of difficulty in accepting the life changes the illness necessitates. He may show progress in learning how to give himself insulin one day and not be able to remember how the next. Nurses who become frustrated when patients' progress toward self-care is not smooth must realize that reverting to former behaviors often precedes periods of positive behavioral change.

It is difficult to make and sustain change. Patience, self-awareness, and maturity on the part of the nurse are required during the working phase. Continued trust building, use of active listening, and other helpful communication responses facilitate the patient's expression of needs and feelings during the working phase.

The Termination Phase

The termination phase includes those activities that enable the patient and the nurse to end the relationship in a therapeutic manner. The process of terminating the nurse-patient relationship begins in the orientation phase when participants estimate the length of time it will take to accomplish the desired outcomes. This is part of the informal contract.

As in any relationship, positive and negative feelings often accompany termination. The patient and nurse feel good about the gains the patient has made in accomplishing goals. They may feel sadness about ending a relationship that has been open and trusting. People tend to respond to the end of relationships in much the same way they have responded to other losses in life. Feelings of anger and fear may surface, in addition to sadness.

Feelings evoked by termination should be discussed and accepted. Summarizing the gains the patient has made is an important activity during this phase. The importance of the relationship to patient and nurse can be shared in a caring manner.

Box 19–3 Professional Versus Social Relationships

PROFESSIONAL	SOCIAL
Limited in time	Not time limited
Goal directed	Not usually goal directed
Patient centered	Centered on both parties
Obligation to problem solve	No obligation to problem solve
Nonjudgmental acceptance	May or may not be nonjudgmental
Aim is improved health	Aim is pleasure
Planned and purposeful	Spontaneous

The giving and receiving of gifts at termination has different meanings for different people. The meaning of such behavior should be explored in a sensitive manner and discussed with the nurse's supervisor.

Because termination is often painful, participants are sometimes tempted to continue the relationship on a social basis, and requests for addresses and phone numbers are not uncommon. The nurse must realize that professional relationships are different from social relationships. It is not helpful to stay in touch with patients following termination of a professional nurse-patient relationship. Several other differences between social and professional relationships are outlined in Box 19–3.

Every nurse will experience countless nurse-patient relationships of differing lengths and meanings during the course of a professional career. If nurses can view each new relationship both as an opportunity to assist another human being to grow and change in a positive, healthful way as well as a challenge to grow and change themselves, the rewards of nursing will be even richer.

Communication with Professional Colleagues

This chapter has focused on nurse-patient communication as the core of the nursing process and foundation of the therapeutic use of self. In addition to patients and their families, however, nurses must also communicate effectively with a variety of professional and ancillary personnel such as physicians, other nurses, and nursing assistants. Health care delivery suffers when the members of the health care team experience communication breakdown.

As a general rule, nurses can use the same communication skills with colleagues that have been discussed as part of nurse-patient communication. The attitude of respect for others, regardless of position, is essential. Active listening, acceptance, and nonjudgmentalism are key elements, as are the conscious use of feedback, appropriateness, efficiency, and flexibility.

Wise nurses do not leave their communication skills at the patient's bedside but use them throughout their personal and professional lives. Using clear, simple messages and clarifying the intent of others constitute a positive goal in all personal and professional communication. As with patients, trust must exist before communication with coworkers can be effective.

CHAPTER SUMMARY

The "therapeutic use of self" means using one's personality and communication skills effectively while implementing the nursing process to help patients improve their health status. Communication is the core of nurse-patient relationships and is the primary instrument through which desired change is effected in others.

Acceptance of others' values, beliefs, and life-styles is important in nursing. Developing awareness of biases can help nurses to prevent the intrusion of these biases into nurse-patient relationships.

Communication is both verbal and nonverbal and consists of a sender, a receiver, a message, feedback, and context. Perception, evaluation, and transmission are the three major operations in communication.

Communication develops sequentially. It may be successful or unsuccessful. Successful communication meets four major criteria: feedback, appropriateness, efficiency, and flexibility. Active listening is a key factor in successful communication. Unsuccessful communication is caused by a variety of factors that can be identified and eliminated.

There are three identifiable phases of the nurse-patient relationship—the orientation, working, and termination phases. Certain tasks occur during each phase.

In addition to communicating well with patients, nurses use communication skills to improve working relationships with physicians, other nurses, ancillary workers, and other members of the health care delivery team.

REVIEW/DISCUSSION QUESTIONS

1. Explain why nonverbal communication often is more revealing than verbal communication.
2. List as many factors as you can that can influence the communication process.
3. Identify a recent interaction you have had in which communication was incongruent. Analyze what effect the incongruence had on the communication. When are you likely to use incongruent communication?
4. Think of a person with whom you have experienced difficult communication. Identify which of the barriers to successful communication are functioning in that person's communication with you and analyze your responses to that person.

5. Identify the tasks that must be accomplished in each phase of the nurse-patient relationship.

6. Initiate a class debate on the topic "Nurses should not accept gifts from patients."

REFERENCES

Barke, J. (Ed.). (1955). *Burns' poems and songs.* London: Collins.

Gardner, M. (1990). Where did all the listeners go? *Christian Science Monitor*, April 27, 1990, 14.

McCabe, B. W. (1989). Ego defensiveness and its relationship to attitudes of registered nurses toward older people. *Research in Nursing and Health*, 12(2), 85–91.

Peplau, H. (1952). *Interpersonal relations in nursing.* New York: G.P. Putnam's Sons.

Ruesch, J. (1972). *Disturbed communication: The clinical assessment of normal and pathological communicative behavior.* New York: W.W. Norton.

SUGGESTED READINGS

Brammer, L. M. (1985). *The helping relationship: Process and skills* (3rd ed.). Englewood Cliffs, NJ: Prentice-Hall.

Collins, M. (1983). *Communication in health care: The human connection.* St. Louis: C.V. Mosby.

Davis, A. J. (1984). *Listening and responding.* St. Louis: C.V. Mosby.

Grensing, L. (1990). A formula to avoid miscommunicating. *Nursing*, 20(9), 122–124.

Jungman, L. B. (1979). When your feelings get in the way. *American Journal of Nursing*, 79, 1074–1075.

Lloyd, A. (1991). Stop, look and listen. *Nursing Times*, 87(12), 30–31.

Severtsen, B. M. (1990). Therapeutic communication demystified. *Journal of Nursing Education*, 29(4), 190–192.

Chapter

20

Nursing Ethics

Pamela S. Chally

CHAPTER OBJECTIVES

What students should be able to do after studying this chapter:

1. Differentiate between morals and ethics.

2. Discuss the importance to nursing of having a code of ethics.

3. Identify basic theories and principles central to ethical dilemmas and moral development.

4. Describe ethical dilemmas resulting from conflicts between patients, health care professionals, and institutions.

5. Describe models for ethical decision making.

6. Discuss the impact of ethical issues on nurses and other health care professionals.

VOCABULARY BUILDING

Terms to know:

autonomy	ethical decision making	nonmaleficence
beneficence	ethics	patients' rights
bioethics	justice	personal value system
code of ethics	moral development	utilitarianism
deontology	morals	veracity

*T*o understand ethics and its relationship to health care, the terms *morals, ethics,* and *bioethics* must first be clarified. It is important to realize that there are conflicting viewpoints by philosophers and scholars on how to define these terms, however.

"Morals" refer to established rules in situations where a decision about right and wrong must be made. Morals provide standards of behavior. These standards guide the behavior of an individual or social group. Morals reflect the "is" or reality of how individuals or groups behave. An example of a moral standard is "Good people do not lie."

If morals reflect the "is" of human behavior, then **ethics** is a term used to reflect the "should" of human behavior. Ethics identify what should be done to live with one another. Ethics are process oriented and involve critical analysis of actions. If ethicists, people who study ethics, reflected on the moral statement "One should not lie," they would clarify definitions of lying and explore the circumstances under which lying might be acceptable.

Despite the fact that differences between ethics and morals are noted by several authors (Davis and Aroskar 1991; Silva 1990; Thompson and Thompson 1985), in everyday usage the terms are often used interchangeably.

When ethical theories and principles are applied to problems in health care, the field of study is called **bioethics**. Bioethics as an area of ethical inquiry came into existence around 1970 when health care began to shift its focus from curing disease toward concern for the total patient (Husted and Husted 1991). A new term, *Clinical ethics,* is increasingly being used.

Advances in medicine, science, and technology sometimes create ethical dilemmas. For example, people can now be kept "alive" even when brain dead. But should they be kept alive under these circumstances just because we now have the technology to do so? This kind of issue mandates that nurses be concerned with what "should" be done for patients they care for. It is important that actions be critically analyzed for their appropriateness, since health care professionals possess a good deal of power over those in their care.

It is within this context that nurses need to study codes of ethics, ethical theories and principles, moral development, ethical dilemmas, and ethical decision-making models. Such knowledge will increase nurses' ability to participate in the resolution of ethical dilemmas.

Nursing Codes of Ethics

As you learned in Chapter 6, an essential characteristic of professions is that they have a code of ethics. A **code of ethics** is an implied contract through which the profession informs society of the principles and rules by which it functions.

Ethical codes help with professional self-regulation. They serve as guidelines to the members of the profession who then can meet the societal need for trustworthy, qualified, and accountable care givers. It is important to remember that codes are useful only if they are upheld by the members of the profession.

The American Nurses Association's Code for Nurses

The need for a code of ethics was expressed by the Nurses' Associated Alumnae (forerunner of the American Nurses Association [ANA]) as early as 1897 (Veins 1989). It was 1950, however, before a written code was actually adopted. During that 53-year time span, nursing was emerging as a profession in its own right.

The 1950 *Code* consisted of 17 short, succinct statements depicting the nurse in action—e.g., "The nurse accepts . . . ," "The nurse sustains . . ." (Veins 1989). Even in 1950 the broad spectrum role of the nurse—in illness, prevention, and health promotion—was stressed. In addition, this code encouraged nurses to participate in lifelong learning activities. Minor revisions to the first *Code* were agreed upon by delegates to the ANA's conventions throughout the 1950s.

In 1958, the ANA's Committee on Ethical Standards began reviewing the entire *Code*, and in 1960, major revisions were suggested (Veins 1989). The 1960 *Code* also contained 17 statements, but new statements were added and some were deleted. The new statements addressed nurses' responsibilities to participate in the professional organization and the necessity of identifying and upholding professional standards. Another new statement addressed nurses' participation in negotiating terms of employment. This opened the way, in later years, for the ANA to function as a collective-bargaining agent for nurses. An earlier statement, describing nurses' obligations to physicians, was eliminated from the 1960 *Code* (Veins 1989).

The next major revision of the *Code*, completed in 1976, resulted in 11 statements. The emphasis of the 1976 *Code* was the nurse's relationship to the client. No longer was the word *patient* used. *Client* was adopted in the belief that it was a more inclusive term than *patient*. All gender-related language was eliminated. A paragraph dealing with consequences of breaking the *Code* was also added. Accordingly, the nurse who violated the *Code* could be censured, suspended, or expelled from the ANA. Any violations of civil law would subject the nurse to legal action as well (American Nurses Association 1976). Clarifying statements were added to each point in the *Code* in the 1976 revision. These interpretations provided definitions of key terms and elaborated on the meaning of each statement.

In 1985, the *Code* was again reviewed. All 11 statements remained the same, but the interpretations were updated. In particular, more emphasis was placed on clients' rights. The 1985 *Code for Nurses* is the latest version of nursing's ethical code. The statements of the *Code for Nurses* (American Nurses Association 1985) are found in Chapter 4.

International Council of Nurses Code for Nurses

The International Council of Nurses (ICN) (1973) also has a code of ethics for the profession. This document discusses the rights and responsibilities of nurses around the world.

Box 20–1   International Code for Nurses

The fundamental responsibility of the nurse is fourfold: to promote health, to prevent illness, to restore health, and to alleviate suffering.

The need for nursing is universal. Inherent in nursing is respect for life, dignity, and rights of man. It is unrestricted by considerations of nationality, race, creed, color, age, sex, politics or social status.

Nurses render health services to the individual, the family and the community and coordinate their services with those of related groups.

NURSES AND PEOPLE

The nurse's primary responsibility is to those people who require nursing care.

The nurse, in providing care, promotes an environment in which the values, customs and spiritual beliefs of the individual are respected.

The nurse holds in confidence personal information and uses judgment in sharing this information.

NURSES AND PRACTICE

The nurse carries personal responsibility for nursing practice and for maintaining competence by continual learning. The nurse maintains the highest standards of nursing care possible within the reality of a specific situation.

The nurse uses judgment in relation to individual competence when accepting and delegating responsibilities.

The nurse when acting in a professional capacity should at all times maintain standards of personal conduct which reflect credit upon the profession.

NURSES AND SOCIETY

The nurse shares with other citizens the responsibility for initiating and supporting action to meet the health and social needs of the public.

NURSES AND CO-WORKERS

The nurse sustains a cooperative relationship with co-workers in nursing and other fields. The nurse takes appropriate action to safeguard the individual when his care is endangered by a co-worker or any other person.

NURSES AND THE PROFESSION

The nurse plays the major role in determining and implementing desirable standards of nursing practice and nursing education.

The nurse is active in developing a core of professional knowledge.

The nurse, acting through the professional organization, participates in establishing and maintaining equitable social and economic working conditions in nursing.

(From International Council of Nurses. (1973). *International Council of Nurses code for nurses.* Geneva, Switzerland: Author. Used by permission.)

The ICN first adopted a code of ethics in 1953. Its last revision in 1973 represents agreement by 80 national nursing associations that participate in the international association (Grippando and Mitchell 1989). Inherent in the *International Council of Nurses Code for Nurses* is nursing's respect for the life, dignity, and rights of all people unmindful of nationality, race, creed, color, age, sex, politics, or social status. Box 20–1 contains this code.

Ethical Theories

There is no single ethical theory ascribed to by all philosophers or ethicists. Instead, numerous theories have been developed. We will discuss two of the primary ethical theories that nurse ethicists have identified as useful.

Utilitarianism

Utilitarianism theory was first described by David Hume (1711–1776) and was developed further by many notable philosophers including Jeremy Bentham (1748–1826) and John Stuart Mill (1806–1873). Mill had a significant influence on utilitarian ethics as we know it today.

According to Mill (1985; originally published in 1863), a "right action" conforms to the "greatest happiness principle." In other words, it is right to maximize the greatest good for the happiness or pleasure of the greatest number of people. Utilitarian ethics calculates the effect of all alternative actions on the general welfare of present and future generations. Thus, this position is also referred to as "calculus morality" (Davis and Aroskar 1991).

The utilitarian approach to ethics assumes that it is possible to balance good and evil. The goal is that most people will experience good rather than evil. Benefits are to be maximized for the greatest number of people possible. In this approach, each individual counts as one.

Professional health care personnel employ utilitarian theory in many situations. The concept of triage, where the sick or injured are classified by the severity of their condition to determine priority of treatment, is an example of utilitarianism. In triage, those who are so gravely ill or injured that they cannot possibly recover are not treated at all. Although this seems cruel, when there are many more sick and wounded than available facilities to care for them, triage is accepted worldwide as an ethical basis for determining treatment.

Frequently, utilitarianism is the basis for deciding how health care dollars will be spent. Money is more likely to be spent on research for diseases that affect large numbers of people than for research on diseases that affect only a few. A difficulty of this approach is that while the appeal is made to the happiness of the majority, the individual or minority, who also deserves help, may be overlooked.

Deontology

The major proponent of deontology was Immanuel Kant (1724–1804). Kant (1985; originally translated in 1959) believed that the rightness or wrongness of an action depended on the inherent moral significance of the action. He believed that an act was moral if it originated from goodwill. Ethical action consisted in doing one's duty. To do one's duty was right; not to do one's duty was wrong.

Deontology can be further divided into either act or rule deontology. Act deontologists determine the right thing to do by gathering all the facts and then making a decision. Much time and energy are needed to carefully judge each situation in and of itself. Once a decision is made, there is commitment to universalizing it. In other words, if one makes a moral judgment in one situation, the same judgment will be made in any similar situation.

Rule deontologists emphasize that principles guide our actions. Examples of rules might be "Always keep a promise" or "Never tell a lie." In all situations, the rule is to be followed. Deontologists are not concerned with the consequences of always following certain rules or actions. If the principle believed in is "Always keep a promise," the deontologist will keep promises, even if circumstances have changed. For example, if a father has promised that he will take his son to a baseball game and then a close family member becomes critically ill, the baseball game promise will be kept regardless of the changed circumstances.

In nursing, there are many rules and duties that nurses follow. One such rule is "Do no harm" (beneficence). Another justifiable rule is "The patient should be allowed to make his or her own decisions" (autonomy). But consider the situation of a severely depressed young man who wishes to end his life by committing suicide and asks the nurse's assistance. Clearly the rule about doing no harm conflicts with allowing the young man to make his own decisions. You can see that dilemmas cannot always be resolved using theoretical approaches alone.

Ethical Principles

Justice

The principle of *justice* states that equals should be treated the same and that unequals should be treated differently (Beauchamp and Childress 1989). In other words, patients with the same diagnosis and health care needs should receive the same care. Those with greater or lesser needs should receive different care.

In health care, the most common concern about justice relates to allocation of resources. How much of our national resources should be appropriated to health care? Which health care problems should receive the most financial resources? Which clients should have access to health care services? According to the principle of justice, the answer to these questions is based on treating all individuals equally.

Numerous models have been developed for distributing health care resources. These models include:

1. To each equally.
2. To each according to merit. This may include past or future contributions to society.

3. To each according to what can be acquired in the marketplace.
4. To each according to need (Jameston 1984).

All of these suggestions for distribution have merit and make it very difficult to decide who should be treated for what. It would be ideal if all patients could receive all available treatment for their health needs. Unfortunately, this is not possible because of the cost involved.

Justice as a principle often leaves us with more questions than answers. It raises our consciousness about making ethical decisions but certainly does not determine what the answer should be.

Autonomy

The principle of **autonomy** is the claim that individuals are "permitted personal liberty to determine their own actions according to plans they themselves have chosen" (Veatch and Fry 1987, p. 101). Freedom to make one's own decisions is respected under the principle of autonomy. The principle refers to the control individuals have over their own lives. Respect for the individual is the cornerstone of this principle.

Autonomy applies to both decisions and actions. Autonomous decisions have several characteristics. They

1. Are based on individuals' values.
2. Utilize adequate information.
3. Are free from coercion.
4. Are based on reason and deliberation.

An autonomous action is one that results from an autonomous decision (Wright 1987).

The concept of autonomy has featured prominently in ethics and philosophy since the time of the ancient Greeks. Philosophers and lawyers agree that people have a right to make decisions for themselves. It was established in health care settings over 75 years ago that professionals should not act against the wishes of an adult human being of sound mind (*Schoendorf* v. *Society of New York Hospital* 1914).

It is almost impossible to disagree with autonomy. Autonomy is a basic principle of the United States Constitution. Throughout this nation's history, people have fought and died for the right of individual autonomy. However, disregard for autonomy is glaringly evident in the health care system.

Health care professionals often take actions that profoundly affect patients' lives without adequate consultation with the patients. Incorporating the principle of autonomy in all health care situations is difficult, if not impossible. Patients cannot always make their own choices. Examples of those unable to participate in decisions include infants or small children, mentally incompetent patients, and unconscious patients. Other patients may be unable to participate in decision making because of external constraints such as financial limitations, lack of necessary information, or the norms of their culture.

Beneficence

Beneficence is commonly defined as "the doing of good." According to Frankena (1973), there are several duties involved with this principle. They include:

1. Not to inflict harm or evil (**nonmaleficence**).
2. To prevent harm or evil.
3. To remove harm or evil.
4. To promote or do good.

The first duty, not to inflict harm, takes priority over the three following duties. Even so, all four duties are obligations that must always be taken into account. Additional considerations may take precedence when there is conflict about the appropriate course of action. For example, a surgical procedure will inflict harm on the body but potentially has long-term benefits. The procedure may be lifesaving, or it may diminish pain or increase mobility. In this sense, even though it inflicts harm in the short term, it is justified because of the long-term good that will result.

Virtually everyone would agree that causing good and avoiding harm are important to all human beings—and certainly to health care professionals. It is therefore surprising how often conflicts center around this principle. In addition to consideration of both short-term and long-term benefits, the principle of beneficence conflicts with other ethical principles. Consider the elderly patient who has just broken her hip for the second time and refuses to eat. Should she be allowed to autonomously decide for herself not to eat even though it will harm her? The principles of autonomy and beneficence are in conflict.

Veracity

Veracity is defined as "telling the truth." Truth telling has long been identified as fundamental to the development and continuance of trust among human beings. Telling the truth is expected. It is necessary to basic communication, and societal relationships are built on the individual's right to know the truth.

All communication between individuals has the potential to be misleading. It is easy for information to be misunderstood, misinterpreted, or not comprehended. Usually these misunderstandings are unintentional. *Intentional* deception, however, is considered morally wrong.

Despite that well-established fact, much intended deception occurs between health professionals and people seeking health care. Persons seeking health care often are not truthful when giving their health histories. An example that commonly occurs relates to truthfulness concerning use of drugs and alcohol.

At the same time, health care professionals are not always truthful in responding to patients' questions. The nurse may choose to answer only part of a question, rather than giving all the known facts. A long tradition of a double standard in truth telling exists in health care (Wright 1987). Health care professionals are not responsible for false information given to them by their patients. They *are* responsible for information that they give *to* patients, however.

A number of reasons have been proposed to justify deception by health care professionals. For the most part, the justifications are related to the idea that patients would be better off not knowing certain information or that they are not capable of understanding the information. Based on these justifications, health care professionals often believe they have the right to decide what people should know and should not know about their illnesses. If both patient and health care provider are respectful of one another as individuals, it is difficult to accept that deception between two human beings is ever justified.

Theories of Moral Development

How does a person become moral or able to make decisions about right and wrong? Answering this question moves us into the realm of moral development. **Moral development** describes how a person learns to deal with moral dilemmas from childhood through adulthood. Two major theorists who have worked at understanding this area of human development are Lawrence Kohlberg (1973, 1986) and Carol Gilligan (1982, 1987).

Kohlberg's Levels of Moral Development

Kohlberg (1976, 1986) proposed three levels of moral development:

1. Preconventional.
2. Conventional.
3. Postconventional.

In the preconventional level, the individual is inattentive to the norms of society when responding to moral problems. Instead, the individual's perspective is self-centered. At the preconventional level, what the individual wants or needs takes precedence over right or wrong. Kohlberg saw this level of moral development in most children under nine years of age, as well as in some adolescents and adult criminal offenders.

The conventional level is characterized by making moral decisions that conform to the expectations of one's family, group, or society. When confronted with a moral choice, people functioning at the conventional level follow family or cultural group norms. According to Kohlberg, most adolescents and adults generally function at this level.

The postconventional level involves more independent modes of thinking than previous stages, so that the individual is able to define his or her own moral values. People at the postconventional level may ignore both self-interest and group norms in making moral choices. They create their own morality, which may differ from society's norms. Kohlberg believed that only a minority of adults achieve this level.

Each of Kohlberg's levels is subdivided into two stages. Progression through the stages occurs over varying lengths of time, but each stage is sequential and is characterized by higher capacity for logical reasoning than the preceding stage.

Kohlberg (1976) suggested that certain conditions may stimulate higher levels of moral development. Intellectual development is one necessary characteristic. Individuals at higher levels intellectually are generally more advanced in moral development than those operating at lower levels of intelligence.

An environment that offers people opportunities for group participation, shared decision-making processes, and responsibility for the consequences of their actions also promotes higher levels of moral reasoning. Further moral development is stimulated by the creation of conflict in settings where the individual recognizes the limitations of present modes of thinking. Students have been stimulated to higher levels of moral reasoning through participating in courses on moral discussion and ethics (Kohlberg 1973).

Gilligan's Levels of Moral Development

Gilligan (1982) was a student of Kohlberg who was concerned that Kohlberg did not give adequate acknowledgment to the experiences of women in moral development. She recognized that Kohlberg's theories had largely been generated from research with men and boys. When women were finally tested regarding their moral development, they scored lower than men.

Gilligan believed that this was due not to poor moral development in women but to the fact that women's identities are largely dependent on relationships with others. Because of the basic difference in the way men and women feel about relationships, Gilligan believed that Kohlberg's theory was inadequate to explain women's moral development.

She suggested that women view moral dilemmas in terms of conflicting responsibilities. The sequence she described included three levels and two transitions, with each level representing a more complex understanding of the relationship of self and others and each transition resulting in a crucial reevaluation of the conflict between selfishness and responsibility. Gilligan's levels of moral development are:

1. Orientation to individual survival.
2. A focus on goodness as self sacrifice.
3. The morality of nonviolence.

She believed that the moral person is one who responds to need and demonstrates a consideration of care and responsibility in relationships. She therefore described a moral development perspective focused on care. This perspective differed from the orientation toward justice described by Kohlberg (1973, 1976).

Recent work by Gilligan and her associate (Gilligan and Attanucci 1988) has attempted to define the relationship between the two moral orientations of justice and care. They determined that both perspectives were present when people faced real-life moral dilemmas, but people generally tended to focus on one set of concerns and paid only minimal attention to the other perspective. As expected, the care focus was more often exhibited by women, and the justice focus was more often exemplified by men.

The justice and care perspectives in themselves are not competing theories but are two separate moral perspectives that organize thinking in different ways.

The justice perspective strives to treat others fairly, whereas the care perspective endeavors not to turn away from someone in need.

Gilligan, Brown, and Rogers (1988) described a combined care/justice perspective that incorporates both viewpoints as moral deliberations are made. This is an area that continues to develop. Moral development theory must incorporate all perspectives, some of which may not yet be identified (Chally 1990).

Understanding Ethical Dilemmas in Nursing

Ethical dilemmas occur frequently in nursing practice. This is to be expected since nurses focus on life and death issues involving human beings. Many ethical dilemmas arise in nursing because of conflicts between patients, health care professionals, and/or institutions. In order to understand these conflicts, the following areas will be explored:

1. Personal value systems.
2. Peers' and other professionals' behaviors.
3. Patients' rights.
4. Institutional and societal issues.

The Role of Personal Value Systems

Rokeach (1973) defined a value system as "an enduring organization of beliefs concerning preferable modes of conduct or end-states of existence along a continuum of relative importance" (p. 5). Value systems are learned beliefs that help a person choose between difficult alternatives.

As discussed in Chapter 9, each person has a value system. This value system has a beginning foundation in beliefs, purposes, attitudes, qualities, and objects that are important to one's parents. In time, we develop our own value systems. Our **personal value system** is a rank ordering of values with respect to their importance to one another.

Value systems vary from individual to individual. Something important to one individual may hold greater or lesser significance to someone else. For example, a clean, neat home means more to some individuals than others.

Variations in value systems become highly significant when dealing with critical issues such as health and illness or life and death. Value systems enable people to resolve conflicts and decide on a course of action based on a priority of importance.

Value systems are not the same as ethical principles. It is not enough to recognize and act on one's values. In addition, one must determine if the value system is ethical (Uustal 1987). Only after careful reflection concerning how ethical our value systems are can we as nurses take actions based on our personal or professional values.

Identifying your value system and its influence on decision making will help you understand your behavior more clearly. In addition, it will also give you clues as to why other people behave differently. The "Childhood Value Mes-

Box 20-2   Childhood Value Messages

By the time we were ten, most of our values had already been "programmed." Remember the values you learned as a child? They were taught to you by family members and friends, through the media, in religious classes, and by observing others. What are the value messages you remember learning as a child? Recall as many of them as you can and write them in the spaces provided. Here are a few examples to get you going: "Clean your plate—don't you know children in other parts of the world are starving?" "Finish your work first, then you can play." "Whatever you do, do well." Now it's your turn to write some of the value messages you heard in childhood.

1.
2.
3.
4.
5.
6.
7.
8.

How many of these values still influence the way you think and act today? Which ones influence you professionally?

If you want to explore further:

1. Next to at least half of the values on your list, write the person's name who taught or modeled that value.
2. Put a star next to those messages that are your values today.
3. Put a check next to those that seem to be liabilities.
4. Talk with your colleagues about the childhood values you've identified and how they influence you today.

(From Uustal, D. B. (1987). Values: The cornerstone of nursing's moral art. In M. Fowler and J. Levine-Ariff, *Ethics at the bedside* (pp. 136–170). Philadelphia: J.B. Lippincott, pp. 155–156. Used by permission.)

sages" exercise in Box 20–2 will help you identify values learned as a child that may still influence you today.

To see how values conflicts can affect health care delivery, consider the following patient vignette:

> Mrs. Hamid has recently relocated to the United States from Iran. It is important in her religious faith that males not be present during labor and delivery or at anytime when a female's body is exposed. A female obstetrician is delivering Mrs. Hamid, but complications develop. Her baby's heart rate drops abruptly, and a Caesarean delivery is indicated. The only anesthesiologist available in the hospital for this emergency surgery is a male. What action should the nurse take?

Dilemmas Involving Peers' and Other Professionals' Behavior

All practicing nurses participate as members of the health care team. This involves cooperation and collaboration with other professionals. As is true in all situations between human beings, conflicts can easily develop, particularly in stressful circumstances. These conflicts may be between two nurses, the nurse and physician, the nurse and hospital administration, or the nurse and any other health care professional.

As discussed in the section on personal values systems, conflicts can evolve because of differing value systems. One nurse may feel that assisting with abortions is wrong, whereas the institution performs many abortions daily. Some conflicts develop because individuals are not respectful of the human rights of other individuals.

Conflicts in human rights often center around one of the ethical principles discussed earlier in the chapter: justice, autonomy, beneficence, or veracity. In some circumstances the ethical dilemma may result from a violation of even more basic human rights, those guaranteed by the United States Constitution.

A serious issue today is the large number of nurses and other health care professionals impaired by drug dependence or other addictions. Deciding how and when to confront a suspected drug user may result in an ethical dilemma. Fortunately, some employers and state nurses associations have developed plans to assist impaired nurses in getting the help they need and make provisions for them to return to the profession once they are far enough along in their recovery process. Your state nurses association can provide information on specific programs for impaired nurses in your state.

To understand the ethical dilemmas that can result from conflict between peers, consider the following vignette:

> Miss Corbin, R.N. [registered nurse], works on a surgical floor. She is waiting to care for Mr. Hudson, who is expected back from the postanesthesia unit after surgery. Miss Corbin sees a nurse colleague drawing up a pain medication. She notes that the medication has Mr. Hudson's name on it and that the narcotic record lists Mr. Hudson as the patient for whom this medication was prepared. The nurse colleague returns to the medicine room ten minutes later with an empty syringe. Miss Corbin asks, "Who needed pain medication?" "Mr. Hudson," the colleague replies. "He was in pain after surgery." Confused, Miss Corbin checks Mr. Hudson's room and finds he has not returned from the recovery room yet. What should Miss Corbin do?

Conflicts Regarding Patients' Rights

Years ago, health professionals, particularly physicians, were considered "all-knowing" experts. Very few patients questioned the physician, let alone demanded their basic human rights. Now consumers of health care are increasingly demanding to have a say in matters affecting their health care. *A Patient's Bill of Rights* (American Hospital Association 1972) outlines the rights believed to be important to patients. The patient's relationship with the physician as well as the relationship between the patient and hospital are discussed. You may want to review this document, found in Box 3–2.

Many other specialty groups have developed published lists of rights. Examples include *Declaration of the Rights of Mentally Retarded Persons, Dying Person's Bill of Rights, Pregnant Patient's Bill of Rights, Rights of Senior Citizens,* and the *United Nations Declarations of the Rights of the Child.* As consumers have become more aware of their rights, conflicts between patients, health care professionals, and institutions have developed. Many of the rights demanded by consumers are their legal as well as moral rights and have been upheld by the judicial system.

It is beyond the scope of this chapter to discuss all rights due patients. Many have been identified, however, including informed consent, the right to die, privacy, confidentiality, respectful care, and information concerning their medical condition and treatment. In addition, the patient has the right to be informed if any aspect of treatment is experimental. Based on that knowledge, the patient can refuse to participate in any research project.

The following case illustrates a conflict related to **patients' rights**:

> A 28-year-old quadriplegic male is admitted to the hospital with pneumonia and severe pressure ulcers. He asks not to be given antibiotics and to be allowed to die with dignity. At the insistence of the hospital administration, the physician orders intravenous antibiotics. What is the nurse's responsibility?

Conflicts Created by Institutional and Societal Issues

Nurses experience ethical dilemmas when conflicts develop between policies of their employing institution and themselves. Controversial health care policies at the local, state, or national level can also interfere with the nurse's ability to implement care safely and effectively.

In recent years, grave concerns over health care have centered around the cost of care. The rising cost of health care over the past quarter century is a matter that has prompted worry for individuals, groups, and communities, as well as governmental officials. All health care agencies are stressing cost containment measures in order to survive. At times, cost containment policies conflict with the nurse's value system, whose goal is to provide high-quality, individualized patient care.

Other institutional and societal concerns can result in ethical dilemmas for the nurse whose personal value system does not support the policies set forth by those in authority. Examples include policies concerning access to health care for the elderly, children, and persons with acquired immunodeficiency syndrome (AIDS).

Nurses are employed today by many types of institutions. The scope and complexity of these institutions vary significantly from large multiservice medical complexes to small clinics or offices. All institutions, however, that receive governmental funds are subject to public scrutiny and accountability. Ethical dilemmas may develop between nurses and the institutions that employ them concerning policies dictated by the institution or mandated by governmental agencies.

Ethics committees have been created to deal with ethical dilemmas in institutional settings. Ethics committees are usually multidisciplinary groups charged with the responsibility of making difficult ethical choices. Cases needing consideration are referred to the committee.

The following vignette illustrates an ethical conflict between a nurse and the employing institution:

Research Note

The purposes of this descriptive study were to (1) explore the degree to which nurses are formally involved in ethical decision making by virtue of their membership on institutional ethics committees, (2) describe their perceptions of the role of these committees, and (3) assess the nurses' preparation for functioning on these committees.

The study was completed in two phases. The goal of the first phase was to determine the number of acute care hospitals in a midwestern state that have ethics committees and also to obtain the names of the nurses who serve as members of these committees. In the second phase, individual nurses were contacted to assess how involved they were in ethical decision making and their perceptions of the role the ethics committee plays in their institutions.

In the state surveyed, 45 percent of acute care hospitals reported having an ethics committee. All hospitals with ethics committees reported that nurses served on the committees. The number of nurses serving on an ethics committee reportedly averaged 2.19.

Respondents indicated that the committees provided consultation and emotional support, were active in the area of education and multidisciplinary discussion, and made recommendations on ethical policy. In addition, 87 percent of the respondents indicated that their committees had developed specific policies and procedures regarding patient care in ethically ambiguous situations. The greatest number of policies had been developed around issues of resuscitation, living wills, and withdrawal of treatment. Nurses perceived that their contributions were valued by other committee members.

(From Oddi, L. F., and Cassidy, V. R. (1990). Participation and perception of nurse members in the hospital ethics committee. *Western Journal of Nursing Research,* 12(3), 307–317.)

Dina Cook is a nurse working in intensive care. All beds in the unit are full. For the past three days, Miss Cook has been assigned to care for a 92-year-old woman critically ill with heart failure. The patient has no financial resources of her own, and no family member has seen her since she was admitted from a nursing home. Her condition has changed very little over the course of her hospitalization, and she remains in very critical condition. Suddenly, orders come for the elderly woman to be transferred to a bed on a regular hospital unit. As she is being moved out of the intensive care unit, a state senator's son who was injured in an automobile accident is admitted to her recently vacated bed. What is the nurse's responsibility?

Ethical Decision Making

Nurses encounter situations daily that require them to make professional judgments and act on those judgments. The judgments or decisions are often made in conjunction with other persons involved in the situation: patients, families, and other health care professionals. Whether involved in a collective or individual decision, nurses need to be knowledgeable about the steps in **ethical decision making**.

Various models of ethical decision making have been developed. Two frameworks will be discussed.

Thompson and Thompson's Model of Ethical Decision Making

Thompson and Thompson (1985, p. 99) identified ten steps necessary for making ethical decisions. The steps include:

1. Review the situation to determine health problems, decisions needed, ethical components, and key individuals.
2. Gather additional information.
3. Identify the ethical issues in the situation.
4. Identify personal and professional values.
5. Identify the values of key individuals.
6. Identify any existing value conflicts.
7. Determine who should decide.
8. Identify the range of actions and anticipated outcomes.
9. Decide on a course of action and carry it out.
10. Evaluate the results.

Silva's Model of Ethical Decision Making

Silva (1990, p. 109) drew from components of several ethical decision-making frameworks to present a five-part model. This model will be described in some detail, and a case study will be analyzed using Silva's model of ethical decision making.

1. Data collection and assessment.
   A. Situational considerations.
   B. Health team considerations.
   C. Organizational considerations.

Collection and assessment of data related to an ethical dilemma are integral to the decision-making process. In regard to step A, situational considerations, one must determine if a situation is an ethical dilemma or another type of dilemma. Concerning health team considerations, it is important to determine what persons will be affected by the decision and how they will be affected. Regarding organizational considerations, one must identify how the organization, particularly its procedures and policies, may affect the resolution of an ethical dilemma.

2. Problem identification.
   A. Ethical considerations.
   B. Nonethical considerations.

A clear understanding of the ethical problem is crucial to resolving a dilemma. Both ethical and nonethical considerations must be identified. In the nurse's professional role, the *Code for Nurses* (American Nurses Association 1985) clearly outlines the nurse's first priority as the patient.

3. Consideration of possible actions.
   A. Utilitarian thinking.
   B. Deontological thinking.

Once the ethical problem is identified, possible actions must be considered. Serious consideration should only be given to those actions that are reasonable to implement.

4. Decision and selection of course of action.
   A. Contribution of internal/group factors.
   B. Contribution of external factors.
   C. Quality of decision and course of action.

It is now time to make a decision. Both internal (people-related) and external (legal, institutional, and social) factors should be considered.

5. Reflection on decision and course of action.
   A. Reflection on decision.
   B. Reflection on course of action.

After a decision is implemented, the result must be evaluated for its effectiveness. If the action accomplished its purpose, resolution of the ethical dilemma will presumably have occurred. If the dilemma is not resolved, additional problem-solving approaches will need to be implemented.

Case Study: Ethical Decision Making Using Silva's Model

Eleanor Gift, age 68 years, is scheduled for triple bypass surgery. Martha Blake, R.N., is the nurse doing her preoperative teaching the evening before the procedure is scheduled. It is apparent to Miss Blake that Mrs. Gift does not want to have surgery. She expresses much apprehension about the surgery and generally feels quite negative about the outcome. The surgeon, however, has convinced Mrs. Gift and her family that she must undergo the surgery in order to survive. Although far from happy about the situation, Mrs. Gift is resigned to the impending surgery. What is Miss Blake's nursing responsibility in this situation?

1. Data collection and assessment.

   Situational considerations. The situational factors contributing to the ethical dilemma include:

   A. Mrs. Gift is apprehensive and feels quite negative about the surgery. Despite these negative feelings, Mrs. Gift and her family feel that there is no other option but to go ahead with the surgery.

   B. It is not clear what options the physician has presented to Mrs. Gift concerning the necessity of her surgery.

Health team considerations. Persons most involved with this situation are Mrs. Gift, the patient's family, the surgeon, and Miss Blake, R.N. Relevant information for those most involved includes:

A. Mrs. Gift is in her late sixties and apparently has a history of cardiovascular disease. She is from a generation that frequently does not question the authority of a physician.

B. The physician is not present but apparently has talked to the patient and her family about the procedure.

C. Miss Blake has recognized that Mrs. Gift does not feel positively about the surgery scheduled for tomorrow.

Organizational considerations. Little information is given as to the specifics of this situation. It seems appropriate to assume, however, that the surgeon may not be as aware of the patient's concerns as the nurse is. As is the case in most hospital organizations, it also seems safe to assume that the physician holds more prestige and authority than the others who are involved. Since the procedure is scheduled for tomorrow, time is of the essence.

2. Problem identification.

Ethical considerations. Major ethical considerations in the case are:

A. Mrs. Gift: Does she have all the information she needs to make an informed decision? Has she been forced to make a decision that she feels is not the right one? Or is she simply experiencing presurgical anxieties, which would be expected the night before a scheduled operation?

B. The surgeon: Has the physician given Mrs. Gift all the necessary information she needs to make an informed decision? On the other hand, has the information been presented so matter-of-factly that the patient does not recognize she has an option concerning the surgery?

C. The nurse: Was it Miss Blake's responsibility to delve into Mrs. Gift's concerns the evening before surgery was scheduled? It seems possible that just as Mrs. Gift agreed to surgery earlier, she probably can be talked into following through without a thorough exploration of all her concerns.

Nonethical considerations. The major nonethical consideration seems to center around the limited amount of time before surgery is scheduled.

This case study involves the principle of autonomy. A question exists as to whether or not Mrs. Gift was allowed to make her own decision concerning the surgery. It is not clear that Mrs. Gift made the decision based on her individual values, with adequate information, free from any coercion (external or internal), and grounded in rational reason and deliberation.

3. Consideration of possible actions.

The following actions are options in this situation:

- Continue with the teaching under the assumption that surgery will take place as scheduled.
- Inform the physician about the concerns.
- Inform the supervisor about the concerns.
- Advise the patient to refuse to have surgery tomorrow.
- Encourage Mrs. Gift to include her family in the decision.
- Explore Mrs. Gift's concerns thoroughly and help her to deal with her apprehension and fears.

Box 20–3   Comparison of Models of Ethical Decision Making

NURSING PROCESS	THOMPSON AND THOMPSON (1985)	SILVA (1990)
Assess	Review the situation Gather additional data	Data collection and assessment
Analyze	Identify the ethical issues Identify the values of key individuals Identify value conflicts	Problem identification
Plan	Determine who should decide Identify the range of actions and anticipated outcomes	Consideration of possible actions
Implement	Decide on a course of action and carry it out	Decision and selection of course of action
Evaluate	Evaluate the results	Reflection on decision and course of action

---

- Determine to the best of your ability if Mrs. Gift has autonomously consented to have surgery.

In this case study, the ethically justifiable action can be arrived at by using deontological thinking. A deontologist might consistently follow a rule that promotes patient autonomy in decision making.

4. Decision and selection of course of action.

Contribution of internal/group factors.   Mrs. Gift is the focus of the decision that must be made. She certainly is the one who is most affected by the outcome of the decision.

Contribution of external factors.   In this case, time is of some significance since surgery is scheduled in the morning. Of more importance, however, is the fact that a patient has the right to make decisions related to his or her care. No one can be forced to undergo a procedure.

Quality of decision and course of action.   The decision made was to explore as thoroughly as possible Mrs. Gift's true feelings concerning the surgery. It is critical to determine if Mrs. Gift truly feels the surgery is in her best interest and has made an autonomous decision.

5. Reflection on decision and course of action.

Once the decision is implemented, it should be evaluated to determine if the action accomplished its purpose.

As can be identified in Box 20–3, the steps identified in both Thompson and Thompson's and Silva's models are similar to the nursing process framework. As the nurse is attempting to resolve an ethical dilemma, it may be helpful to recognize the universality of the problem-solving process whether it is applied to a patient care situation or an ethical dilemma.

CHAPTER SUMMARY

The terms *morals* and *ethics* are often used interchangeably. Technically, however, morals reflect what is done in a situation, whereas ethics are concerned with what should be done. It is important that nurses are familiar with ethical theories and principles, moral development, and decision-making models in order to actively participate in resolving ethical dilemmas affecting the members of our profession. Codes of ethics, developed by the profession's members, are important to the development of professional status. The ANA *Code for Nurses* (1985) serves as a guideline for nurses regarding ethical behavior. The history of the *Code for Nurses* is reflective of nursing's history as a profession. Ethical dilemmas occur in all areas of nursing practice. Often dilemmas are present because of conflicts between patients, health care professionals, and/or institutions. Ethical decision-making models are helpful in determining the best action to take concerning an ethical dilemma.

REVIEW/DISCUSSION QUESTIONS

1. What is the difference between morals and ethics? Give an example of each from your own value system.
2. How is nursing's code of ethics important to the bedside nurse?
3. Compare the American Nurses Association's *Code for Nurses* with the *International Council of Nurses Code for Nurses*. How are they similar, and how are they different?
4. Select an ethical theory or principle that is most congruent with your approach to ethical dilemmas. Use it as a basis for resolving the ethical dilemmas in this chapter. How well does it hold up under these test conditions?

REFERENCES

American Hospital Association. (1972). *A patient's bill of rights.* Chicago: Author.

American Nurses Association. (1976). *Code for nurses with interpretive statements.* Kansas City, MO: Author.

American Nurses Association. (1985). *Code for nurses with interpretive statements.* Kansas City, MO: Author.

Beauchamp, T. L., and Childress, J. F. (1989). *Principles of biomedical ethics* (3rd ed.). New York: Oxford University Press.

Chally, P. S. (1990). Theory derivation in moral development. *Nursing & Health Care,* 11(6), 302–306.

Davis, A. J., and Aroskar, M. A. (1991). *Ethical dilemmas and nursing practice* (3rd ed.). Norwalk, CT: Appleton & Lange.

Frankena, W. K. (1973). *Ethics* (2nd ed.). Englewood Cliffs, NJ: Prentice-Hall.

Gilligan, C. (1982). *In a different voice: Psychological theory and women's development.* Cambridge, MA: Harvard University Press.

Gilligan, C. (1987). Moral orientation and moral development. In E. Kittay and D. Meyers (Eds.), *Women and moral theory* (pp. 19–33). Totowa, NJ: Rowman and Littlefield.

Gilligan, C., and Attanucci, J. (1988). Two moral orientations: Gender differences and similarities. *Merrill-Palmer Quarterly, 34*(3), 223–231.

Gilligan, C., Brown, L., and Rogers, A. (1988). *Psyche embedded: A place for body, relationships, and culture in personality theory* (Monograph No. 4). Cambridge, MA: Harvard University, Laboratory of Human Development.

Grippando, G. M., and Mitchell, P. R. (1989). *Nursing perspectives and issues* (4th ed.). Albany, NY: Delmar.

Husted, G. L., and Husted, J. H. (1991). *Ethical decision making in nursing.* St. Louis: C.V. Mosby.

International Council of Nurses. (1973). *International Council of Nurses code for nurses.* Geneva, Switzerland: Author.

Jameston, A. (1984). *Nursing practice: The ethical issues.* Englewood Cliffs, NJ: Prentice-Hall.

Kant, I. (1985). The categorical imperative. In J. Feinburg (Ed.), *Reason and responsibility: Readings in some basic problems of philosophy* (6th ed.)(pp. 540–547). Belmont, CA: Wadsworth. (Reprinted from Kant, I. (1959). *Foundations of the metaphysics of morals,* trans. L. W. Beck. Indianapolis: Bobbs-Merrill, pp. 31–49.)

Kohlberg, L. (1973). Continuities and discontinuities in childhood and adult moral development revisited. In L. Kohlberg (Ed.), *Collected papers on moral development and moral education.* Cambridge, MA: Moral Education Research Foundation.

Kohlberg, L. (1976). Moral stages and moralization: The cognitive developmental approach. In T. Lickona (Ed.), *Moral development and behavior* (pp. 31–53). New York: Holt, Rinehart & Winston.

Kohlberg, L. (1986). A current statement on some theoretical issues. In S. Modgil and C. Modgil (Eds.), *Lawrence Kohlberg: Consensus and controversy* (pp. 485–546). Philadelphia: Falmer Press.

Mill, J. S. (1985). Utilitarianism. In J. Feinburg (Ed.), *Reason and responsibility: Readings in some basic problems of philosophy* (6th ed.) (pp. 503–515). Belmont, CA: Wadsworth. (Original work published in 1863.)

Oddi, L. F., and Cassidy, V. R. (1990). Participation and perception of nurse members in the hospital ethics committee. *Western Journal of Nursing Research, 12*(3), 307–317.

Rokeach, M. (1973). *The nature of human values.* New York: Free Press.

Schoendorf v. *Society of New York Hospital,* 105 N.E. 92 (N.Y. 1914).

Silva, M. C. (1990). *Ethical decision making in nursing administration.* Norwalk, CT: Appleton & Lange.

Thompson, J. B., and Thompson, H. O. (1985). *Bioethical decision making for nurses.* Norwalk, CT: Appleton-Century-Crofts.

Uustal, D. B. (1987). Values: The cornerstone of nursing's moral art. In M. Fowler and J. Levine-Ariff (Eds.), *Ethics at the bedside* (pp. 136–170). Philadelphia: J.B. Lippincott.

Veatch, R., and Fry, S. T. (1987). *Case studies in nursing ethics*. Philadelphia: J.B. Lippincott.

Veins, D. C. (1989). A history of nursing's code of ethics. *Nursing Outlook*, 37(1), 45–49.

Wright, R. A. (1987). *Human values in health care: The practice of ethics*. New York: McGraw-Hill.

SUGGESTED READINGS

Aroskar, M. A. (1980a). Anatomy of an ethical dilemma: The theory. *American Journal of Nursing*, 80, 658–660.

Aroskar, M. A. (1980b). Anatomy of an ethical dilemma: The practice. *American Journal of Nursing*, 80, 661–663.

Brody, H. (1981). *Ethical decisions in medicine* (2nd ed.). Boston: Little, Brown.

Curtin, L. (1982). No rush to judgment. In L. Curtin and M. J. Flaherty (Eds.), *Nursing ethics: Theories and pragmatics* (pp. 57–63). Bowie, MD: Brady.

Francoeur, R. T. (1983). *Biomedical ethics: A guide to decision making*. New York: Wiley.

Legal Aspects of Nursing

Virginia Trotter Betts and Frances I. Waddle

CHAPTER OBJECTIVES

What students should be able to do after studying this chapter:

1. Describe the components of a model nursing practice act.

2. Discuss the authority of state boards of nursing.

3. Explain the conditions that must be present for malpractice to occur.

4. Identify nursing concerns related to delegation, assault and battery, informed consent, and confidentiality.

5. Describe strategies nurses can use to protect themselves from legal actions.

VOCABULARY BUILDING

Terms to know:

advance directives	criminal law	licensure by
assault	delegation	endorsement
battery	documentation	licensure
"captain of the ship"	duty of care	malpractice
doctrine	duty to report	negligence
civil law	expert witness	Patient Self-
common law	informed consent	Determination Act
competency	law	privileged
confidentiality	legal authority	communication

proximate cause
respondeat superior
risk management

standard of care
standard of nursing
practice

statutory law
tort

*P*rofessional nurses have many complex and interesting relationships with the law that are important to identify and understand. This is an area that is both extremely important and constantly changing. Therefore, schools of nursing sometimes offer required or elective courses in law as applied to nursing. "Nursing and the law" is also one of the most popular continuing education topics for nurses. The purpose of this chapter is to highlight key issues in the law for professional nurses and to develop interest in further study, which is essential to maintain a working knowledge of the law as it relates to professional nursing practice.

The American Legal System: A Review

The purpose of the law in the United States is found in the Preamble to the United States Constitution: to assure order, protect the individual person, resolve disputes, and promote the general welfare. In order to achieve these broad objectives, the law concerns itself with the legal relationships between persons and the government.

U.S. law evolved from centuries-old English **common law**. Common law is decisional or judge-made law. Every time a judge makes a legal decision, the body of common law expands.

In addition to common law, there are **statutory laws**, which are laws established through formal legislative processes. Every time the U.S. Congress or state legislatures pass legislation, the body of statutory law expands.

An important distinction to understand is the difference between civil and criminal law. **Civil law** involves issues between individuals, whereas **criminal law** involves public concerns against unlawful behavior that threatens society.

All law in the United States flows from the U.S. Constitution and must conform to its principles. The Constitution provides for division of powers through the establishment of three branches of government—the judicial, executive, and legislative branches. The chief functions of the judicial branch are to resolve legal disputes, interpret statutory laws, and amend the common law. The executive branch implements laws through governmental agencies. The legislative branch makes statutory laws and speaks most directly for the people.

The word **law** is defined as the sum total of man-made rules and regulations by which society is governed in a formal and binding manner (Hemelt and Mackert 1982). It encompasses the actions of the legislative branch in enacting statutes, the executive branch in administering the statutes through rules, and the judicial branch in interpreting statutes and rules.

Professional nurses need to be aware of a wide array of legal issues. Of particular importance to nurses are: the statutory authority governing nursing practice, executive authority of state boards of nursing, the civil law areas of torts, privacy rights, and the evolving common law related to health care. The remainder of this chapter will focus on these key concerns.

Nursing as a Practice Discipline

Disciplines such as nursing, medicine, dentistry, law, and many others are regulated by the individual states. The practitioners of these disciplines cannot legally practice without a license. The purpose of licensing certain professions is to protect the public safety. The statute that defines and controls nursing is called a nursing practice act. All 50 states and several U.S. territories have nursing practice acts.

Statutory Authority of State Nursing Practice Acts

Nurses, as health care providers, have certain rights, responsibilities, and recognitions through various state laws, or statutes. The nursing practice act in each state does at least four things:

1. Defines the practice of professional nursing.
2. Identifies the scope of nursing practice.
3. Sets the educational qualifications and other requirements for licensure.
4. Determines the legal titles and abbreviations nurses may use.

In many states, nursing practice acts also define the responsibilities and authorities of the state board of nursing. Thus, the nursing practice act of each state is the most important statutory law affecting nurses.

Once the law regarding nursing practice is established, the legislative branch delegates authority to an executive agency, usually called the state board of nursing. State boards of nursing are responsible for enforcing the nursing practice acts in the various states. The state board of nursing promulgates rules and regulations that flesh out the law. It is the statutory law plus the rules and regulations promulgated by the state board of nursing that give full meaning to the nursing practice act in each state.

Nursing practice acts are revised from time to time to keep up with new developments in health care and the changing practice of nursing. State nurses associations are usually instrumental in lobbying for appropriate updating in nursing practice acts.

Because of the importance of practice acts to professional nurses, the American Nurses Association (ANA) has developed suggested language for the content of state nursing practice acts. The document *A Guideline for Suggested State Legislation* was published in 1990 to guide state nurses associations seeking revisions in their nursing practice acts (American Nurses Association 1990). The guidelines encourage consideration of the many issues inherent in a nursing practice act and the political realities of each state's legislative and regulatory processes.

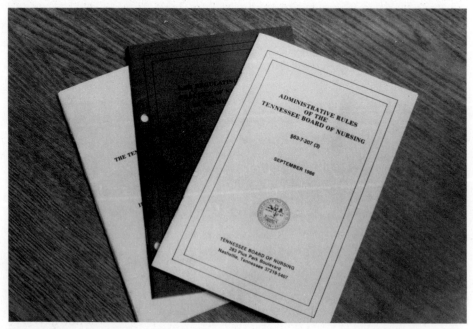

The nursing practice act and other state rules and regulations are vital documents that affect the legal practice of nursing.

Through this document, the ANA recognizes the great importance of the nursing practice act and urges that the following content be included:

1. A clear differentiation between professional and technical nursing practice.
2. Authority for boards of nursing to regulate advanced nursing practice including prescription-writing authority.
3. Authority for boards of nursing to oversee unlicensed assistive personnel.
4. Clarification of nurses' responsibilities for delegation and supervision of other personnel.
5. Support for mandatory licensure for nurses while retaining sufficient flexibility to accommodate the changing nature of nursing practice.

The ANA document provides a broad definition of the practice of professional nursing and appropriate professional practice activities. It also defines technical nursing practice and identifies appropriate activities (American Nurses Association 1990).

The guidelines provide sample language recognizing the baccalaureate degree with a major in nursing, commonly called the B.S.N. (bachelor of science in nursing), as the minimum educational credential for the professional nurse and the associate degree in nursing, commonly called the A.D.N., as the appropriate minimum educational credential for the technical nurse. However, the document does not specify the names of these two levels of nurses.

There has been extensive debate about the need to change the minimum educational qualifications for professional nursing practice. In the early 1980s, the ANA reaffirmed its long-standing position that in the future the baccalaureate (B.S.N.) should be the minimum educational qualification for professional nursing practice and the associate degree (A.D.N.) the minimum educational qualification for technical nursing practice.

To date, only North Dakota has implemented these changes in the minimum educational qualifications for nurses. However, many state nurses associations consider such changes a priority for future nursing practice act modifications.

Executive Authority of State Boards of Nursing

Both federal and state laws provide for the executive branch of government to administer and implement laws. The state executive, or governor, generally delegates the responsibility for administering the nursing practice statutes to an executive agency, the state board of nursing. In most states the state board of nursing consists of registered nurses (R.N.s), licensed practical nurses (L.P.N.s), and consumers, all of whom are generally appointed by the governor.

The state board of nursing's authority is limited. It can adopt rules that clarify general provisions of the nursing practice act, but it does not have the authority to enlarge the law.

State boards of nursing usually have three functions:

1. Quasi-executive—authority to administer the nursing practice act.
2. Quasi-legislative—authority to adopt rules necessary to implement the act.
3. Quasi-judicial—authority to deny, suspend, or revoke a license or to otherwise discipline a licensee or to deny an application for licensure.

Each of these state board of nursing functions is as broad or as limited as the state legislature specifies in the nursing practice act and other related laws.

Establishing Rules Regulating Nursing Practice

The federal government and each state have administrative procedures acts (APAs) that specify the process executive branch agencies such as the state board of nursing must use in promulgating rules to implement a specific law. Though one state's APA may differ in certain areas from others', there are recommended principles for all APAs. The principles for promulgation of rules include:

1. Written notice and publication of the proposed rules.
2. Opportunity for oral and written comments about the proposed rules.
3. A public hearing or forum for response to the proposed rules.
4. Identification of options the executive agency may exercise to withdraw, modify, or adopt the proposed rules.

5. Review of the adopted rules by a legislative committee or legal review, such as by the office of the state attorney general.
6. Publication of the final rules in an official governmental document.
7. Codification of the adopted rules in an official publication such as the *Code of Federal Regulations (CFR)* or a state administrative code.

In some states, rules may be proposed through a petition to the executive agency.

An executive agency may have the authority to suspend a license or a permit to practice if there is evidence of a threat to the public health and welfare if the license or permit remains in effect while the action is pending. The APA also specifies a process that executive agencies like state boards of nursing must follow when considering action on a specific professional or occupational license or permit. This process is consistent with individuals' constitutional rights to due process. The process usually includes:

1. Notice of a complaint or cause of the proposed action.
2. Notice of the date, time, and place of a hearing on such complaint.
3. Right of the applicant or licensee to legal counsel.
4. Right of the applicant or licensee and the agency to subpoena witnesses and records and to examine and cross-examine such witnesses.
5. The agency's authority in such matters.
6. Right of either party to appeal the decision.
7. Final decision and notice to applicant or licensee.

State boards of nursing may be independent agencies in the executive branch of state government or part of a department or bureau such as a department of licensure and regulation. Some state boards have authority to carry out the nursing practice act without review of their actions by other state officials. Others must recommend action to another department or bureau and receive approval for the recommendation before they can act.

LICENSING POWERS

The legal regulation of nursing practice is accomplished primarily through state licensure of nurses. The *Report of the National Advisory Commission on Health Manpower* concluded: "The first requirement for assuring that health care approaches its potential quality is to make licensure effective to the limit of its capabilities" (U.S. Department of Health, Education and Welfare 1968).

The accepted definition of individual **licensure** is: "The process by which an agency of government grants permission to persons to engage in a given profession or occupation by certifying that those licensed have attained the minimal degree of competency necessary to ensure that the public health, safety and welfare will be reasonably well protected" (U.S. Department of Health, Education and Welfare 1971).

The licensure process is a police power of the state. The state, through the legislative branch, determines what groups are to be licensed and the limitations of such licenses. Licensure laws may be either mandatory or permissive. A mandatory law requires any person who practices the profession or occupation to be licensed. A permissive law protects the use of the title granted in the law but does not prohibit persons practicing the profession or occupation if they do not use the title. All states now have mandatory licensure for nursing practice.

In most states, state boards of nursing have the authority to enforce minimum criteria for nursing education programs. Nursing practice acts generally specify that candidates for licensure must graduate from a state-approved nursing education program as a prerequisite for writing the licensure examination.

State approval is different from accreditation; many nursing education programs achieve accreditation by the nationally recognized accrediting agency, the National League for Nursing. While many other professions and occupations require graduation from a nationally accredited educational program as a prerequisite for licensure, only state approval is required in nursing.

LICENSING EXAMINATIONS

Since 1944, most state boards of nursing have participated in a cooperative effort to develop an examination for licensure of R.N.s and L.P.N.s that can be adopted by each state and assist in the interstate mobility of nurses. In describing this system, Schorr (1975, p. 1131) wrote:

> Ours was the first health profession to have an examination that is used nationwide in judging a candidate's basic competence and right to be licensed. Because of this, the State Board Test Pool Examination (SBTPE) facilitates endorsement of a nurse's license by a state to which he or she is moving, providing the score on the SBTPE in the original state meets the required minimum score set by the board in the new state. Although the examination is used nationally and the questions on it are developed by nurses from all over the country, so that the tests really mirror practice nationwide, the principle of states' rights has also been worked into the system.

Until 1978, the SBTPE was developed by the ANA's Council of State Boards of Nursing and the National League for Nursing served as the testing service. In 1978 the National Council of State Boards of Nursing (NCSBN) was established and continued the activities of the ANA Council of State Boards. Through the NCSBN, each state still participates in the licensing process through test development and adoption of a minimum passing score.

Licensing examinations in nursing are now called the National Council Licensure Examination for Registered Nurses (NCLEX-RN) and the National Council Licensure Examination for Practical Nursing (NCLEX-PN). They are each administered twice yearly. Although the tests have traditionally been administered by paper and pencil, the SBNs and the NCSBN plan to administer them by computerized adaptive testing (CAT) beginning in 1994.

Since nursing licensing examinations are national examinations, they facilitate the system of **licensure by endorsement**. Endorsement means that R.N.s or L.P.N.s/L.V.N.s (licensed vocational nurses) can move from state to state without having to sit for another licensing examination. If they submit proof of licensure in another state and pay a licensure fee, they can receive licensure from the new state by endorsement. Licensure by endorsement is not available to all practice disciplines. Nursing's plan serves as a national model for other licensed professions and occupations.

Special Concerns in Professional Nursing Practice

Nurses make decisions daily that affect the well-being of their patients. They often know very personal information about patients and are in a position of great trust. Several areas of nursing practice are particularly fraught with legal risk. They include malpractice, delegation, assault and battery, informed consent, and confidentiality. Each of these concerns will be discussed.

Malpractice

Malpractice is the greatest legal concern of health care practitioners. In order to understand malpractice, it is necessary first to understand the legal concepts of torts and negligence.

Torts are civil wrongs against a person and may be either intentional or unintentional. There must be harm resulting from the action, but the harm does not have to be physical. Emotional or economic harm may also result in a tort.

Negligence is the failure to act as a reasonably prudent person would have in specific circumstances. For example, if in burning yard debris on a windy day a man sets fire to his neighbor's garage, the neighbor may charge negligence. A reasonably prudent person would not have started a yard fire on a windy day and an injury (the burned garage) can be shown to be a direct result of his failure to act prudently.

Malpractice is negligence applied to the acts of a professional. In other words, malpractice occurs when a professional fails to act as a reasonably prudent professional would under specific circumstances. Malpractice is classified as an unintentional tort. This means that it is not necessary to prove that the professional intended to be negligent. In malpractice, both *doing* things that should *not* be done (commissions) and *not doing* things that *should* be done (omissions) may be the basis of legal actions.

When a patient brings a malpractice claim against a nurse defendant, evidence is presented to the jury to determine if the elements of liability are present. At question is whether the nurse met the prevailing **standard of care**.

The nursing standard of care is what the reasonably prudent nurse, under similar circumstances, would have done. It is a peer standard of care that reflects not excellence but a minimum standard of "do no harm." The nursing standard of care is decided by the jury on a case-by-case basis and is developed through use of **expert witness** testimony; documents, including national standards of nursing practice; the patient record; and other pertinent evidence such as the direct testimony of the patient, the nurse, and others.

The prerequisite for a malpractice action is that the defendant (nurse) has specialized knowledge and skills and through the practice of that specialized knowledge caused the plaintiff's (patient's) injury. In order for a plaintiff patient to prove that the nurse defendant is liable for the injury, all elements of a cause of action for negligence must be proved. The elements are the same for any professional accused of malpractice. The elements necessary for a malpractice action are as follows:

1. The professional nurse has assumed the **duty of care** (responsibility for the patient's care).
2. The professional nurse breaches the duty of care by failing to meet the standard of care.
3. The failure of the professional nurse to meet the standard of care *proximately caused* the injury.
4. The injury is proved.

Setting forth all elements of a malpractice action requires a high degree of proof. Money damages are awarded when a patient plaintiff prevails. The money damages are based on proven economic losses, such as time missed from work, out-of-pocket health care costs, and remuneration for pain and suffering caused by the injury. In the case of a death, the next of kin can become the plaintiff on behalf of the deceased patient.

In the past, malpractice lawsuits have involved nurses, but the defendants called on to pay damages were traditionally physicians and hospitals, even when the substandard care was provided by nurses. Physicians were implicated through the **"captain of the ship" doctrine**. This doctrine implies that the physician is in charge of all patient care and thus should be responsible financially. Hospitals were implicated through the legal theory of "**respondent superior**," which attributes the acts of employees to their employer. However, as nurses increase their expertise, autonomy, credentials, and authority for nursing practice, liability for nursing care will correspondingly be increased. Nurses are expected to be defendants more often in the future (Sweeney 1991).

A review of malpractice cases where the liability of the nurse has been successfully litigated showed the categories of cases as follows:

a. The nurse failed to carry out the medical order (*Dobrzeniecki* 1984).
b. The nurse carried out an order incorrectly (*Holbrooks* 1983).
c. The nurse implemented a faulty medical order (*Doerr* 1985).
d. The nurse failed to make an accurate assessment (*Harris* 1985).
e. The nurse failed to act on an assessment (*Duren* 1985).
f. The nurse failed to report inadequate patient care (*Utter* 1977).
g. The nurse failed to secure adequate care for a patient (*Goff* 1958).
h. The nurse abandoned a patient needing care (*Hiatt* 1974).

The lesson to be learned from such malpractice cases is that professional nurses must carefully consider the legal implications of practice and be willing and capable of conforming that care to legal expectations.

Delegation

Delegation, that is, "empowering one to act for another," is an issue gaining increasing importance in nursing practice. The ability to delegate has generally been reserved for professionals since they hold licenses that sanction the entire scope of practice for a particular profession. Professional nurses, for example, may delegate independent nursing activities and delegated medical functions to other nursing personnel.

State nursing practice acts do not give delegatory authority to licensed practical/vocational nurses. Professional nurses retain accountability for acts delegated to another person and are responsible for determining that the delegatee is competent to perform the delegated act. Likewise, the delegatee is responsible for carrying out the delegated act safely. The professional nurse is legally liable for the nursing acts delegated to others. This is an important liability and one not fully appreciated by many practicing nurses.

Delegatory acts must also be considered from the standpoint of their ethical implications. The *Code for Nurses* states, ''The nurse exercises informed judgment and uses individual competence and qualifications as criteria in seeking consultation, accepting responsibilities, and delegating nursing activities to others'' (American Nurses Association 1985). This statement makes reference to accepting delegated responsibilities as well as making them. An important point is that nurses are ethically bound to refuse to accept acts that are not within their area of expertise, even if physicians or hospital authorities request that they accept them.

The professional nurse's primary legal and ethical consideration must be the patient's right to safe and effective nursing care.

Assault and Battery

Assault and battery is an intentional tort that is often the basis for legal action against a nurse defendant. **Assault** is a threat or an attempt to make bodily contact with another person without the person's consent. Assault precedes battery; it causes the person to fear that a battery is about to occur. **Battery** is the assault carried out, the unpermissible, unprivileged touching by one person of another. Actual harm may or may not occur as a result of assault and battery.

If, for example, a nurse threatens a patient with a vitamin injection if he doesn't eat his meals, the patient may charge assault. Actually giving the patient a vitamin injection against his will would leave the nurse open to charges of battery, even if there is a physician's order. It is important to remember that patients have the right to refuse treatment, even if the treatment would be in their best interest.

Both by common law and by statute, informed consent is required in the health care context as a defense to battery (*United States Code* 1990).

Informed Consent

All patients should be given an opportunity to grant **informed consent** prior to treatment unless there is an emergency that is life-threatening. Northrup and Kelly (1987) described three major elements of informed consent:

1. Consent must be given voluntarily.
2. Consent must be given by an individual with the capacity and competence to understand.

3. The patient must be given enough information to be the ultimate decision maker.

Informed consent is a full, knowing authorization by the patient for care, treatment, and procedures and must include information about the risks, benefits, side effects, costs, and alternatives. In today's world, consumers of health care need a great deal of information and should be told everything that they consider significant (Canterbury 1972).

In order for informed consent to be legally valid, elements of completeness, competency, and voluntariness are evaluated. Completeness refers to the quality of the information provided. **Competency** takes into account the capability of a particular patient to understand the information given and make a choice. Vol-

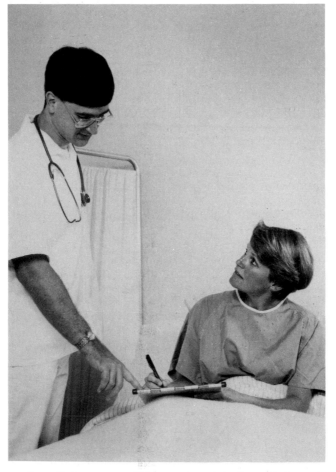

Nurses may be called upon to witness patients' signing of informed consent documents.

untariness refers to the freedom the patient has to accept or reject alternatives. When clients are minors, under the effects of drugs or alcohol (including preoperative medications), or have other mental deficits, there is frequently a problem proving competency to consent.

The role of nurses in informed consent, unless they are themselves primary providers, is to collaborate with the primary provider, most often a physician and/or surgeon. Nurses can witness patients' signing of informed consent documents but are not responsible for explaining the proposed treatment. Nor are they responsible for evaluating whether the physician has truly explained the significant risks, benefits, and alternative treatments.

Professional nurses *are* responsible for determining that the elements for valid consent are in place, providing feedback if the patient wishes to change consent, and communicating the patient's need for further information to the primary provider.

Confidentiality

Confidentiality is both a legal and an ethical concern in nursing practice. Confidentiality is the protection of private information gathered about a patient during the provision of health care services. The *Code for Nurses* states: "The nurse safeguards the client's right to privacy by judiciously protecting information of a confidential nature" (American Nurses Association 1985).

In the *Code* there are acknowledged exceptions to the obligation of confidentiality. They include discussing the care of patients with others involved in their direct care, quality assurance activities, and when the law demands disclosure (American Nurses Association 1985). The *Code* also recognizes the need to disclose information without the patient's consent when the safety of innocent parties is in question (*Tarasoff* 1976).

While some professions have statutorily protected **privileged communication**, nurses are usually not included in such statutes. Thus, nurses may be ordered by the court to share information without the patient's consent. The principle of confidentiality is protected by state and federal statutes, but there are exceptions and limitations. It is essential for the professional nurse to understand these legal limitations.

In certain situations, through statute and common law, there has developed the antithesis of confidentiality—the **duty to report** or disclose. These laws require nurses and other health professionals to report child abuse, gunshot wounds, certain communicable diseases, and threats toward third parties. These laws vary by state and may be the responsibility of institutions providing health care services and not of individuals.

Evolving Legal Issues and the Nurse

Because of the dynamic nature of nursing and health care, legal issues affecting nursing practice are also evolving. Four legal issues that illustrate the changing nature of nursing practice are related to role changes, supervision of assistive personnel, payment mechanisms, and a new law, the Patient Self-Determination Act. Each of these issues will be briefly discussed.

Role Changes in Health Care

Just as nursing's knowledge base and nurses' accountability for nursing practice have increased over time, so has the need to expand the **legal authority** for nursing practice. Even though the definitions and parameters of nursing outlined in nursing practice acts may seem to be an issue of concern only to nurses, this is not the case.

Nurses have found that as they worked through their state nurses associations to modify and update these acts, they met significant political resistance. This is due, in part, to the defensiveness of organized medicine, which often views an expansion of nurses' domain as a diminishment of physicians' roles. It is also due to the historical perceptions by some legislators, employers, and even some nurses that change is not necessary to meet the public's need for nursing care.

Professional nurses realize that it is important for state nursing practice acts to accurately reflect nursing practice and to keep up with changes as they occur. Otherwise, nurses have no legal basis for practice. Health care is becoming more and more specialized, so nursing specialties and subspecialties are increasing. Advanced practice nurses set the pace for evolving nursing practice, and the nursing practice act must support their ability to offer nursing services to consumers in various settings.

In some states, nurses in advanced practice, such as nurse midwives, nurse practitioners, and nurses in private practice have not been supported by changes in the nursing practice act but instead have faced lawsuits (*Fein* 1985). Such activity is intimidating and requires nurses who wish to pursue advanced practice roles to be risk takers. For example, nurses in Missouri were sued for practicing medicine without a license in a women's health practice. After intense litigation, their practice was supported by the Missouri Supreme Court. The court found "legislative intent" in the nursing practice act not to limit nursing practice except to protect the public. The nurses in question were well credentialed and were practicing with the knowledge and support of the Missouri Board of Nursing and the Missouri Nurses Association; so the safety of the public was not in question (*Sermchief* 1983). This is only one example of the legal exposure nurses face when their state's nursing practice act is not updated periodically to explicitly support their expanded scope of practice.

Supervision of Assistive Personnel

Another issue in the 1990s is the role expansion of nonlicensed or limited licensed (L.P.N./L.V.N.) nursing personnel within institutions. There is concern that nurse aides/nursing assistive personnel are increasingly being substituted for nurses, thus creating greater risks to patients and enlarging the liability of nurses, who supervise nursing care. Court decisions indicate that lack of professional nurses poses a significant risk to institutions and nurses alike (Politis 1983).

The Tricouncil of Nursing, a group consisting of representatives of major nursing associations, issued a *Statement on Assistive Personnel to the Registered Nurse* (1990) to guide nurses in the appropriate use of nurse aides/nursing assistive personnel. This statement is included in Box 4–3. The American Nurses Association and the American Organization of Nurse Executives are working to resolve these concerns before health care is compromised.

Historically, organized nursing has opposed the licensure or legal recognition of nurse aides and other nursing support personnel. However, this position needs further study following congressional action mandating training and state registration of nurse aides in Medicaid- and Medicare-certified nursing facilities and Medicare-certified home health agencies. This is a legal issue to watch in the 1990s.

Payment Mechanisms for Nurses

You will recall from Chapter 5 that nurses are increasingly practicing in nontraditional roles and settings. Many professional nurses are both capable of and interested in offering nursing services as independent practitioners, but payment mechanisms limit such activities. Nurses are concerned about offering services for which consumers are unable to obtain reimbursement from their insurance carriers, and third-party reimbursement has traditionally been limited to care provided by physicians.

Over the years, nurses have supported state and federal legislation to provide direct and indirect payments to nurses for nursing services rendered (American Nurses Association 1991a). Changes in state insurance laws were enacted in many states to achieve direct payment for nursing services from private insurance companies. This means that consumers of health care can choose to receive services from physicians, nurses, or other qualified health professionals and receive insurance reimbursement for the chosen professional's fees. Nurses are concerned that these changes are often not implemented or nurses are paid less for similar services provided by other health care professionals.

It is not commonly known that laws can be passed and not implemented. This occurs when the group affected by the law, for example, the insurance industry, is unwilling to implement the changes and no "watchdog" agency is created to make sure that they do. For example, federal legislation was enacted requiring state Medicaid agencies to pay certain nurses (nurse practitioners, nurse midwives, and nurse anesthetists) directly for services provided to Medicaid recipients. As with the laws affecting private insurers, these requirements have not been implemented uniformly. Nurses may need to seek legal remedies to require implementation of policies mandated by federal law (*Nurse Midwifery Associates* 1990).

The Patient Self-Determination Act

Congress enacted the **Patient Self-Determination Act** (PSDA), effective December 1, 1991. The PSDA applies to acute care and long-term care facilities that receive Medicare and Medicaid funds. This act encourages patients to consider which life-prolonging treatment options they desire and to document their preferences in case they should later become incapable of participating in the decision-making process. Written instructions recognized by state law that describe individuals' preferences in regard to medical intervention should they become incapacitated are called "**advance directives**."

This act was passed partly in response to the U.S. Supreme Court's decision in *Cruzan* v. *Director* (1990), which was viewed as limiting individuals' abilities to direct their health care when they become unable to do so. It requires the health care facility to document whether the patient has completed an advance directive. The advance directive provides a process for protecting vulnerable patients, reasonable decision making, and resolving conflicting decisions.

The PSDA's basic assumption is that each person has legal and moral rights to informed consent about medical treatments with a focus on the person's right to choose (ethical principle of autonomy). The act does not create any new rights, and no patient is required to execute an advance directive.

According to the PSDA, acute care (hospitals) and long-term care facilities must:

1. Provide written information to all adult patients about their rights under state law.
2. Ensure institutional compliance with state laws on advance directives.
3. Provide for education of staff and the community on advance directives.
4. Document in the medical record whether the patient has an advance directive.

The health care facility may not refuse to provide care to or otherwise discriminate against patients based on the existence of an advance directive.

Tragic situations, such as the widely publicized cases where families wished to terminate life-support mechanisms for brain-dead relatives and were not allowed to do so, can be prevented. It is hoped that widespread education of the public about advance directives will result in fewer such legal and ethical dilemmas in the future.

Preventing Legal Problems in Nursing Practice

While the range of potential "hot spots" for health care litigation may seem enormous, there are a number of effective strategies that professional nurses can use to limit the possibility of legal action.

Practice in a Safe Setting

In order to be truly safe, facilities in which nurses work must be committed to safe patient care. The safest situation is one in which the agency:

1. Employs an appropriate number and quality of personnel to address the numbers and acuity of patients.

2. Has policies, procedures, and personnel practices that promote quality improvement.
3. Keeps equipment in good working order.
4. Provides orientation to new employees, supervises all levels of employees, and provides opportunities to learn new procedures consistent with the level of health care services provided by the agency.

In addition to an active quality improvement program, each health care institution should have a **risk management** program. Risk management seeks to identify and eliminate potential safety hazards, thereby reducing patient and staff injuries. Common institutional risks are medication errors, falls, assessment errors, and failure to communicate (Campazzi 1980).

Communicate with Other Health Professionals

The professional nurse must have open and clear communication with nurses, physicians, and other health care professionals. Safe nurses trust their own assessments, inform physicians and others of changes in patients' conditions, and question unclear or inaccurate physicians' orders.

A key aspect of communication essential in preventing legal problems is keeping good patient records. This written form of communication is called "**documentation**." Current and descriptive documentation of patient care is essential, not only to quality care but to protecting the nurse. Assessments, plans, interventions, and evaluation of the patient's progress must be reflected in the patient's clinical record if malpractice is alleged.

The clinical record, particularly the nurse's notes, provides the core of evidence about each patient's nursing care (Kerr 1975). No matter how good the nursing care, if the nurse fails to write it in the clinical record, in the eyes of the law the care did not take place.

Meet the Standard of Care

The single-most important protective strategy for the nurse is to be a knowledgeable and safe practitioner of nursing and to meet the **standard of care** with all patients. Meeting the standard of care involves being technically competent, keeping up-to-date with health care innovations, being aware of peer expectations, and participating as an equal on the health care team.

In addition to being current with the nursing literature, professional nurses must use national standards of practice as parameters for care giving, care planning, and care evaluation (American Nurses Association 1991). The ANA has promulgated generic and specialty standards of nursing practice. These national standards can be used by quality improvement programs in individual hospitals in establishing their own "local" standards of nursing care (Betts 1978).

Carry Professional Liability Insurance

Despite the efforts of dedicated professionals, at times mistakes are made, and unfortunately, patients are injured. It is essential for nurses to carry professional

---

Box 21–1   Guidelines for Preventing Legal Problems in Nursing Practice

- Practice in a safe setting.
- Communicate with other health professionals.
- Meet the standard of care.

- Carry professional liability insurance.
- Promote positive interpersonal relationships.

---

liability insurance to protect their assets and income, should they be required to pay monetary compensation to injured patients. Nursing students should also carry insurance, and most schools of nursing require that they do so.

Professional liability insurance policies vary. Generally, they provide up to $1 million coverage for a single incident and up to $3 million total. The amount of coverage depends on the nurse's specialty. Nurse midwives, for example, pay much higher liability insurance premiums than do psychiatric nurses because the midwives' potential for suit is greater. Most policies also provide the defendant nurse with a defense attorney (The American Association of Nurse Attorneys 1984).

Professional liability insurance is available through most state nurses associations, nursing students' associations, and private insurers. Group policies, such as those available through professional associations, are less expensive than individual policies and are an important benefit of association membership.

Promote Positive Interpersonal Relationships

Even in the face of untoward outcomes from a health care provider, it is usually only the unhappy patient that sues. Therefore, the best strategy for the professional nurse is prevention of legal actions through positive interpersonal relationships.

Prevention includes giving personalized, concerned care, including the patient and the family in planning and implementing care, and promoting positive and open interpersonal relationships that value the psychosocial aspects of care. The professional nurse who uses self as a therapeutic agent and acknowledges the holism of the patient is likely to prevent most legal problems. Box 21–1 summarizes the important steps nurses can take to avoid legal problems in nursing practice.

CHAPTER SUMMARY

There are many legal issues for professional nurses. First, nurses must recognize that the law is a system of rules that governs conduct and attaches consequences to certain behavior. Such consequences include civil or criminal action or both. Nursing practice is limited by the definition of practice in the state nursing practice act and the qualifications for licensure to practice nursing in that state. Like nursing practice, the law is dynamic and must be responsive to society's needs. Advances in technology have increased the possibility for legal actions involving nurses. Technology has also increased concern about informed consent and patients' right to direct the care they choose to receive or refuse. Many nurses possess only a cursory knowledge of legal issues that affect nursing practice every day. These issues deserve increased attention by nurses in all areas of practice.

REVIEW/DISCUSSION QUESTIONS

1. Using your state's nursing practice act, describe the scope of practice of the registered nurse. When was the last time the law was modified? Does it accurately reflect current nursing practice?
2. Read the section of the nursing practice act relating to advanced practice. What parameters do nurses have in the areas of independent practice and prescription writing in your state?
3. Go to the college library and browse through back issues of the *Regan Report on Nursing Law*. What kinds of legal issues do you find involving nurses?
4. Explain the Patient Self-Determination Act to your family and friends. What questions do they have about advance directives? Find out what the laws regarding advance directives are in your state.
5. When interviewing for a position in a hospital, what questions should you ask to determine if it is a legally safe setting in which to practice?

REFERENCES

American Nurses Association. (1985). *Code for nurses.* Kansas City, MO: Author.

American Nurses Association. (1990). *A guideline for suggested state legislation.* Kansas City, MO: Author.

American Nurses Association. (1991a). *Pacesetter,* 18(2), Kansas City, MO: ANA Council of Psychiatric/Mental Health Nursing.

American Nurses Association. (1991b). *Standards of practice.* Kansas City, MO: Author.

Betts, V. T. (1978). Using psychiatric audit as one aspect of a quality assurance program. *Current Perspectives in Psychiatric Nursing, 2,* 202–208.

Campazzi, M. (1980). Nurses, nursing, and malpractice litigation, 1967–1977. *Nursing Administration Quarterly,* 5(3), 1–8.

Canterbury v. *Spense,* 464 F²772 (1972).

Cruzan v. *Director Missouri Department of Health,* 110 Supreme Court 2841 (1990).

Dobrzeniecki v. *University Hospital of Cleveland,* 27 ALTA Law Rpt. 425 (1984).

Doerr v. *Hurley,* 28 ALTA Law Rpt. 42 (1985).

Duren v. *Suburban Community Hospital,* 28 ALTA Law Rpt. 168 (1985).

Fein v. *Permanente Medical Group,* 474 U.S. 892 (1985).

Goff v. *Doctors General Hospital,* 333 $P^2$29 (1958).

Harris v. *Skrocki,* 28 *ALTA Law Rpt.* 420 (1985).

Hemelt, M., and Mackert, M. E. (1982). *Dynamics of law in nursing and health care.* Reston, VA: Reston Publishing.

Hiatt v. *Groce,* 523 $P^2$320 (1974).

Holbrooks v. *Duke Hospital, Inc.,* 305 $SE^2$69 (1983).

Kerr, K. (1975). Nurses notes: That's where the goodies are. *Nursing,* 75(2), 34–41.

Northrup, C., and Kelly, M. (1987). *Legal issues in nursing.* St. Louis, MO: C.V. Mosby.

Nurse Midwifery Associates v. *Hibbett,* 918 $Fed^2$605 (1990).

Politis, E. (1983). Nurses' legal dilemma: When hospital staffing compromises professional standards. *University of San Francisco Law Review,* 3, 109–126.

Schorr, T. M. (1975). Securing licensure. *American Journal of Nursing,* 75(7), 1131.

Sermchief v. *Gonzales,* 660 SW^2 683 (1983).

Sweeney, S. (1991). Medical negligence: Proving nursing negligence. *Trial,* 91(5), 34–40.

Tarasoff v. *Board of Regents of the University of California,* 551 $P^2$334 (1976).

The American Association of Nurse Attorneys. (1984). *Demonstrating financial responsibility for nursing practice.* Baltimore, MD: Author.

Tricouncil for Nursing. (1990). *Statement on assistive personnel to the registered nurse.* Washington, D.C.: Author.

42 *United States Code* 1395 cc. (1990).

U.S. Department of Health, Education and Welfare. (1968). *Report of the National Advisory Commission on Health Manpower. II.* Washington, D.C.: Government Printing Office.

U.S. Department of Health, Education and Welfare. (1971). *Report on licensure and related health personnel credentialing* (DHEW Publication No. [HSM] 72–11). Washington, D.C.: Government Printing Office.

Utter v. *United Hospital Center, Inc.,* 236 $SE^2$213 (1977).

SUGGESTED READINGS

American Nurses Association. (1989). *Nurses and hospitals: Partners in prevention.* Kansas City, MO: Author.

Cournoyer, C. (1989). *The nurse manager and the law.* Rockville, MD: Aspen.

Havinghurst, C., and King, N. (1983). Private credentialing of health care personnel: An antitrust perspective. Part one. *American Journal of Law and Medicine,* 9, 140.

Chapter

Nurses and Political Action

Judith K. Leavitt and Virginia Trotter Betts

CHAPTER OBJECTIVES

What students should be able to do after studying this chapter:

1. Differentiate between politics and policy.

2. Explain the concept of personalizing the political process.

3. Cite examples of sources of power.

4. Describe how nurses can become involved in politics at the levels of citizen, activist, and politician.

5. Explain how organized nursing is involved in political activities designed to improve nursing and health care.

VOCABULARY BUILDING

Terms to know:

adjudicate	judicial branch	nurse politician
balance of power	knowledge-based	pay equity
electoral process	power	policy
executive branch	legislative branch	policy development
general election	nurse activist	policy outcomes
inherent power	nurse citizen	

political action
    committees (PACs)
politics
position power

power grabbing
powers of
    appointment
power sharing

primary election
referendum
separation of powers
sex-role stereotyping

*H*ave you ever known a nurse member of Congress? How about a nurse mayor? Did you know that a nurse was responsible for developing the federal system for health care financing?

Nurses have served as head of the American Association of Retired Persons, as head of Planned Parenthood of America, and as chief of staff for the Minority party leader in the U.S. Congress. Nurses have major leadership roles in government, professional, and community organizations and in the workplace. This chapter discusses the political process, describes how nurses can become politically active, and explains some of the ways nurse leaders have achieved their positions.

Politics: What It Is and What It Is Not

Most people tend to think of politics as what is happening in Washington. People tend to think of politics as part of what is wrong with government and believe that it is something removed from everyday life. But politics is a part of daily life, both personal and professional. Politics is not simply what happens in government. Ultimately, politics refers to anything that influences the outcome of decisions among people.

Politics is defined as the allocation of scarce resources (Kalisch and Kalisch 1982). *Allocation* implies that someone is making decisions about how to use these scarce resources. Who distributes the resources, the amount of resources allocated, and who receives the allocated resources are all based on who has the power.

Scarce connotes limits. There are not enough resources for everyone who wants or needs them. *Resources* usually means money. However, resources can also be people, time, status, power, programs—any number of precious assets that are limited.

People often speak of politics with negative overtones. In reality, politics is neither good nor bad. It is the outcome of the political process that may be judged as positive or negative.

Policy is defined as the principles and values that govern actions directed toward given ends; policy statements set forth a plan, direction, or goal for action. Although it is different from politics, policy is *shaped* by politics (Mason, Talbott, and Leavitt 1993). Policies may be laws, regulations, or guidelines that govern behavior in government, workplaces, schools, organizations, and communities.

Politics, that is, decisions about how to allocate scarce resources, influences the development and implementation of policies. If, for example, a state had a budgetary shortfall and policymakers had to decide which programs to cut, political influence could be brought to bear to protect certain programs. Policymakers might, for instance, be influenced by lobbyists for paving contractors to spare highway construction budgets. And in the absence of lobbying on behalf of libraries, they might choose to cut library funding to balance the budget.

Politics has significant impact on the practice of nursing. The ability of the individual nurse to provide care is affected by innumerable policy *and* political decisions. As you learned in Chapter 21, state licensure as a registered nurse derives from legislation that defines the scope of nursing practice. The defined scope determines what a nurse can and cannot do. For instance, giving intravenous medication, performing physical assessments, and taking blood pressures are now well accepted as falling within the scope of nursing practice. Yet 25 years ago these activities were within the scope of the medical practice act rather than the nursing practice act.

Decisions about acceptable professional scope and practices are defined by state laws. Questions that refine these laws depend on a particular state's regulatory structure and can be decided by either boards of nursing, boards of medicine, the attorney general, or the courts. Politics affects appointments to these various regulatory boards, as well as the selection of attorneys general and judges. It also affects the legislation that defines the scope of practice.

Regulations developed to carry out legislation also impact the practicing nurse. For instance, the protocols for administering and documenting the administration of narcotic drugs are promulgated by a regulatory agency of the federal government. The rules that define nurses' authority to order or administer narcotics depend on who writes the regulations. If nurses do not have a part in developing the regulations, the outcome is likely to restrict rather than enhance nursing authority for this aspect of patient care.

Broader issues affecting the nursing profession are also political. Issues of **pay equity**, or equal pay for work of comparable value, are of concern to organized nursing because nurses have historically been underpaid for services. One of the first cases demonstrating the inequality of nursing salaries involved public health nurses in Colorado. They brought a case against the city of Denver, stating that they were paid considerably less than city tree trimmers and garbage collectors. The nurses demanded just compensation for their work by demonstrating that nursing requires more complex knowledge and is of greater value to society than tree trimming.

As a result of this suit, recognition of nursing's low pay was brought to public attention in such a way that support was mobilized for increasing nursing salaries. This was an example of political action by nurses that resulted in both **policy development** (supporting regulations that expanded comparable pay issues to other jobs) and **policy outcomes** (salary increases for the individual nurse).

"The Personal Is Political"

Women involved in the feminist movement in the 1960s coined the phrase "The personal is political." Those who invented this statement recognized that each individual, woman or man, could utilize personal experience to understand and become involved in broader social and political issues.

Prior to the social movements of the 1960s, most people believed that politics was impersonal. People were thought of as being political only if they joined a political group or became a politician. Defining politics on a personal level encouraged individuals to develop their own insights into how the world should be, what is fair or unfair, what can be contributed, and what can be changed. A personal view of politics gives people power to contribute to the community, the workplace, and the school.

This premise of personalizing the political process has become a foundational belief for organized nursing. The American Nurses Association (ANA) has been increasingly involved in legislation and electoral politics for the last 20 years. Not only do the ANA and its members, the state nursing associations, have government relations experts on their staffs, but most of the other major nursing organizations—such as the National League for Nursing, the American Association of Colleges of Nursing, and specialty nursing organizations—also engage in lobbying to advocate for the needs of their members and the public. Nursing leaders now recognize that "being political," both through professional associations and as individuals, is essential to the practice and promotion of nursing and is the responsibility of all professional nurses.

Politics and Power

All politics involve the concept of power. The questions, "Who makes decisions?" "How are those decisions made?" and "Who is impacted by the decisions?" could be rephrased as, "Who has the power?" "How is it used?" and "Who is affected?"

The word *power* has many meanings and, like **politics**, has had negative overtones. Power usually connotes influence, strength, and control. It involves a relationship between individuals or groups.

There are numerous kinds of power. There is **position power**, such as that inherent in being a dean, director of nursing, or chief executive of a company. There is **knowledge-based power**, such as the way information can be used by an expert to affect an outcome. There is power in numbers; a group is always more effective in creating influence than an individual. There is power related to wealth. And there has always been power accorded to whomever belongs to the dominant race, gender, or class of a community or nation.

Individuals who do not use the **inherent power** in a position are said to have latent power, because it is untapped. Nurses have latent power in terms of numbers. Although there are over 2 million nurses in the United States, nurses have traditionally not used the power of their numbers effectively. One in 44 women voters is a nurse. Just imagine how powerful nursing's voice could be if that power were used in a coordinated way in the voting booth.

The power of nursing knowledge has also been underused. No other group of health care providers spends as much time in direct patient contact as do nurses. Nurses know what patients need and can use this knowledge to develop policy for meeting those needs. Unfortunately, nurses have been slow to use their power. Nurses have gradually begun to believe in their expertise and are now participating in the development of health policies, sharing knowledge with legislators, and serving in community organizations to develop health services.

Historically, power has tended to connote a negative quality involving force and domination, particularly when related to women. Because of this, many women and many nurses resisted using the latent power they have always had. Yet power associated with maleness is usually perceived as a positive quality. This concept of linking positive or negative characteristics to males or females is known as **sex-role stereotyping.**

Power is neither good nor bad. It is how it is used that gives it value. If nurses use the power of persuasion to motivate patients to take prescribed medication, they are using the power of position and knowledge positively. If, on the other hand, they urge patients who are not well enough to get out of bed, they are using the power of position negatively.

Power is not given; it must be taken. It is the taking of power that converts latent power into action. Nurses are beginning to recognize that they can have power, that they must want it, and that they must use it. Use of power is a hallmark of political activity.

Just as there are sex-role differences in the perception of power, there are differences in the way women and men have traditionally used power. Miller (1976) notes that the traditional male model of power is called **power grabbing**. It involves hoarding power and control, taking it from others, or wielding it over others. Women more often use **power sharing**, which is a process of equalizing resources, knowledge, or control.

It is important to recognize that these two ways of using power are neither good nor bad. The most effective power brokers are those who can use both methods and know which is most effective for a particular situation.

The power of the media as a political tool is being used more effectively by the nursing profession. Because of the increased need for nurses in all aspects of health care delivery, the major nursing organizations in 1991 launched a national recruitment campaign through the print and electronic media. The ads depicted positive images of nursing and resulted in thousands of inquiries about nursing education programs. This instance of using the media to promote nursing's positive qualities provided political clout to the nursing profession. When nursing is viewed as a valuable but scarce commodity, the result has traditionally been increased government support. The power of positive images affects legislators as well as prospective students who are attracted to nursing.

Miss America of 1988, Kaye Lonnie Rae Rafko, was the first nurse to receive this title. In appearances throughout the country, she shared stories about her nursing practice in which she cared for people with cancer. She discussed her desire to return to school to become an oncology clinical specialist. She testified before Congress in support of increased funding for nursing education. This type of powerful image can result in increased power for nursing.

A Lesson in Civics Comes Alive

No American student escapes secondary school without one or more courses in civics or American government. Many students find these courses uninteresting and not relevant to their lives. To many adults, however, American government is vibrant and fascinating. Government is important to nursing and the other health professions and therefore deserving of a quick review.

The Three Branches of Government

The framers of the U.S. Constitution had a major objective—the **separation of powers**—to prevent the aggregation of power in any one person or branch of government. Thus, they set out a government with three branches—the legislative, executive, and judicial—and a mechanism of checks and balances for each. History reveals a waxing and waning of the powers of each branch over time, depending on the personalities of incumbents, contemporary social problems, and world events.

Under the Constitution, each branch of the federal government has separate and distinct functions and powers. The function of the **legislative branch** is to enact laws. Legislative powers include setting and collecting taxes, overseeing commerce, declaring war, defining criminal offenses, coining money, and amending the Constitution (just to name a few). The legislative branch is assumed to be closest to the people and more susceptible to change through social pressure (Congressional Quarterly 1983).

The **executive branch** of government's chief function is to administer the laws of the land. At the federal level, power is vested with the president, who has a wide variety of governmental departments and employees (the bureaucracy) to carry out executive functions. The president has extensive **powers of appointment** (judges, ambassadors, agency heads) and is commander in chief of the armed forces. The president can recommend legislation, give the State of the Union report, and most important as a balance, can approve or veto the legislation of Congress (Cournoyer 1989).

The role of the **judicial branch** is to **adjudicate,** or decide, "cases or controversies" on particular matters. The greatest power of the courts is to provide judicial review over governmental activities to uphold the privileges of the Constitution. The Supreme Court is the ultimate legal authority of the land and can review decisions from lower courts.

The **balance of power** among the three branches of government is illustrated in Figure 22–1. Notice that all three branches are involved in the legislative process.

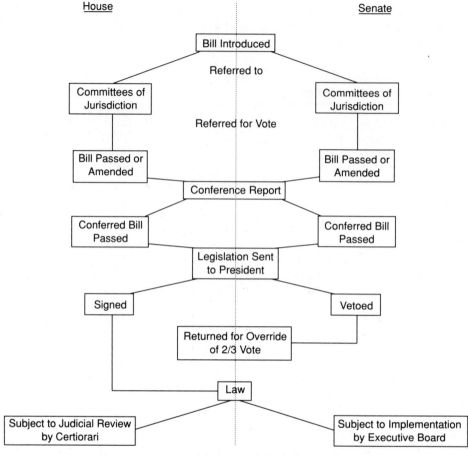

Figure 22–1 Legislation and the balance of power.

Three Levels of Government

Government in the United States is organized at federal, state, and local levels. The Constitution established the relative powers of federal and state governments and the rights of the individual person. The Constitution identified specific powers of the federal government (matters of national interest needing uniform policies) while reserving all other powers for the states. States in turn have developed their own constitutions and delineated power relationships with local communities and between branches of state government.

Exclusive powers of the federal government include declaring war, making treaties, administering postal services, and developing foreign relationships. State and local governments can tax and spend, maintain internal order, regulate domestic relationships, and promote health and safety.

All levels of government are expected to maintain their activities within the parameters of the Constitution. The Bill of Rights serves to promote and protect the rights of the individual from governmental intrusion.

The Electoral Process

The process of electing public officials to office is known as the **electoral process.** Governmental elections for the most part focus on selecting local, state, and federal legislators and executive branch leaders such as the president, governor, and mayor. Federal judgeships are appointed, although some state judges are elected by the people in certain jurisdictions.

Lack of voter participation is a source of frustration for anyone helping to support candidates get elected. In 1988, only half of the eligible voters voted in the presidential election. In 1990, only 36 percent of voters cast a vote. One of the reasons suggested for the low turnouts is the obstacle of registering to vote. As a result, new laws are being passed at the state and federal levels that would make the process easier and more accessible. The convenience of "motor-voter registration," which is automatic registration at the same time as car registration; on-site registration at the time of voting; and mail registration at social service and health centers are some of the solutions used in different states.

The process of getting elected to office occurs primarily through the two major parties—the Democratic and Republican parties. There are third parties that have become active in different regions at different times. Some of the more familiar third parties are the Liberal, the Right to Life, Conservative, Green, Socialist, Communist, and Rainbow Coalition parties. None have yet played a major role in electing candidates.

In most states, citizens must declare party affiliation when registering to vote. U.S. electoral politics is largely dominated by a two-party system consisting of the Democrats and the Republicans. There are three major types of elections: primary elections, general elections, and referendums.

Primary elections are those in which a party is choosing among several internal candidates for a particular office. The outcome of primary elections is that a party's candidate for a particular office is selected. In most states, voters may only vote in the primary of the party in which they registered.

In **general elections**, all registered voters may vote. They need not vote a "straight party ticket"; that is, the voter can choose a candidate from any party on the ballot. Unless there is a tie or a challenge to the general election, the outcome is the selection of a governmental official such as a governor, senator, or president.

A **referendum** occurs when the registered voters are asked to express a preference on a policy issue that has been referred to the public by a legislative body. For example, a local city council may seek a referendum on raising property taxes to support school reform.

It is essential to know the basic electoral rules if one is working on a campaign, raising money for a candidate, or considering running for office. Rules vary from locality to locality. Information is available through local boards of election.

Health Care Legislation/Regulating Issues

Impact for Nursing

Many issues facing nursing professionals can best be addressed through government. The key questions for nurses to ask when seeking governmental intervention to improve nursing practice and health care are: "Where can I play?" and "Where can I win?" There are local, state, and federal courts, all of which require standing (a *material* interest in the outcome of a case) in order to seek a judicial remedy. There are mayors, governors, presidents, their staffs, and department heads who make key decisions about how to implement (or not implement) health policy.

Historically, nurses have sought legislative remedies for changes in health care policy. This is because nurses have learned to be effective with legislative branch relationships. We need to broaden our focus to include the other two branches more effectively.

There have been three major eras in health policy development in the United States. As you learned in Chapter 14, the era extending from post–World War II through the 1960s served to dramatically increase health services and expand capacity. The 1970s and 1980s focused on concerns about escalating costs, and the current era, the 1990s, is focusing on attempts to enhance or ensure quality while attending to access and cost issues.

Unfortunately the nursing profession was not well organized politically during the time of expanding capacity and access. Despite being the only health provider group in favor of the Medicare/Medicaid programs of the 1960s, nurses were not included as reimbursable providers. Times have changed, however. Women and nurses have increased their political savvy, and through the well-orchestrated efforts of the ANA, state nurses associations (SNAs), and their **political action committees** (PACs), nurses are now participating effectively in both governmental and electoral politics (Goldwater and Zusy 1991). PACs raise and distribute money to candidates who support the organization's stand on certain issues.

IMPACTING LEGISLATION

Nurses can make a difference in health policy outcomes. Through governmental politics, nurses impact the policy process by identifying health problems as policy problems, by developing policy formulations through suggested legislation and formal testimony, by lobbying governmental officials both in the executive and legislative branches for making certain health policies a priority for action, and by filing suit as a party or as a friend of the court in order to implement health policy strategies on behalf of consumers.

Capitol Update, a newsletter published by the ANA, reports on the progress in nursing's influence with members of Congress, their staffs, and the regulatory agencies that set policy for health programs. Such activity reflects the work of both paid nursing lobbyists and nurses' volunteer efforts. The activity in Washington, D.C., is mirrored throughout the nation as state nurses associations conduct similar work with state governments.

Organized activity in identifying, financially supporting, and working for candidates who are committed to nursing and "nurse-friendly" issues has dramatically increased in the last decade. Again, this is a combined staff and volunteer function of the professional association.

Individual nurses can make a difference in policy development, in elections, and in many other effective ways but in no way more crucially than in becoming a policymaker himself or herself. Either by election or by appointment, nurses need to be *making* health decisions—not just influencing them. Getting elected or getting appointed requires visibility, expertise, energy, risk taking, and also a view of how very important policy and politics are to achieve nursing's health objectives.

Getting Nurses Appointed

Becoming a policymaker involves either running for office or being appointed to office. Appointments are made by the chief executive of a city, county, state, or the nation. They are usually made in response not only to the expertise and visibility of the individual appointee but also as a result of that appointee's membership in an organization active in the election of the particular chief executive making the appointment (Kalisch and Kalisch 1982).

Many boards, commissions, and government posts are open to executive appointment, and nurses who are active in their professional organization's political activities should seek such appointments. State boards of nursing, through rules and regulations, make definitive health and nursing policy. They are usually appointed by governors.

Working in a gubernatorial campaign through the state nurses association or through the candidate's party is an avenue to board of nursing appointments. Boards of health, health care facilities, human services, and others all use similar processes of appointment and could benefit from nursing expertise.

Getting Involved

Nurses can become involved in the political process in a variety of ways. Three levels of involvement can be termed involvement as a nurse citizen, as a nurse activist, or as a nurse politician. Each level will be discussed briefly.

The Nurse Citizen

A **nurse citizen** is not just any citizen. The nurse citizen brings the perspective of health care to the voting booth, to public forums that advocate for health and human services, and to involvement in community activities. For example, budget cuts to a school district might involve elimination of school nurses. At a school board meeting, nurses can effectively speak about the vital role that school nurses provide to the health of children and the cost-effectiveness of maintaining the position.

Nurses tend to vote for candidates who advocate for improved health care. Here are some examples of how nurses can be politically active:

Box 22–1   Communication Is the Key to Influence

Cultivate a relationship with policymakers from your home district.

Communicate by visits, telephone, letters.

Letters need these elements:

- Use personal stationery.
- State who you are (a nurse and a voter).
- Identify the issue by a file number, if possible.

- Be clear on where you stand and why.
- Be positive when possible.
- Be clear.
- Give your return address and phone number to urge a dialogue.
- Follow up with calls or letters.

Be quick to thank and praise when policymakers do something you like.

- Register to vote.
- Vote in every election.
- Keep informed about health care issues.
- Speak out when services are inadequate.
- Participate in public forums.
- Know your local, state, and federal elected officials.
- Join professional nursing organizations.
- Participate in community organizations that need health experts.
- Join a political party.

Once nurses make a decision to become involved politically, they need to learn how to get started. One of the best ways is to form a relationship with one or more policymakers. Box 22–1 contains several pointers for influencing policymakers.

The Nurse Activist

The **nurse activist** takes a more active role than the nurse citizen and often does so because an issue arises that directly impacts the nurse's professional or personal life. It is the need to respond that moves the nurse to a more active level of participation. For example, a nurse in private practice who has difficulty getting private insurance companies to honor patients' claims for reimbursement may become active in lobbying state legislators for changes in insurance regulations.

Nurse activists can make changes by:

- Contacting a public official through letters, telegrams, or phone calls.
- Registering people to vote.

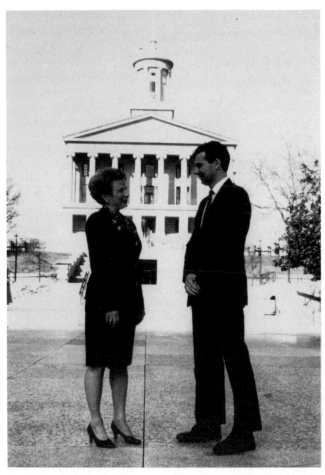

The nurse activitist has a high level of involvement in selected political issues.
(Courtesy of *Tennessee Nurse, photograph by Chip Powell.*)

- Contributing money to a political campaign.
- Working in a campaign.
- Becoming an active party member.
- Lobbying decision makers.
- Forming or joining coalitions that support an issue of concern.
- Writing letters to the editor of local papers.
- Inviting legislators to visit the workplace.
- Holding a media event to publicize an issue.
- Providing or giving testimony.

Some pointers on how to make a difference in health policy development are included in Box 22–2.

Box 22–2 Key Questions for Nurses Who Want to Make a Difference in Health Policy

1. *Know the system.* Is it a federal, state, or local issue? Is it in the hands of the executive, legislative, or judicial branch of government?
2. *Know the issue.* What is wrong? What should happen? Why is it not happening? What is needed: leadership, a plan, pressure, data?
3. *Know the players.* Who is on your side and who is not? Who will make the decision? Who knows whom?

Will a coalition be effective? Are you a member of the nursing professional organization?
4. *Know the process.* Is this a vote? Is this an appropriation? Is this a policy procedure? Is this a committee or subcommittee report?
5. *Know what to do.* Should you write, call, go to lunch, organize a petition, show up at the hearing, give testimony, demonstrate, file a suit?

The Nurse Politician

Once a nurse realizes and experiences the empowerment that can come from political activism, some choose to run for office. No longer satisfied to help others get elected, the **nurse politician** desires to develop the legislation, not just influence it.

In 1992, there were more than 50 nurse legislators in state government, 3 nurses running for Congress, numerous local mayors, city council members, and hundreds of nurses appointed to governmental regulatory agencies. These include 4 nurses heading state health departments in Hawaii, Oregon, Michigan, and Washington.

Nurse politicians utilize their knowledge about people, their expertise about health, their ability to communicate effectively, and their superb organizational skills in running for office. Because the public places a high value on nurses, nurse politicians are trusted. If nurses know how to run a campaign, they stand a good chance of being elected.

Once nurses are elected, they can be expected to sponsor legislation that reflects their professional experiences. Many of the laws that expand reimbursement for nursing services, funding for services to women and children, occupational and safety issues, and research on women's health have been sponsored by nurse legislators and supported by nurses working as key legislative staff members.

The nurse politician must be ready to sacrifice a regular schedule and personal privacy as well as have adequate financial resources to run for office.

Research Note

How politically active are nurses? Theresa Gesse, a certified nurse-midwife and professor of nursing wondered how active her fellow midwives were in the political arena, so she designed a study to answer that question. Dr. Gesse conducted a national survey of the members of the American College of Nurse-Midwives (ACNM). She randomly selected a 600 person sample and sent them a questionnaire about their political activities. Nearly 60 percent returned the questionnaires. Their answers indicated that nurse-midwives tended to be Democrats, liberal in their beliefs, and that they believed people like themselves can influence the political process. They were particularly in-terested in women's issues. Nearly three-quarters were involved in the statewide chapters of ACNM. They tended to feel that the ACNM should increase its political activity, but were not heavily involved in political activity themselves, except for voting. Gesse wondered if these nurses were depending on professional associations instead of being individually involved. She recommended that nurse-midwives assume responsibility for political involvement as individuals "beginning at the local, grassroots level."

(From Gesse, T. (1991). Political participation behaviors of nurse-midwives. *Journal of Nurse-Midwifery,* 36(3), 184–191. Reprinted by permission.)

Fortunately, more nurses are willing to make this commitment because they believe in their own power and ability to enhance the well-being of the public.

The nurse politician can:

• Run for an elected office.
• Seek appointment to a regulatory agency.
• Be appointed to a governing board in the public or private sector.

We Were All Once Novices

Nurses who have achieved success as leaders started with no knowledge of the political process and no expectation of the greatness they would achieve. Instead, they became involved because some issue, some injustice, or some abuse of power impacted on their lives. Instead of complaining or feeling helpless, they responded by taking an active role in bringing about change.

The mark of a leader is the ability to identify a problem, have a goal, and know how to join others in reaching that goal. A leader must know how to ask the right questions, analyze the positive and restraining forces toward meeting the goal, and know how to get and use power. A leader must know how to ask for help and how to give support to those who join the effort. These are the marks of nursing leaders who have been political experts.

A Nurse Who Knew How to Use Political Power

Florence Nightingale, the mother of modern nursing, was the consummate political woman. Her story exemplifies how she learned to use her skills and power to bring about revolutionary change to health care in the nineteenth century. She never anticipated that she would achieve greatness, least of all as a nurse, a life-style society considered demeaning to a woman of her intellectual and social standing.

Florence Nightingale received an exemplary education in the classics but was frustrated and depressed by the prospect of a life of parties and social restrictions accorded to upper-class women of her time. She sought the advice of family friend and physician Dr. Samuel G. Ridley Howe about how to fulfill her desire to serve humanity. He believed that women should be able to achieve what men could and encouraged her to seek an apprenticeship as a nurse at a hospital in Germany. After a three-month educational program, she was asked to serve as superintendent of two hospitals in London.

When the Crimean War broke out, she was asked by her friend Sir Sidney Herbert, the secretary of war, to organize a contingent of nurses and travel to Scutari, Turkey, to supervise a military hospital. Overcoming the distrust and incredible obstacles placed in her path by military physicians, she was able to revolutionize the military sanitation system and health care of British soldiers, proving the value of nurses in wartime.

After the war, using money raised to honor her achievements, she established the Nightingale Training School for Nurses in London. This was the first independent and formal nursing curriculum in the Western world.

Although ill health meant that she never again appeared in public, she completed reform of the British health care system, reformed the Indian health care system, established public health nursing, and continued to oversee the Nightingale schools of nursing—all from her bed.

You might wonder how she did this. The answer is that she did it through her own incredible determination and the support of powerful friends in government. She was a strong-willed person, with social and financial power. She had an excellent education and sought theoretical knowledge as well as practical experience to learn about care of the sick. She developed and nurtured connections to powerful men, since there were few powerful women at the time, other than Queen Victoria. She sought their support and in turn supported them when they needed her help.

Nightingale's goals changed as new problems arose because she recognized that being adaptable is also a characteristic of leadership. In essence, she used her public support, her connections to people in powerful positions, and her intellectual skills to reach an unparalleled position of leadership. As a result, she was able to gain personal power and move health care into the modern era.

Nursing Awaits Your Contribution

You can apply the skills discussed in this chapter. Look to teachers, family, friends, and community leaders whom you admire. What are the qualities they possess that you wish to have? Your role models can serve as inspiration for you to imitate.

You may also choose to form a relationship with a political mentor. A mentor is not only a role model but actively teaches, encourages, and critiques the process of growth and change in the learner. All nurses who have become political leaders have found mentors along the way to guide and support their growth. Your mentor could be a faculty member, such as the adviser to the student nurse organization or honor society, who can teach you leadership skills. Ask for help in running for a class office or student council president. If elected office doesn't appeal to you, use your political skills to develop a school or community project with other nursing students.

You may have a relative or friend involved in a political campaign who could help you learn about the political process. You might find a problem during a clinical experience that inhibits your ability to provide necessary care or the level of care that you wish. Seek a faculty member or nurse in the clinical facility who can guide you through the process of change.

Watch the communication skills of your role models or mentors. How does your own behavior compare with theirs? What enhances or impedes your progress? Get your friends and peers to join your activity. Seek their help and support. Always thank them and be ready to offer your help and support when they need it.

CHAPTER SUMMARY

Professional organizations and professional nurses have much to offer in formulating policy decisions at all levels of government and in each branch. Nursing—once called "the sleeping giant of the health care industry"—is no longer sleeping. Today organized nursing is involved in politics at many levels in promoting:

1. *Nursing's Agenda for Health Care Reform*, discussed in Chapter 4.
2. Reimbursement for professional nurses at federal, state, and local levels.
3. Expanding the scope of nursing practice.
4. Protection of the civil and privacy rights of clients, for example, in the areas of abortion rights, HIV/AIDS (human immunodeficiency virus/acquired immunodeficiency syndrome), and the terminally ill.
5. Prevention services and primary care services for women, children, and the elderly.

The list is almost limitless. The roles and opportunities for women and nurses in the field of policy development and politics are changing, and nursing can benefit from this "window of opportunity." Having more nurses involved in policy development and politics will be good for nursing and for the nation.

Once you realize that becoming politically active is as easy as signing your name in support of an issue, registering to vote, organizing a project, or speaking out on an issue, you will have started your political education. You will feel empowered. You will realize how important you can be—how *you* can make a difference. All of us, as nurses and as recipients of health care, will be better for your involvement.

REVIEW/DISCUSSION QUESTIONS

1. Conduct a class poll. Of those in the class who are eligible to vote, how many are registered? How many voted in the last local, state, or national election? Challenge those not registered to become registered before the end of the current school term.
2. List three types of power. How can nurses use these types of power in behalf of their profession and the health care system?
3. Since nurses have differing personal and political values, it has been a challenge to get them all united behind a single issue or candidate. If you were the president of the American Nurses Association, what techniques would you use to persuade the 2 million American nurses of the power of their numbers?
4. What types of political issues should nurses take a particular interest in? Do you see signs that nurses are actively involved in these issues in your community?
5. Find out whether the members of your state board of nursing are elected or appointed. What is the makeup of the board (how many registered nurses, licensed practical nurses, consumers, and so forth)? Do nurses hold most of the seats on the state board? Are there any other health professionals such as physicians on the board of nursing? If so, are there any nurses on the state board of medicine?

REFERENCES

Congressional Quarterly, Inc. (1983). *How Congress works.* Washington, D.C.: Author.

Cournoyer, C. (1989). *The nurse manager and the law.* Rockville, MD: Aspen.

Goldwater, M., and Zusy, M. J. (1991). *Prescription for nurses: Effective political action.* St. Louis: C.V. Mosby.

Kalisch, B., and Kalisch, P. (1982). *Politics of nursing.* Philadelphia: J.B. Lippincott.

Mason, D., Talbott, S., and Leavitt, J. (Eds.). (1993). *Policy and politics for nurses: Action and change in the workplace, government, organizations, and community* (2nd ed.). Philadelphia: W.B. Saunders.

Miller, J. B. (1976). *Towards a new psychology for women.* Boston: Beacon Press.

SUGGESTED READINGS

Mason, D. J., Becker, B., and Georges, C. (1991). Towards a feminist model for the political empowerment of nurses. *Image*, 23(3), 72–77.

Northrup, C., and Kelly, M. (1987). *Legal issues in nursing.* St. Louis: C.V. Mosby.

Chapter

23 *Nursing's Future Challenges*

Kay K. Chitty

CHAPTER OBJECTIVES

What students should be able to do after studying this chapter:

1. Review societal influences on the nursing profession anticipated during the next decade.

2. Recognize the impact that changes in the health care system will have on the practice of nursing.

3. Explain trends in nursing education needed to meet society's future nursing needs.

VOCABULARY BUILDING

Terms to know:

birthrate	epidemiologist	morbidity rate
centenarian	euthanasia	mortality rate
cultural diversity	futurist	nursing informatics
demography	heterogeneous	shared governance
differentiated practice	homogeneous	urbanization
disenfranchised	managed care	

*A*s seen throughout this textbook, the profession of nursing is profoundly affected by changes in society and in the world. As we look toward the twenty-first century, it seems clear that nursing again faces many challenges, as it has in the past. The challenges nurses face relate to a variety of factors: changes in demographics, unhealthy life-styles of many Americans, the deterioration of the environment, a maturing economy that can no longer support rapidly increasing health care costs, and the politicizing and regulation of health care.

The World Health Organization (WHO) has set an idealistic goal: health for all by the year 2000. Even though the United States is the wealthiest of the industrialized nations, it falls far short of this goal. Millions of Americans have no health insurance, and most have less than enough. Infant mortality rates are unacceptably high; among industrialized nations, the United States ranked twenty-fourth in 1989, just behind New Zealand (MacDorman 1992). We spend the highest percentage (12 percent) of our gross national product (GNP) for health of any nation in the world. As a rule, however, Americans are disgruntled with the health care system as it exists and believe it requires a complete over-haul to correct its shortcomings (Styles 1990).

Chapter 3 reviewed the high levels of respect and public confidence that nurses currently enjoy. Chapter 4 described the remarkable unified effort of 65 nursing organizations that led to the development of *Nursing's Agenda for Health Care Reform*. And Chapter 14 reviewed past and present methods of funding the nation's health care. This chapter will explore some of nursing's challenges and opportunities in the twenty-first century.

A challenge to nursing was articulated by Emily Friedman in a 1990 article in the *Journal of the American Medical Association*:

> The history of American nursing is not an entirely happy story, yet it is anything but a tale of failure. . . . Without all [its] battles, nursing would not now be in the position it holds: that of a profession in heavy demand, with more autonomy than ever, in an age more receptive to women [*editor's note*: and to men in nursing] than any in history. Nursing, more than at any point in its history, has the chance to exercise enormous power in society. The question is whether it can or will. (p. 2858)

Societal Challenges

At least five societal influences are expected to have major impact on the future of the nursing profession: demographic changes, environmental deterioration, unhealthy life-styles and resulting illnesses, economics of health care, and the politicization and regulation of health care. Each of these influences will be examined briefly.

Demographic Challenges

Demography is the science that studies vital statistics and social trends. Demographers look at **birthrates** (births per thousand people), **morbidity** (illness)

rates, mortality (deaths) **rates**, marriages, the ages of various populations, and migration patterns. From this wealth of information, **futurists,** people who predict what will occur, draw conclusions about what these trends mean for the future.

Four trends detected by demographers are particularly important to the future of nursing: rising numbers of elderly people, continuing increase in poverty in America, an increase in cultural diversity in the population, and a continuing trend toward urbanization. Each has implications for nursing.

RISING NUMBERS OF ELDERLY

Estimates vary, but demographers have predicted that the number of people between the ages of 65 and 74 in the United States by the year 2000 will exceed 18 million. The number of elderly people over age 75 is expected to exceed 16 million more, for a total of more than 35 million people aged 65 or older (U.S. Bureau of the Census 1990). **Centenarians**, that group of people over 100 years of age, is one of the fastest-growing groups in the nation. Many older people are healthy, but the likelihood of illness becomes greater as people age. Clearly, nurses of the future must be prepared to work effectively with rising numbers of elderly patients. Ethical issues such as **euthanasia** (mercy killing) will become increasingly important as technology enables people to sustain life far beyond the point of useful and meaningful existence.

CONTINUING POVERTY

The number of Americans living below the poverty line is increasing, particularly among children and the elderly. When basic needs for food, clothing, and shelter are unmet or uncertain, health care becomes a luxury. Children's immunizations, prenatal care for pregnant women, nutritious meals, and a variety of other health-maintaining factors are neglected. Poor people tend to put off seeking care until illness is advanced—and thus harder to treat. Preventable conditions are often not prevented due to lack of education, lack of sanitation, crowded living conditions, improper shelter, homelessness, and a host of other poverty-related factors. Poverty will continue to create increasing numbers of **disenfranchised** people, that is, people who have no power in the political system, with limited access to health care. Nursing, as a profession, is committed to providing nursing care to all people, regardless of social and economic factors. The combination of the shortage of nurses and increasing numbers of medically disenfranchised people threatens to make that commitment an unrealistic one.

INCREASING CULTURAL DIVERSITY

Cultural diversity refers to the array of people from different racial, religious, social, and geographic backgrounds who make up a particular entity. Some countries, such as Japan, are very **homogeneous** in culture. This means the citizens have very similar cultural beliefs and practices. Others, such as the United States, have a very **heterogeneous** cultural mix. This means the cultural beliefs and practices of the citizens are quite different.

Immigration to the United States from Southeast Asia, Central America, Mexico, and the Caribbean Islands has increased in recent years as a result of civil unrest, wars, and poor economic conditions. This is but the latest wave of newcomers to the United States in addition to European Americans, African Americans, and others whose ancestors came to this country earlier. Each group has its own health beliefs, folk remedies, and conventional wisdom about health and sickness. Nurses increasingly need to take these beliefs into consideration when planning and implementing nursing care for individuals of diverse cultural backgrounds. The nursing profession itself will become increasingly diverse as its members reflect the diversity of the larger society.

CONTINUING URBANIZATION

Urbanization, that is, people moving from rural, farming areas to cities, has increased since the time of the industrial revolution. That trend continues today and is expected to continue in the future. As cities grow, suburbs flourish, and most people who can afford to do so move away from the industrial centers of cities. Decaying inner cities with large populations of poor people create major social problems such as homelessness, drugs, gangs, single-parent households, mental illness, violence, and crime. These phenomena spill over into the suburbs and rural areas, creating further social change. Nurses of the future will be increasingly confronted with the health problems created by these social phenomena.

Environmental Deterioration

Every newspaper, news magazine, and television news program brings new and disturbing reports of the deterioration of our environment. Major environmental tragedies, such as the nuclear power plant accident at Chernobyl and 200 burning oil wells in Kuwait, overshadow the less dramatic but insidious gradual decline in the quality of the world's air, water, plant, and animal life. Acute and chronic respiratory diseases are increasing, as are cancers of all types. Stories about the depletion of the ozone layer, accidental lead and mercury poisonings, pesticides spilling into streams and rivers, and the accidental release of radioactive steam from nuclear power plants are commonplace. **Epidemiologists** (people who study how diseases are caused) believe there is a relationship between environmental decline and increases in certain diseases.

Humans are responsible for destroying the environment, and the more human beings there are, the faster the environment will decline. Overpopulation contributes to the deterioration of the world's environment, yet few countries are dealing effectively with issues of overpopulation. The related problems of environmental deterioration and overpopulation are health care issues that future nurses will undoubtedly have to face.

Unhealthy Life-Styles

In spite of the focus on wellness in modern American society, unhealthy life-styles still predominate; this trend is expected to continue. There are more obese

Americans than ever before, even though obesity is known to predispose people to a number of illnesses. Futurists predict that Americans will eat more meals in restaurants in the future, but ordering a nutritious, well-balanced meal in a fast-food restaurant is a major challenge, even to those people with a working knowledge of nutritional science.

As a result of pressure from health-conscious consumers, some of the larger restaurant chains have introduced salads, grilled chicken sandwiches, and other "low-fat" items. On close examination, however, the fat content of some of these foods is still unacceptably high. And the majority of the regular menu items are still loaded with animal fats, long known to cause cardiovascular disease, and sodium, known to aggravate a variety of health conditions.

Yet another life-style issue is tobacco use. Smoking will increase among the young, especially young females and minorities, both of whom are targeted for increased marketing by the tobacco companies. For years, smoking has been known to cause lung cancer, emphysema and other chronic lung diseases, low birthweight babies, and a host of other health problems. In the next decade the incidence of lung cancer in older women will exceed breast cancer as years of smoking take their inevitable toll. Smokeless tobacco use will rise, creating unhealthy oral mucous membranes and predisposing users to oral cancer.

Lack of exercise is another life-style issue for Americans of the future, particularly the young. The ready availability of entertainment on television is at least partly to blame. Studies show the more television people of all ages watch, the more they are likely to gain weight. Snacking and television watching go hand in hand. Entire generations of Americans, raised watching several hours of television each day, are unlikely to give up the habit in the future.

Lack of exercise is not limited to the young, however. For every middle-aged jogger seen pounding the roadways, legions of sedentary adults remain unseen at home, gradually becoming less and less fit and more susceptible to disease. Browsing through mail-order catalogs aimed at the affluent middle-aged population reveals a plethora of labor-saving devices being developed and marketed to make Americans even less active in the future.

Advertising affects yet another life-style risk factor. With the emphasis on thinness in fashion advertising, many girls and young women resort to unhealthy habits such as starving or binging and purging. Rather than eating sensibly and engaging in exercise to maintain normal weights, they assume bizarre eating habits in the pursuit of the fashionable, if unnatural, degree of gauntness. Barring a dramatic change in the fashion industry, eating disorders and their resulting health hazards will continue to increase.

Another life-style issue is stress. The rapid pace of modern life creates stress, yet Americans continue to step up the pace with cellular telephones, fax machines, satellite communications, personal computers, paging devices, "call-waiting" options, and all the other fruits of modern technology. Although many Americans mourn the loss of leisure time, indications are that when given more leisure time, many people spend it working. This evidence indicates that stress-related diseases will increase in the next decade and beyond.

The twin epidemics of acquired immunodeficiency syndrome (AIDS) and drug abuse are two related life-style issues that will profoundly affect the future of nursing. When the AIDS epidemic began in this country in the early 1980s, most of those affected were homosexual men. A few years later, infection rates among intravenous drug users began to rise. By the mid-1980s AIDS moved into the general population of heterosexual adults, a trend already seen in other countries and certain to rise in the United States. Another trend, already beginning, is the spread to adolescents. Although optimists in the medical community predict a vaccine against human immunodeficiency virus (HIV) in the next decade, millions of Americans are already infected, and no cure is on the horizon. Substance-abusing people suffer more accidents and illness than their non-abusing counterparts, thus requiring more medical and nursing care. People with AIDS also require intensive nursing care, particularly during outbreaks of opportunistic infections such as pneumonias.

Nurses' own life-style choices will come under scrutiny as the issue of HIV infection in physicians, dentists, nurses, and other health care workers will become a larger focus of public concern. Nurses will be involved in the development of sound public policies concerning these issues.

Given the predominance of these unhealthy life-style factors, it is clear that nurses will play an increasingly important role in educating people about wellness and self-care in the decade ahead. Nurses will also be instrumental in educating the public about how to be informed consumers of health care services. And nurses will provide nursing care in acute care settings, such as hospitals, to those who choose not to listen.

Rising Costs of Health Care

Every year for several decades the federal budget deficit has reached "an all-time high." There is apparently no end in sight to the nation's spendthrift habits. At federal, state, and local levels, governments are spending more money than is generated through taxes. The pressure for health care creates a significant part of these budgetary problems.

Society's poor, homeless, elderly, substance abusers, AIDS patients, and mentally ill are increasing in number, and all need care. How can we pay for it now and in the future when the numbers are expected to increase?

In many states, Medicaid is already the largest and fastest-growing single state expense. If the nation's economy continues to be flat, more and more families will become eligible for Medicaid coverage, compounding the problem.

The aging of America will continue to create huge numbers of Social Security— and Medicare-eligible citizens. The decrease in the ratio of these individuals to the number of those working and paying Social Security and income taxes will place an additional burden on the federal government's budget in the foreseeable future.

The next decade will see hospitals closing in record numbers, pressure from the business community forcing changes in health care, and the institution of some form of national health insurance. The nursing profession stands to benefit from these phenomena, since nursing has been shown to be a cost-conscious yet high-quality alternative to traditional medical care (Maraldo 1991). In addition, nurses are well equipped to provide **managed care** (making sure that certain people get certain services at the best price). As a profession, nursing is expected to benefit from the nation's health care woes by expanding roles in prevention and community health centers (Maraldo 1992).

One cost-effective method of providing basic health care to children is through school nurses. As the burden of providing care continues to shift from federal agencies to state and local agencies, local school boards will recognize the economies to be realized through school nursing. The 1990s will see a dramatic rise in state-mandated health services for schoolchildren. These services will be delivered largely by school nurses (Moccia 1992).

Politicization and Regulation of Health Care

Spiraling health care costs will force increasing regulation of health care in the future, and nurses will become increasingly active in developing health policy. *Nursing's Agenda for Health Care Reform* (see Chapter 4) is one example of how nurses will use their political activism to improve access, guality, and value in the delivery of health services. Legislation mandating the direct reimbursement of nurses for their services will become commonplace, despite the opposition of organized medicine and hospital administration.

Nursing, through its professional associations, will become a powerful player in the nation's health care politics. Nurses will form coalitions with consumer groups, such as the American Association of Retired Persons (AARP), to influence consumer-friendly legislation at state and national levels. As described in Chapter 22, individual nurses will become politically active as voters, campaign workers, community health activists, and political candidates.

As nursing's public profile becomes higher, public scrutiny of the profession will increase. Consumers of nursing services will exercise *their* political power to pressure nursing to provide first-class health care.

Challenges in Nursing Practice

The societal changes just reviewed will necessarily create changes in nursing practice. Nurses in the next decade will face an ever-widening array of practice opportunities both within and outside traditional health care settings, such as hospitals.

Continued Shortages

Home care will continue to expand as cost-effective home care technologies come on stream. School nurses will be needed in large numbers. The demand for nurses will continue to outstrip the supply. There is no end in sight to the increasing opportunities for nurses; therefore, the supply of nurses will remain inadequate to meet the demand.

The Bureau of Labor Statistics predicts that by the year 2000, 350,000 new jobs for registered nurses will be created. As opportunities for nurses increase, employment benefits and the conditions under which nurses work also will improve as employers compete with each other for nurse employees. Flexible scheduling and job sharing will become commonplace. These initiatives will enable nurses who have not been practicing due to the demands of family life to return to practice and will attract to the profession others seeking such flexibility.

Cost Containment

Cost containment initiatives in hospitals will eliminate layers of middle management, creating a stronger voice for nurses involved in direct patient care. Cost containment measures will also require nurses to demonstrate the cost-effectiveness of nursing care. The "bottom line" will be an increasing focus of concern in the nursing office as well as in the financial affairs office.

Autonomy and Accountability

Shared governance (participation by nurses on strong policy-making hospital committees) is a trend already seen and mandated by accreditation bodies such as the Joint Commission on the Accreditation of Healthcare Organizations (JCAHO). Along with the empowerment of nurses, however, will come increased demand for accountability. Effective nursing care will be measured by patient outcomes. Continuous quality improvement of nursing care will be emphasized more than ever. Nurses must be ready to show evidence that the care they provide makes a demonstrable difference in patient outcomes.

As middle management declines and nursing becomes a stronger voice in hospitals, nursing administrators will become more closely aligned with nursing and less dependent on the nonnursing administrative bureaucracy for power. This reunification of nursing managers and bedside nurses will strengthen the profession even further.

Technology

Technology will continue to advance at a dizzying pace. **Nursing informatics,** the organization and use of nursing data, will change nursing practice dramatically. Portable intelligence devices (computers) will be used by all professional nurses. These devices will allow immediate access to all patient data needed in refining the plan of care. In addition, voice-activated bedside computers will allow nurses to record patient information literally "at the bedside," rather than making written notes and transferring them to the patient's chart at a later time.

Nurses will continue to fight the tendency technological advances, such as patient monitoring devices, have of dehumanizing patients. Nurses will continue to value and provide a humanizing, "high-touch" environment.

Nurses will realize that advanced technology and traditional nursing values are not mutually exclusive. Patients can have both if nurses stay patient centered rather than machine or monitor centered.

Advances in technology will continue to bring new ethical dilemmas. Nurses will be more active in exploring ethical aspects of patient care and will sit on ethics committees in hospitals, formerly the exclusive domain of physicians and health care ethicists.

Differentiated Practice

Levels of nursing practice will become more clearly differentiated. **Differentiated practice** means that nurses prepared in associate degree, baccalaureate degree, and higher degree programs will have different, well-defined roles. The competencies of nurses at each level will be clearly demonstrated. Employers will understand the differences, and patient care delivery systems will be reorganized to capitalize on the strengths of each.

Practice in Nontraditional Settings

More nurses will practice in the community and in nontraditional settings such as nurse-managed clinics. Nurse entrepreneurship will flourish in the future owing to the resourcefulness and self-confidence of nurses and to the trust the public places in the nursing profession. Increasing numbers of nurses will own clinics and other health-related businesses, such as free-standing wellness programs, dialysis care services, and worksite health programs.

Challenges in Nursing Education

As the next decade sees nursing practice become more exciting and autonomous than ever, the need for strong, differentiated educational preparation of nurses at all levels will be crucial. More nurses will recognize the value of bachelor's degrees for beginning professional practice and master's degrees for specialty practice. More will pursue doctoral degrees to prepare for research and theory development. In response, colleges of nursing will expand flexible educational programs to improve access. They will also develop differentiated levels of nursing education that correspond to differentiated levels of practice.

Outcome-Based Education

Just as nursing practice will be challenged to measure patient outcomes, nursing education will be challenged to develop student competencies. The quality of educational programs will be judged by student outcomes, that is, what students actually can do as a result of education. Schools of nursing will monitor their graduates' activities and achievements as practicing nurses to determine how successful their educational programs have been. The emphasis on accountability of schools of nursing will increase as measures of competence in graduates are refined. Substandard schools will be closed (Maraldo 1992).

Diversity

Nursing students will reflect the nation's demographics and become more diverse than ever before. More minorities, men, older students, and students with degrees in other fields will come into nursing because of the emotional rewards, financial security, and professional image it offers. Access to education for nontraditional and traditional students will become an issue. Schools will expand nontraditional curricula that enable adults to work and go to school simultaneously. Nursing courses delivered via telecommunications and satellite linkages will increase access for students living in remote areas.

Changes in demographics will impact the content of school curricula as well as the methods by which it is delivered. As school nurse programs in the nation's public schools expand, the need for nurses prepared in this long-neglected specialty will give rise to new programs at both the undergraduate and graduate levels. Schools of nursing will develop and expand multicultural courses. International educational opportunities will increase as boundaries between nations blur in the first post–cold war decade.

Technology and the Knowledge Explosion

Technological advances, combined with the growth of nursing theories, will create a knowledge explosion in nursing. Computer competence will not suffice for nurses of the future. They will need to master sophisticated information systems in order to use the wealth of available knowledge to improve patient care. Nursing faculty will be required to actively practice the profession to keep up with rapidly changing technologies.

Nurses of the future will need to be well versed in health care costs, budgeting, and financing of health care. Business education will be increasingly emphasized, particularly at the graduate level, as nurses pursue entrepreneurial and intrapreneurial roles.

Nursing schools will be hard-pressed to include in their curricula everything nurses of the future need to know, and no single nurse will be able to know all there is to know. Licensing examinations will change to reflect the expansion of nursing knowledge. Licensure at multiple levels will become a reality. Employers of new graduate nurses will create internships designed to enable novices to make the transition from student to practicing nurse effectively.

Collaboration

More education and resulting self-confidence will enable nurses to develop collaborative relationships on an equal footing with physicians and other highly educated health care professionals. This will further strengthen the profession.

Nursing faculty, nurse administrators, and practicing nurses will join forces to strengthen educational experiences for tomorrow's nurses and to collaborate on clinical research.

Resource and Faculty Shortages

Higher education in the United States suffers from underfunding. As a result, budgetary constraints have been felt all over the nation. A number of schools of nursing have been closed as a result of funding shortfalls. This means that budgets for operating expenses, equipment, and faculty salaries are under par in many locations.

As the demand for nursing education increases, the shortage of nursing faculty will also increase. Many longtime nursing faculty will retire in the next decade. Younger nurses are not entering teaching because salaries for faculty in schools of nursing have not kept pace with those in practice settings.

Federal subsidies for schools of nursing, eliminated in the late 1970s, must be reintroduced to keep faculty salaries competitive and to supplement state and private funding. Even so, the nation's nursing schools will have long waiting lists of prospective students.

Hospitals will increasingly support nursing education with financial aid to students, subsidies of faculty salaries, joint appointments of faculty, and other forms of assistance.

CHAPTER SUMMARY

Predicting the future is an occupation fraught with peril in a society and world that are changing rapidly. This chapter has highlighted some of the societal changes that seem likely to occur in the next decade leading us into the twenty-first century: changes in demographics, the deteriorating environment, risky life-styles, economics of health care, and governmental regulation of health care. These changes will be accompanied by changes in both nursing practice and nursing education.

Nursing practice will become more autonomous and entrepreneurial. More nurses will practice in nontraditional settings. They will be able to demonstrate that the care they provide makes a positive difference in patient outcomes, and they will continue to provide a warm, humanizing influence on patient care in potentially dehumanizing "high-tech" environments.

The major challenge for nursing education in the next decade will be to produce a steady supply of well-prepared graduates in the face of an aging faculty, rapidly changing technology, increasing cultural diversity of students and patients, and budgetary constraints in higher education.

REVIEW/DISCUSSION QUESTIONS

1. As the number of elderly Americans rises, the rate of chronic illness also rises. What challenges does this present for nurses of the future?
2. Take a position on the statement, "Nurses of the future will have an impact on the environment that exceeds that of the ordinary citizen." Be prepared to defend your position.
3. Describe economic issues that nurses of the future will be concerned about that today's nurses are not.
4. Initiate a classroom debate on the issue "HIV-positive nurses should not be limited in how they practice nursing."
5. What, in your opinion, would it take to attract sufficient numbers of students into nursing to meet the nursing needs of Americans in the year 2000? Could there ever be a danger of producing too many nurses? Give a rationale for your answer.

REFERENCES

Friedman, E. (1990). Troubled past of "invisible" profession. *Journal of the American Medical Association,* 264(22), 2851.

MacDorman, M. F. (1992). Centers for Disease Control, Center for Health Statistics. Personal communication.

Maraldo, P. J. (1991). *Executivewire.* New York: National League for Nursing, January 1991.

Maraldo, P. J. (1992). *Executivewire.* New York: National League for Nursing, January/ February 1992.

Moccia, P. (1992). In 1992: A nurse in every school. *Nursing and Health Care,* 13(1), 14–18.

Styles, M. M. (1990). Challenges for nursing in this new decade. *Maternal Child Nursing,* 15(6), 347.

U. S. Bureau of the Census. (1990). *Current population reports* (Series P.25, No. 1018). Washington, D.C.: Author.

SUGGESTED READINGS

Barnum, B. J. (1991). Whither nursing? *Nursing and Health Care* 12(1), 3.

Carter, M. A. (1989). And the beat goes on. *Journal of Professional Nursing,* 5(6), 299.

Hurley, M. L. (1991). What do the new JCAHO standards mean for you? *RN,* June 1991, 42–46

Orlando, I. J. (1987). Nursing in the 21st century: Alternate paths. *Journal of Advanced Nursing,* 12, 405–412.

Radke, K. J., et al. (1991). Curriculum blueprints for the future: The process of blending beliefs. *Nurse Educator,* 16(2), 9–13

Epilogue

You, our readers, are inheriting a rich legacy of achievement and progress in the nursing profession. Much remains to be done. You will be challenged to lead the way in your communities and regions in addressing the issues of health care costs and access to health care for the elderly, the poor, and others who are disenfranchised. You will be part of the solution.

It is the hope of all the nurses who have participated in writing this textbook that through this book you were stimulated to develop values, beliefs, knowledge, professionalism, and desire to be a nursing leader of the future and a positive force for change in the nursing profession.

Glossary

Acceptance See "nonjudgmental acceptance."

Acceptance stage The stage of illness in which people come to acknowledge the presence of an illness.

Accountability Responsibility for one's own behavior.

Accreditation A voluntary review process of educational programs or service agencies by professional organizations.

Action language A developmental phase in language development of older infants that consists of reaching for or crawling toward a desired object, or of closing the lips and turning the head when an undesired food is offered.

Active collaborator Engaged as a participant with another.

Active listening A method of communicating interest and attention using such signals as good eye contact, nodding, and encouraging the speaker.

Acuity Degree of illness.

Adaptation A change or response to stress of any kind.

Adaptation theory A conceptual framework that focuses on the patient as an adaptive system; that is, one that strives to cope with both the internal and external demands of the environment.

Adjudicate To decide or sit in judgment, as in a legal case.

Advance directives Written instructions recognized by state law that describe individuals' preferences in regard to medical intervention should they become incapacitated.

Advanced practice Nursing roles that require either a master's degree or specialized education in a specific area.

434

Aesthetics   The study of the nature of beauty.

Affective goal   Effort directed toward a change in a patient's values or belief system.

Alternative educational programs   Programs other than basic nursing programs, such as baccalaureate programs for registered nurses and the New York Regents' External Degree Program.

Altruism   Unselfish concern for the welfare of others.

Ambulatory care   Health services provided to those who visit a clinic or hospital as outpatients and depart after treatment on the same day.

ANA Position Paper   A 1965 paper published by the American Nurses Association concluding that baccalaureate education should become the basic foundation for professional practice.

Analysis   The second step in the nursing process during which various pieces of patient data are analyzed. The outcome is one or more nursing diagnoses.

Ancillary workers   Nonprofessional auxiliary health care workers, such as nursing assistants.

Androgyny   Developing both feminine and masculine characteristics.

Anxiety   A diffuse, vague feeling of apprehension and uncertainty.

Applied science   Use of scientific theory and laws in a practical way that has immediate application.

Appropriateness   A criterion for successful communication in which the reply fits the circumstances, matches the message, and the amount is neither too great nor too little.

Articulation   An educational mobility system providing for direct movement from a program at one level of nursing education to another without significant loss of credit.

Assault   A threat or an attempt to make bodily contact with another person without the person's consent.

Assessment   The first step in the nursing process involving the collection of information about the patient.

Associate degree program   The newest form of basic nursing education program leading to the associate degree (AD), consisting of three or fewer years, and usually offered in technical or community colleges.

Autonomy   Self-governing; freedom from the influence of others.

Baccalaureate degree program   Basic nursing education offered in four-year colleges and universities leading to the bachelor's degree in nursing (BSN).

Balance of power   A distribution of forces among the branches of government so that no one is strong enough to dominate the others.

Ball, Mary Ann (1817–1901)   A Civil War woman who cared for the wounded and was known by them as "Mother Bickerdyke."

Barton, Clara (1821–1912)   A famous Civil War nurse and founder of the American Red Cross.

Basic program   Any nursing education program preparing beginning practitioners.

Battery   The unpermissible, unprivileged touching of one person by another.

Belief   The intellectual acceptance of something as true or correct.

Beneficence   The ethical principle of doing good.

Mother Bickerdyke   Affectionate nickname given by soldiers to Mary Ann Ball, a Civil War lay nurse.

Biculturalism   A term used to describe nurses who learn to balance the ideal nursing culture they learned about in school and the real one they experience in practice, using the best of both.

Bioethics   An area of ethical inquiry focusing on the dilemmas inherent in modern health care.

Birthrate   The number of births in a particular place during a specific time period, usually given as a quantity per 1000 people in a year.

Breckinridge, Mary   Founder of the Frontier Nursing Service in 1925.

Brown Report   A 1948 report recommending that basic schools of nursing be placed in universities and colleges, and that efforts be made to recruit large numbers of men and minorities into nursing education programs.

"Captain of the ship" doctrine   A legal principle that implies that the physician is in charge of all patient care, and thus, should be financially responsible if damages are sought.

Caring   Watching over, attending to, and providing for the needs of others.

Case manager   An individual responsible for coordinating services provided to a group of patients.

Centenarian   A person who has reached the age of 100 or more years.

Certificate of need (CON)   A cost containment measure requiring health care agencies to apply to a state agency for permission to construct or substantially add to an existing facility.

Certification   Validation of specific qualifications demonstrated by a registered nurse in a defined area of practice.

Change agent   An individual who recognizes the need for organizational change and facilitates that process.

Civil law   Law involving disputes between individuals.

Clarification   A therapeutic communication technique in which the nurse seeks to more clearly understand a patient's message.

Clinical director   Middle management nurse who has responsibility for multiple units in a health care agency.

Clinical ladder   Programs allowing nurses to progress while staying in direct patient care roles.

Clinical specialist   A nurse with an advanced degree who serves as a resource person to other nurses and often provides direct care to patients or families with particularly difficult or complex problems.

Closed system   A system that does not interact with other systems or with the surrounding environment.

Coalition   A temporary alliance of distinct factions.

Code for Nurses   A statement of the nursing profession's code of ethics.

Code of ethics   A statement of professional standards used to guide behavior and as a framework for decision making.

Cognition   Intellectual activity requiring knowledge.

Cognitive goal   Effort directed toward a desired change in a patient's knowledge level.

Cognitive rebellion   A stage in the educational process wherein students begin to free themselves from external controls and to rely on their own judgment.

Collaboration   Working closely with another person in the spirit of cooperation.

Collaborator   A person who cooperatively works with one or more other persons.

Collective action   Activities undertaken by or on behalf of a group of people who have common interests.

Common law   Law that comes about as a result of decisions made by judges in legal cases.

Communication   The exchange of thoughts, ideas, or information; a dynamic process that is the primary instrument through which change is effected in nursing situations.

Competency   Refers to the capability of a particular patient to understand the information given and make an informed choice.

Concept   An abstract classification of data; for example, "temperature" is a concept.

Conceptual framework   A group of concepts that are broadly defined and systematically organized to provide a focus, a rationale, and a tool for the integration and interpretation of information.

Confidentiality   Assuring the privacy of individuals participating in research studies or being treated in health care settings.

Congruent   The form of communication that occurs when the verbal and nonverbal elements of a message match.

Consultation   The process of conferring with patients, families, or other health professionals.

Consumerism   A movement to protect consumers from unsafe or inferior products and services.

Context   An essential element of communication consisting of the setting in which an interaction occurs, the mood, the relationship between sender and receiver, and other factors.

Continuing education   Informal ways, such as workshops, conferences, and short courses, in which nurses maintain clinical expertise during their professional careers.

CEU   The continuing education unit (CEU), created as a method of recognizing participation in nonacademic educational offerings.

Continuous quality improvement (CQI)   A management concept focusing on excellence and employee involvement at all levels of an organization.

Contract Unwritten or written agreement between nurse and patient to work toward mutually developed goals.

Convalescence stage The final stage of illness during which most people are recovering.

Cost containment An attempt to keep health care costs stable or increasing only slowly.

Counselor One who provides basic emotional support.

Criminal law Law involving public concerns against unlawful behavior that threatens society.

Crisis An emotional upheaval that occurs when a problem or situation exists that poses a threat to the individual and is not solved by the usual coping methods.

Cultural diversity Social, ethnic, racial, and religious differences in a group.

Culture The attitudes, beliefs, and behaviors of social and ethnic groups that have been perpetuated through generations.

Culture of nursing The rites, rituals, and valued behaviors of the nursing profession.

Curtis, Namahyoke The first trained Black nurse employed as a military hospital nurse during the Spanish-American War of 1898.

Data Information or facts collected for analysis.

Deaconess Institute A large hospital and planned training program for deaconesses established in 1836 by Pastor Theodor Fliedner at Kaiserswerth, Germany.

Deductible The amount individuals must pay out-of-pocket before their health insurance begins to pay.

Deductive reasoning A process through which conclusions are drawn by logical inference from given premises; proceeds from the general case to the specific.

Delegate To refer a task to another.

Delegation The practice of assigning tasks/responsibilities to other persons.

Demographics The study of vital statistics and social trends.

Demography The science that studies vital statistics and social trends.

Deontology The ethical theory that the rightness or wrongness of an action depends on the inherent moral significance of the action.

Dependency The degree to which individuals adopt passive attitudes and rely on others to take care of them.

Dependent intervention Nursing actions on behalf of patients that require knowledge and skill on the part of the nurse but may not be done without explicit directions from another health professional, usually a physician.

Developmental theory A theory in which growth is defined as an increase in physical size and shape to a point of optimal maturity.

Diagnosis Identification of a disease or condition.

Diagnosis-related groups (DRGs) A method of classifying illnesses according to similarities of diagnosis.

Differentiated practice   Nursing practice at two levels, professional and technical, with differences in both educational preparation and responsibilities.

Diploma program   The earliest form of formal nursing education in the United States, diploma programs are usually based in hospitals, require two to three years of study, and lead to a diploma in nursing.

Disease   A pathological alteration at the tissue or organ level.

Disenfranchised   The state of having no power or no voice in a political system.

Dissonance   Lack of harmony.

Dix, Dorothea L.   A Boston school teacher, devoted to the care of the mentally ill, who served as the first superintendant of the Women Nurses of the Army during the Civil War.

Dock, Lavinia   A well-known early twentieth century nurse who was actively involved in women's rights issues and the suffragette movement.

Documentation   Written communication about patient care, usually found in the patient record.

Duty of care   The responsibility of a nurse or other health professional for the care of a patient.

Duty to report   The requirement, according to state law, for health professionals to report certain illnesses, injuries, and actions of patients.

Economic and general welfare   Employment issues relating to salaries, benefits, and working conditions.

Educative instrument   A tool for increasing the knowledge and power of another.

Efficiency   A criterion for successful communication that consists of using simple, clear words timed at a pace suitable to participants.

Electoral process   The procedures that must be followed to select someone to fill an elected position.

Elliott, Francis Reed   The first Black nurse accepted by the American Red Cross Nursing Service in 1918.

Empathy   Awareness of, sensitivity to, and identification with the feelings of another person.

Entrepreneur   A person who sees a need for, organizes, manages, and assumes responsibility for a new enterprise or business.

Environment   All the many factors, such as physical or psychological, that influence life and survival.

Epidemiologist   A scientist who studies the origins and transmission of diseases.

Epistemology   The branch of philosophy dealing with the theory of knowledge.

Ethical decision making   The process of choosing between actions based on a system of beliefs and values.

Ethics   The branch of philosophy that studies the propriety of certain courses of action.

Euthanasia   The act of putting to death painlessly a person suffering from an incurable disease; mercy killing.

Evaluation   Measuring the success or failure of the output and consequently the effectiveness of a system. It is the final step in the nursing process wherein the nurse examines the patient's progress to determine if a problem is solved, is in the process of being solved, or is unsolved. In communication theory, the analysis of information received.

Executive branch   The branch of government responsible for administering the laws of the land.

Experimental design   Research designs that provide evidence of a cause-and-effect relationship between actions.

Expert witness   An individual called upon to testify in court because of special skill or knowledge in a certain field, such as nursing.

Extended care   Medical, nursing, or custodial care provided to an individual over a prolonged period of time.

Extended family   A term used to describe nonnuclear family members such as grandparents, aunts, and uncles.

External degree program   An alternative program in which learning is independent and is assessed through highly standardized and validated examinations.

External factors   Impact on individuals of the values, beliefs, and behaviors of the significant people around them.

False reassurance   A nontherapeutic form of communication.

Famous trio   Three famous schools of nursing founded in 1873; the Bellevue Training School, the Connecticut Training School, and the Boston Training School.

Feedback   The information given back into a system to determine whether or not the purpose of the system has been achieved. A major element in the communication process.

Flexibility   A criterion for successful communication that occurs when messages are based on the immediate situation rather than preconceived expectations.

Flexible staffing   A mechanism whereby nurses work at times other than the traditional hospital shifts of 7 am to 3 pm, 3 pm to 11 pm, or 11 pm to 7 am and every other weekend.

Flexner Report   A 1910 study of medical education that provided the impetus for much-needed reform.

Formal socialization   The process by which individuals learn a new role through what others purposely teach them.

For-profit agency   A health care agency that is established to make a profit for the owners or stockholders.

Franklin, Martha   Founder, in 1908, of the National Association of Colored Graduate Nurses (NACGN).

Frontier Nursing Service   Founded in 1925, the Frontier Nursing service provided the first organized midwifery service in the United States.

Functional nursing   A system of nursing care delivery in which each worker has a task, or function, to perform for all patients.

Futurist   An individual who studies trends and makes predictions about the future.

Galileo   An Italian physicist and astronomer who lived from 1564 to 1642.

General election   An election in which all registered voters may vote and may choose a candidate from any party on the ballot.

General systems theory   A theory promulgated by Ludwig von Bertalanffy in the late 1930s to explain the relationship of a whole to its parts.

Generalizable   Research findings that are transferable to other situations.

Generic master's degree   An accelerated master's degree in nursing for people with nonnursing bachelor's degrees.

Goldmark Report   A major study of nursing education published in 1923 and named *The Study of Nursing and Nursing Education in the United States.*

Goodrich, Annie   Served as Assistant Professor of nursing at Teachers College, head of the Army School of Nursing (formed in 1918), president of the American Nurses Association, and first dean of the school of nursing at Yale University.

Governmental (public) agency   An agency primarily supported by taxes, administered by elected or appointed officials, and tailored to the needs of the communities served.

Graduate education   Preparation at the master's and doctoral levels.

Hardiness   A personality characteristic that describes being able to manage the changes associated with illness and to have less physical illness resulting from stress.

Health   An individual's physical, mental, and social well-being; a continuum, not a constant state.

Health behaviors   Choices and habitual actions which promote or diminish health.

Health belief model   A conceptual framework designed to predict a person's health behavior, including the use of health services.

Health Care Financing Administration (HCFA)   The federal agency charged with the responsibility of overseeing the Medicare and Medicaid systems.

Health care team   Those individuals, such as nurses, physicians, dieticians, pharmacists, and others, who work together to provide health care services to patients.

Health maintenance   Preventing illness and maintaining maximal function.

Health maintenance organization (HMO)   A network or group of providers who agree to provide certain basic health care services for a single predetermined yearly fee.

Health promotion   Encouraging a condition of maximum physical, mental, and social well-being.

Henderson, Virginia   An influential twentieth century nursing author and theorist who is widely known for her nursing textbooks, insightful definition of nursing, and identification of 14 basic patient needs.

Henry Street Settlement   A clinic for the poor founded by Lillian Wald and her colleague, Mary Brewster, on New York's Lower East Side.

Heterogeneous   Composed of parts of different kinds.

High-level wellness   Functioning at maximum potential in an integrated way within the environment.

High tech nursing   Nursing care that involves the use of technical instruments such as monitors, pumps, and ventilators.

High touch nursing   Nursing care that involves the use of interpersonal skills such as communication, listening, and empathy.

Hill-Burton Act   A 1946 federal law that called for and funded surveys of states' needs for hospitals, paid for planning hospitals and public health centers, and provided partial funding for constructing and equipping them.

Hippocrates (400 B.C.)   A Greek physician who believed that disease had natural, not magical, causes. Known as the father of medicine.

Holism   A school of health care thought that espouses treating the whole patient—body, mind, and spirit.

Home health agency   An organization that delivers various health services to patients in their homes.

Home health nursing   Rapidly growing field of nursing in which nursing care is provided to patients in their own homes.

Homeostasis   A relative constancy in the internal environment of the body.

Homogeneous   Composed of parts of the same or similar kinds.

Hospice   An agency that provides services to terminally ill patients and their families.

Humanistic nursing care   Care that includes viewing professional relationships as human-to-human rather than nurse-to-patient.

Hypothesis   A statement predicting the relationship among various concepts or events.

Illness   An abnormal process in which an individual's physical, emotional, social, and/or intellectual functioning is impaired.

Illness prevention   All activities aimed at diminishing the likelihood that an individual's physical, emotional, social, and intellectual functions become impaired.

Incongruent   Confusing form of communication that occurs when the verbal and nonverbal elements of a message do not match.

Independent intervention   Actions on behalf of patients for which the nurse requires no supervision or direction by physicians.

Inductive reasoning   The process of reasoning from the specific to the general. Repeated observations of an experiment or event enable the observer to draw general conclusions.

Inertia   Disinclination to change.

Informal socialization   The process through which individuals learn a new role by observing how others behave.

Informed consent   The process of asking individuals who are to undergo diagnostic procedures, surgery, or who are asked to be research subjects to sign a consent form after describing the procedures and risks involved and assuring their privacy.

Infrastructure   Basic support mechanisms needed to ensure that an activity can be conducted.

Inherent power   Unused or untapped power.

Input The information, energy, or matter that enter a system.

Institutional review board A committee that ensures that research is well-designed, ethical, and does not violate the policies and procedures of the institution in which it is conducted.

Institutional structure The way in which the workers within an agency are organized to carry out the functions of the agency.

Interdependent intervention Actions on behalf of patients in which the nurse must collaborate or consult with another health professional prior to carrying out the action.

Internal factors Personal feelings and beliefs that influence an individual.

Internalize The process of taking in knowledge, skills, attitudes, beliefs, norms, values, and ethical standards, and making them a part of one's own self-image and behavior.

Internship An apprenticeship under supervision.

Issues management Assisting a group to resolve a particular question to which there are significant differences of opinion.

Job hopping Moving rapidly from job to job.

Judicial branch The branch of government that decides cases or controversies on particular matters.

Justice An ethical principle stating that equals should be treated the same and that unequals should be treated differently.

Knowledge-based power Authority or control based upon the way information is used to effect an outcome.

Law All the rules of conduct established by a government and applicable to the people, whether in the form of legislation or custom.

Legal authority A group of people in whom power is vested by law, such as the powers vested in state boards of nursing by nursing practice acts.

Legislative branch The branch of government consisting of elected officials who are responsible for enacting the laws of the land.

Licensure The process by which an agency of government grants permission to qualified persons to engage in a given profession or occupation.

Licensure by endorsement A system whereby registered nurses or licensed practical/vocational nurses can, by submitting proof of licensure in another state and paying a licensure fee, receive licensure from the new state without sitting for a licensing examination.

Lobby An attempt to influence the vote of legislators.

Logic The study of correct and incorrect reasoning.

Long-term goals Major changes that may take months or even years to accomplish.

Lysaught Report A 1970 report entitled *An Abstract for Action* that made recommendations concerning the supply and demand for nurses, nursing roles and functions, and nursing education.

Mahoney, Mary Eliza (1845–1926) America's first Black "trained nurse."

Malpractice   An unintentional tort that occurs when a professional fails to act as a reasonably prudent professional would under specific circumstances.

Managed care   A process in which an individual, often a nurse, is assigned to review patients' cases and coordinate services so that quality care can be achieved at the lowest cost.

Mandatory continuing education   The requirement that nurses complete a certain number of hours of continuing education as a prerequisite for relicensure.

Maslow, Abraham   An American humanistic psychologist who formulated a theory of human motivation in the 1940s.

Maturational crisis   Emotional disruptions that occur as a response to the stresses associated with predictable events occurring in the lives of most people.

Maximum health potential   The highest level of well-being that an individual is capable of attaining.

Medicaid   A jointly funded federal and state public health insurance that covers citizens below the poverty level and those with certain disabling conditions; established in 1965.

Medicare   A federally funded form of public health insurance for citizens 65 years of age and above; established in 1965.

Mentor   An experienced nurse who shares knowledge with less experienced nurses to help advance their careers.

Message   An essential element of communication consisting of the spoken word, plus accompanying nonverbal communication.

Metaphysics   The consideration of the ultimate nature of existence, reality, and experience.

Milieu   Surroundings or environment.

Model   A symbolic representation of reality.

Modeling   An informal type of socialization that occurs when an individual chooses an admired person to emulate.

Montag, Dr. Mildred   Originator, in 1952, of the concept of associate degree nursing education.

Moonlighting   The practice of working a second job after the regular one.

Moral development   The ways in which a person learns to deal with moral dilemmas from childhood through adulthood.

Morals   Established rules or standards that guide behavior in situations where a decision about right and wrong must be made.

Morbidity rate   The incidence or occurrence of a certain illness in a particular population during a specific period of time, usually given as a quantity of 1000 people in a specific year.

Mortality rate   The number of deaths in a particular population during a specific period of time, usually given as a quantity of 1000 people in a specific year.

Mutuality   Sharing jointly with others.

NCLEX-PN National Council Licensing Examination for Practical Nurses, the examination graduates of practical nursing programs must take in order to become licensed to practice as licensed practical nurses (LPNs) or licensed vocational nurses (LVNs).

NCLEX-RN National Council Licensing Examination for Registered Nurses, the examination graduates of basic nursing programs must take in order to become licensed to practice as registered nurses (RNs).

Negligence The failure to act as a reasonably prudent person would have in specific circumstances.

Neuman, Betty Nursing theorist who developed a systems model of nursing.

Newton, Isaac English philosopher and mathematician who lived from 1642 to 1727.

Nightingale, Florence Nineteenth century English woman known as the founder of modern nursing and nursing education.

Nonexperimental design Research design in which the research subjects are not influenced in any way.

Nonjudgmental An attitude that conveys neither approval nor disapproval of patients' beliefs and respects each person's right to his or her beliefs.

Nonjudgmental acceptance An attitude that conveys neither approval nor disapproval of patients, their personal beliefs, habits, expressions of feelings, or chosen lifestyles.

Nonmaleficence To inflict no harm or evil.

Nontraditional practice settings Nursing practice settings other than hospitals, doctors' offices, and clinics.

Nonverbal communication Communication without words; consists of grooming, clothing, gestures, posture, facial expressions, tone and loudness of voice, and actions, among other things.

North American Nursing Diagnosis Association (NANDA) Group working since 1970 to establish a comprehensive list of nursing diagnoses.

Not-for-profit agency An organization that does not attempt to make a profit for distribution to owners or stockholders. Money made by such organizations is used to operate and improve the organization itself.

Nuclear family Term used to describe a mother, father, and their children.

Nurse activist A nurse who works actively on behalf of a political candidate or certain legislation.

Nurse anesthetist A nurse with specialized advanced education who administers anesthetic agents to patients undergoing operative procedures.

Nurse citizen A nurse who exercises all the political rights accorded citizens, such as registering to vote and voting in all elections.

Nurse executive The top nurse in the administrative structure of a health care organization.

Nurse manager Also known as a head nurse, a nurse manager is in charge of all activities in the unit, including patient care, continuous quality improvement, personnel selection and evaluation, and resource (supplies and money) management.

Nurse midwife A nurse with advanced specialized education who assists women and couples during uncomplicated pregnancies, deliveries, and postdelivery periods.

Nurse-patient relationship The mode of connection between a nurse and patient.

Nurse politician A nurse who runs for political office.

Nurse practitioner A nurse with advanced education who specializes in primary health care of a particular group, such as children, pregnant women, or the elderly.

Nursing The provision of health care services, focusing on the maintenance, promotion, and restoration of health.

Nursing diagnosis A process of describing a patient's response to health problems that either already exist or may occur in the future.

Nursing informatics The branch of nursing that manages knowledge and data through technology with the goal of improving patient care.

Nursing orders Actions designed to assist the patient in achieving a stated patient goal.

Nursing practice act Law defining the scope of nursing practice in a given state.

Nursing process A cognitive activity that requires both critical and creative thinking and serves as the basis for providing nursing care. A method used by nurses in dealing with patient problems in professional practice.

Nursing research The systematic investigation of events or circumstances related to improving nursing care.

Nutting, Adelaide An early 20th century nurse activist, first professor of nursing in the world, and a cofounder of the *American Journal of Nursing.*

Objective data Factual information obtained through observation and examination of the patient, and/or through consultation with other health care providers.

Occupation A person's principal work or business.

Open-ended question An inquiry that causes the patient to answer fully, giving more than a "yes" or "no" answer.

Open posture Bodily position, squarely facing another person, with arms in a relaxed position rather than held tightly across the chest.

Open system A system that promotes the exchange of matter, energy, and information with other systems and the environment.

Orem, Dorothea Nursing theorist known for her model focusing on patients' self-care needs and nursing actions designed to meet patients' needs.

Orientation phase The introductory phase of the nurse-patient relationship during which trust is developed.

Outcome criteria Patient goals.

Out-of-pocket payment Direct payment for health services from individuals' personal funds.

Output The end result or product of a system.

Patient advocate One who promotes the interest of patients.

Patient classification system (PCS) Identification of patients' needs for nursing care in quantitative terms.

Patient interview A face-to-face interaction with the patient in which an interviewer elicits pertinent information.

Patient Self-Determination Act Effective December 1, 1991, this law encourages patients to consider which life-prolonging treatment options they desire and to document their preferences in case they should later become incapable of participating in the decision-making process.

Patients' rights Responsibilities that a hospital and its staff have toward patients and their families during hospitalization.

Pay equity Equal pay for work of comparable value.

Peer review process The process of submitting one's work for examination and comment by colleagues in the same profession.

Perception The selection, organization, and interpretation of incoming signals into meaningful messages.

Person An individual—man, woman, or child.

Personal payment Direct payment for health services from individuals' personal funds.

Personal value system The social principles, ideals, or standards held by an individual that form the basis for meaning, direction, and decision making in life.

Petry, Lucille The first woman appointed to the position of Assistant Surgeon General of the United States Public Health Service in 1949.

Phenomenon An occurrence or circumstance that is observable.

Philosophy The study of the truths and principles of being, knowledge, or conduct.

Planning The third step in the nursing process that begins with the identification of patient goals.

Policy The principles and values that govern actions directed toward given ends. Policy sets forth a plan, direction, or goal for action.

Policy development The generation of principles and procedures that guide governmental or organizational action.

Policy outcome The result of decisions made by governmental or organizational leaders who choose a certain course of action.

Political action committees (PACs) Groups that raise and distribute money to candidates who support their organization's stand on certain issues.

Politics The area of philosophy that deals with the regulation and control of people living in society; in government, the allocation of scarce resources.

Population The entire group of people possessing a given characteristic, such as all brown-eyed people over the age of 65.

Position power Authority and control accorded to an individual who holds an important role in an organization, profession, or government.

Power grabbing Hoarding control, taking it from others, or wielding it over others.

Power sharing   A process of equalizing resources, knowledge, or control.

Powers of appointment   The authority to select the people who serve in positions such as judges, ambassadors, and cabinet officials.

Practical nurse program   A one-year educational program preparing individuals for direct patient care roles under the supervision of a physician or registered nurse (RN).

Preceptor   A teacher; in nursing, usually an experienced nurse who assumes responsibility for teaching a novice.

Preferred provider organization (PPO)   A group of physicians or institutions to which insurance companies direct their policyholders for care.

Premium   The amount paid for an insurance policy, usually in installments.

Primary care   Basic health care including promotion of health, early diagnosis of disease, and prevention of disease.

Primary data source   The patient is considered a primary source of data about him- or herself.

Primary election   An election in which voters who are declared members of a political party choose among several candidates of that same party for a particular office.

Primary nursing   A system of nursing care delivery in which one nurse has responsibility for the planning, implementation, and evaluation of the care of one or more clients 24 hours a day for the duration of the hospital stay.

Private insurance   Insurance obtained from a privately owned company, as opposed to public or governmental insurance.

Private practice   Nursing practice, engaged in by nurses with advanced education, that takes place outside of a health care delivery setting and is usually provided on a fee-for-service basis, similar to medical practice.

Privileged communications   The principle that information given to certain professionals is so confidential in nature as not even to be disclosed in court.

Problem solving   A method of finding solutions to difficulties specific to a given situation and designed for immediate action.

Profession   Work requiring advanced training and usually involving mental rather than manual effort.

Professional   A person who engages in one of the professions, such as law or medicine.

Professional association   An organization consisting of people belonging to the same profession and thereby having many common interests.

Professional boundary   The dividing line between the activities of two professions.

Professional governance   The concept that health care professionals have a right and a responsibility to govern their own work and time within a financially secure, patient-centered system.

Professionalism   Professional behavior, appearance, and conduct.

Professional review organization (PRO)   Organizations that review Medicare hospital admissions and Medicare patients' lengths of stay.

Professional socialization   The process of developing an occupational identity.

Proposition   A statement about how two or more concepts are related.

Prospective payment system (PPS)   A cost containment mechanism wherein providers, such as physicians and hospitals, received payment on a per case basis, regardless of the cost of delivering the services.

Protocol   A written plan specifying the procedure to be followed.

Provider   Any deliverer of health care services, such as a hospital, clinic, nurse, or physician.

Proximate cause   Action occurring immediately before an injury occurred, thereby assumed to be the reason for the injury.

Psychomotor goal   Effort directed toward a change in motor skills or actions by a patient.

Pure science   Summarizes and explains the universe without regard for whether the information is immediately useful; also known as "basic science."

Quality management   See "total quality management."

Qualitative research   Answers questions that cannot be answered by quantitative designs and that must be addressed by more subjective methods.

Quantitative research   Research that is objective and uses data gathering techniques that can be repeated by others and verified. Data collected are quantifiable; that is, they can be counted, measured with standardized instruments, or observed with a high degree of agreement among observers.

Receiver   An essential element of communication consisting of the person receiving the message.

Referendum   An election resulting from the registered voters being asked to express a preference on a policy issue by a legislative body.

Reflection   A communication technique that consists of encouraging patients to think through problems for themselves by directing patient questions back to the patient.

Registered nurse (RN)   An individual who has completed a basic program for registered nurses, and successfully completed the licensing examination.

Rehabilitation services   Those activities designed to restore an individual or a body part to normal or near normal function following a disease or an accident.

Reliable   Yielding the same values dependably each time an instrument is used to measure the same thing.

Reality shock   The feelings of powerlessness and ineffectiveness often experienced by new nursing graduates.

Replication   Repeating a research study as closely as possible.

Research process   Prescribed steps that must be taken in order to properly plan and conduct meaningful research.

Resocialization   A transitional process of giving up part or all of one set of professional values and learning new ones.

Respondeat superior   Legal theory that attributes the acts of employees to their employer.

Retrospective reimbursement Insurance payment made after services are delivered.

Richards, Linda In 1873, she became the first "trained nurse" in the United States.

Risk management A program that seeks to identify and eliminate potential safety hazards, thereby reducing patient injuries.

RN-to-BSN education Programs for registered nurses who hold associate degrees or diplomas in nursing enabling them to acquire baccalaureate degrees in nursing.

Robb, Isabel Hampton An outstanding turn of the century American nurse who was instrumental in forming the forerunners of the National League for Nursing and the American Nurses Association, as well as cofounding the *American Journal of Nursing*.

Role A goal-directed pattern of behavior learned within a cultural setting.

Role model An individual who serves as a model of desirable behavior for another.

Rogers, Martha Nursing theorist who developed a model known as the "science of unitary human beings."

Roy, Sister Callista Nursing theorist who developed an adaptation model based on general systems theory.

Salary compression A phenomenon in which pay increases are limited during an individual's career so that the salary of a veteran nurse may be little higher than the same nurse's salary as a novice.

Sample A subset of an entire population that reflects the characteristics of the population.

Sanger, Margaret Founder of the first birth control clinic in America in 1916 and an ardent proponent of women's rights to use contraception.

Scales, Jessie Sleet She became the first Black public health nurse in 1900.

Scientific discipline A branch of instruction or field of learning based on the study of a body of facts about the physical or material world.

Scientific method A systematic, orderly approach to the gathering of data and the solving of problems.

Secondary care An intermediate level of health care performed in a hospital having specialized equipment and laboratory equipment.

Secondary data source Sources of data such as the nurse's own observations or perceptions of family and friends of the patient.

Self-actualization A process of realizing one's maximum potential and using one's capabilities to the fullest extent possible.

Self-awareness Understanding of one's own needs, biases, and impact on others.

Sender An essential element of communication consisting of the person sending a message.

Separation of powers Under the Constitution, each branch of the federal government has separate and distinct functions and powers.

Set A group of circumstances or situations joined and treated as a whole.

Sex-role stereotyping   The practice of automatically and routinely linking positive or negative characteristics to either males or females.

Shared governance   See "professional governance."

Short-term goals   Specific, small steps leading to the achievement of broader, long-term goals.

Situational crisis   Emotional disruptions that occur as a response to unanticipated, traumatic events.

Skill mix   The ratio of registered nurses to licensed practical nurses and nursing assistants in each hospital unit.

Social crisis   Emotional disruptions that occur as a response to unexpected and uncommon events that do not occur in the everyday lives of most people; generally affect large numbers of people simultaneously.

Socialization   The process whereby values and expectations are transmitted from generation to generation.

Somatic language   Language used by infants to signal their needs to caretakers, such as crying; reddening of the skin; fast, shallow breathing; facial expressions; and jerking of the limbs.

Spellman Seminary   Site of the first nursing program for Blacks, founded in Atlanta, Georgia in 1886.

Standard of care   What the reasonably prudent nurse; under similar circumstances, would have done.

Standard of nursing practice   Those nursing actions that are generally agreed upon, by nurses, as constituting safe and effective patient care.

Statutory law   Law established through formal legislative processes.

Stereotypes   Prejudiced attitudes developed through interactions with family, friends, and others in an individual's social and cultural system.

Stress   Any emotional, physical, social, economic, or other factor that requires a response or change.

Stressors   Stimuli that tend to disturb equilibrium.

Subjective data   Information obtained from patients as they describe their needs, feelings, and strengths, and their perceptions of the problem.

Subjects   The individuals who are studied in a research project.

Subsystems   The parts that make up a system.

Supervision   The initial direction and periodic inspection of the actual accomplishment of a task.

Suprasystem   The larger environment outside a system.

System   A set of interrelated parts that come together to form a whole.

Systems theory   See "general systems theory."

Taylor, Susie (1848–1912)   A young, Black Civil War nurse who knew and was influenced by Clara Barton.

Teacher   The nursing role in which patients receive information from nurses about how to better care for themselves.

Team nursing   A system of nursing care delivery in which a group of nurses and ancillary workers are responsible for the care of a group of patients during a specified time period, usually 8 to 12 hours.

Termination phase   Third phase of the nurse-patient relationship consisting of those activities that enable the patient and the nurse to end a relationship in a therapeutic manner.

Tertiary care   Specialized, highly technical level of health care provided in sophisticated research and teaching hospitals.

Tertiary data source   Sources of data including the medical records and health care providers, such as physical therapists, doctors, or dietitians.

Theory   A general explanation scholars use to explain, predict, control, and understand commonly occurring events.

Theory of human motivation   Abraham Maslow's theory of human needs and their relationship to the stimulation of purposeful behavior.

Third party payment   Payment for health services by an entity other than the patient or the provider of services.

Tort   A civil wrong against a person; may be intentional or unintentional.

Total quality management (TQM)   Management philosophy and activities directed toward achieving excellence and employee participation in all aspects of that goal.

Traditional practice settings   Nursing practice settings in hospitals, doctors' offices, and clinics.

Transition stage   The stage of illness that begins when a person recognizes changes occurring in the body or experiences a symptom.

Transmission   The expression of information, verbally or nonverbally.

Truth, Sojourner (1797–1881)   A famous Black nurse and former slave who was an abolitionist and underground railroad agent during the Civil War.

Tubman, Harriet Ross (1820–1913)   A Black Civil War nurse who helped more than 300 slaves to freedom on the underground railroad.

Urbanization   The process of population migration to cities.

Utilitarianism   An ethical theory asserting that it is right to maximize the greatest good for the happiness or pleasure of the greatest number of people.

Valid   Measuring what it is intended to measure, as in a valid test question or research instrument.

Values   The social principles, ideals, or standards held by an individual, class, or group that give meaning and direction to life.

Ventilation   The verbal "letting off steam" that occurs when people talk about concerns or frustrations.

Veracity   Telling the truth.

Verbal communication   All language whether written or spoken; represents only a small part of communication.

Voluntary (private) agency   An agency supported entirely through voluntary contributions of time and/or money.

Wald, Lillian   Founder of the Henry Street Settlement and public health nursing in the United States. She later formed the National Organization of Public Health Nurses (1912), marking the beginning of specialization in nursing.

Worker's compensation   A federally mandated insurance system covering workers injured on the job.

Work ethic   A belief in the importance of work; an appreciation for the characteristics employers desire in employees and a commitment to providing it.

Working phase   The second phase of the nurse-patient relationship wherein the nurse and the patient tackle tasks outlined in the orientation phase.

Yale School of Nursing   The first school of nursing in the world to be established as a separate university department with an independent budget and its own dean, Annie W. Goodrich.

Index

454